Student Workbook

Health Insurance Today:
A Practical Approach

ELSEVIER

evolve

http://evolve.elsevier.com/Beik/today/

Evolve Student Resources for Beik: Health Insurance Today, Second Edition, offer the following features:

- **Websites to Explore**
  An exciting resource that lets you explore websites carefully chosen to supplement the content of the textbook
- **Content Updates**
  The latest content updates from the author of the textbook to keep you current with recent developments in health insurance billing
- **Image Collection**
  An assembly of all the figures from this text available for download
- **Medisoft Exercises**
  Practice management software exercises are available on the Evolve page to be used with Medisoft Version 14.

Student Workbook

Health Insurance Today: A Practical Approach

Second Edition

Janet I. Beik, AA, BA, MEd
Southeastern Community College (retired)
Administrative Instructor
Medical Assistant Program
West Burlington, Iowa

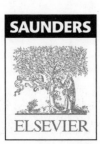

SAUNDERS

ELSEVIER

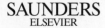
SAUNDERS
ELSEVIER

11830 Westline Industrial Drive
St. Louis, Missouri 63146

Executive Editor: Susan Cole
Associate Developmental Editor: Melissa Gladback
Publishing Services Manager: Patricia Tannian
Senior Project Manager: Kristine Feeherty
Designer: Maggie Reid

Working together to grow
libraries in developing countries

www.elsevier.com | www.bookaid.org | www.sabre.org

ELSEVIER   BOOK AID International   Sabre Foundation

Printed in the United States of America

Last digit is the print number: 9 8 7 6 5 4 3 2 1

Acknowledgments

I would like to express my appreciation and gratitude to those who assisted me in compiling this student workbook, especially those at Elsevier: Susan Cole, Melissa Gladback, Jennifer Presley, Liz Fergus, Kristine Feeherty, and Maggie Reid. Also, I would like to thank all the individuals who reviewed these workbook chapters. Their suggestions and helpful guidance aided in making this workbook a very important ancillary tool to enhance student learning. Last, but not least, I would like to thank several of my former students and peers, now working in healthcare facilities, who so kindly let me run some of these exercises by them to see if the exercises were appropriate for preparing students for their health insurance careers.

Janet I. Beik, AA, BA, MEd

Introduction to the Workbook

OBJECTIVES

After completing the workbook exercises and activities, the student should be able to:

- Define the **terms** used in the chapters.
- Answer the **review questions** within the evaluation criteria set by the instructor.
- Demonstrate the ability to use analytical logic to draw rational conclusions from facts and information in **critical thinking** exercises.
- Use individual/group thinking techniques to reach valid conclusions on **problem-solving** issues and collaborative (group) activities.
- Complete assigned **projects** as directed by the instructor.
- Assume an active and productive role in **group discussions**.
- Analyze hypothetical situations, applying logical concepts for rational decision-making to **case studies** and health insurance scenarios.
- Perform **Internet searches/exploration** to access information needed to complete assigned activities.
- Achieve the required proficiency on all **performance objectives**.
- Complete the **application exercises** as assigned.
  - Generate information and guidelines of major payers for inclusion in the Health Insurance Professional's Notebook.
  - Access the Evolve website for updates.
- Conduct a **self-evaluation** on achievement of successful content mastery and classroom performance.
- Perform basic mathematical computations.
- Generate both paper and electronic CMS-1500 claims in an accurate and timely manner.
- Apply reasoning and problem-solving skills (individually or group) to arrive at practical solutions to common health insurance issues.
- Interpret a variety of computer-generated accounting reports.
- Create appropriate correspondence for fees and collection.
- Abstract relevant information (from health record documents) necessary for completing various forms used in healthcare billing and claims.
- Integrate knowledge necessary for interpreting payer documents, e.g., EOBs and RAs.
- Apply exact processes for accurate coding (ICD-9, CPT, and HCPCS).

TO THE STUDENT

This workbook accompanies the textbook titled *Health Insurance Today: A Practical Approach* and is intended to supplement the material presented in the text. Each chapter follows a precise structure that begins with a short introduction and builds to application activities that allow the student to apply what he or she has learned to today's healthcare environment. The workbook chapters are organized as follows:

- *Introduction to the workbook chapter*. The introduction gives a brief statement regarding what the student can expect in the specific workbook chapter.
- *Workbook Chapter Objectives*. These objectives are different from those listed in the textbook. They are designed to encourage the student to meet the challenges presented in each chapter of the workbook.
- *Defining Chapter Terms*. In this section, the chapter terms are listed and the student is expected to generate clear and precise definitions (in his or her own words) after which a comparison should be made to the correct definitions in the textbook glossary.
- *Assessment*. Each workbook chapter has a review test. These tests may be in the form of multiple choice, true/false, matching, fill-in-the-blanks, or short answer/essay. Generally, tests promote deeper thinking versus "surface" learning, and the benefits are twofold: Tests benefit students, because they provide feedback on discrimination of important material and course relevance; and tests benefit instructors, because they provide feedback on what students have accomplished in the chapter, at course intervals, or at course end. This level of learning is mainly recall; the student, if he or she has read and studied the material in the textbook, should be able to answer the question correctly.

- *Critical Thinking Activities*. These activities require that the student use his or her abilities to analyze and evaluate information and reach a conclusion or answer by using logic and reasoning skills. Each chapter presents anywhere from one to four critical thinking exercises.
- *Problem-Solving/Collaborative (Group) Activities*. In this step, students use thought processes in which previously learned principles are applied to case-specific situations. Problem solving can be accomplished either on an individual basis or collaboratively in groups, as directed by the instructor.
- *Projects/Discussion Topics*. Several topics are listed as suggestions for in-class discussions or oral presentations. As with problem solving, projects and discussion topics will be assigned according to the discretion of the instructor.
- *Case Studies*. Real world "scenarios" are presented to further stimulate critical thinking and problem-solving skills. Like problem solving, case studies allow the student to apply information he or she has learned to resolve a similar situation that may present itself after the student becomes employed in a healthcare facility.
- *Internet Exploration*. Many of today's learners rely heavily on the Internet for research and up-to-date information on a particular subject. In the constantly changing world of healthcare, textbooks are often somewhat outdated by the time they are published. Students must use caution, however, to make sure that the information found on the Internet is not biased or political in nature—this is where critical thinking skills can be used.
- *Performance Objective(s)*. Most workbook chapters present at least one "Performance Objective." A performance (or learning) objective is a statement of what the learners will be expected to do when they have completed a specified course of instruction. It prescribes the conditions, behavior (action), and standard of task performance for the training setting. Performance objectives must be mastered to the predetermined criteria set by the instructor, institution, or organization. If the course is competency-based, performance objectives may be repeated up to three times or until the student successfully meets the predetermined grading criteria.
- *Application Exercises*. Application, a higher level of learning, asks the learner to take the knowledge and skills he or she has acquired and apply them to "real world" situations. In this workbook, there is at least one application exercise per chapter.
- *Creating a Health Insurance Professional's Notebook*. The purpose of this notebook is to allow the student to access information quickly and accurately when preparing insurance claims for some of the major third-party payers.
- *Self-Evaluation*. At the end of each workbook chapter, there are two documents that the student must complete to allow him or her to conduct a self-evaluation. These are:
  - A *Chapter Checklist* to make sure the student has completed all activities and assignments associated with the chapter.
  - A *Performance Evaluation*, which the student will use to evaluate his or her performance in the classroom. This is then compared with the instructor's evaluation. The performance evaluation can also be used by the student to track his or her grade.

TIPS FOR SUCCESSFUL STUDYING

Many students, when they enroll in a college course, don't know how to study effectively. Some tend do too much, while others do too little. The ideal is to find a happy medium. The following are some practical tips on how to get the most out of study time.

Listening in Class

Engage in *active* listening. Involve yourself in the lecture. Research shows that the average college student listens at about 35% efficiency. Here are some tips to maximize active listening:

- Choose a seat where you can see and hear well, away from distractions.
- Have a pen ready to take notes—it helps you focus.
- Watch the instructor as he or she talks. Watch for signals that will help you recognize the difference between important key points and supporting information.
- Think about what the speaker is saying. Think: "What would be a good test question on this material?" or "How could I use this information?" or "What can I ask to clarify what is being said?"
- Try not to let your mind wander. Pull your concentration back when you have a lapse.
- Be open to learning something new—it can be exciting.
- Try to guess what the instructor might say next.

Some experts say it's helpful to use the mnemonic LISAN:

- **L**ead—think ahead, don't just follow.
- **I**deas—watch and listen for the main ideas.
- **S**ignals—be aware of the instructor's nonverbal cues.
- **A**ctive—stay focused.
- **N**otes—they are your summary of the lecture.

Reading, Highlighting, and Taking Notes

Read the assigned material before class. As you read, use a highlighter to mark important points. If you have read the material before class and focused on the key points, you will understand the lecture much better. More important, you will know what questions to ask to clarify any confusing concepts in the reading. Then, as the instructor progresses through the lecture, note any points missed in the reading, paraphrasing (translating to your own words) what the lecturer is saying.

Briefly review your notes from the last class so that you will be able to connect the new material to what you already know. This helps you sort and categorize information mentally and makes information easier to remember.

Some students ask, "Why should I take notes in class?" Here are some good reasons:

- Memory can be unreliable.
- Notes provide a summary from which to study.
- Note-taking encourages you to put the main ideas down on paper, in your own words, making them easier to remember.
- Notes expand on the information in the textbook.
- Instructor lectures and class discussions add current real-life ideas, examples, and explanations.

Many students, especially those new to the college scene, are tempted to write down every word the instructor says. Anyone who has taken a college course knows that this is not practical. What you need to do is distinguish between what is and is not important. This is not an easy task.

Example:

The instructor says: "The goal of the health insurance professional is to submit clean claims—those that can be processed for payment quickly and with the maximum reimbursement allowed without being returned for clarification or omissions or rejected for incorrect information."

The student might note: Goal: Clean claims; complete, no errors, omissions, wrong information = prompt, maximum reimbursement.

The student has reduced a nearly 40-word paragraph to 13 words.

Develop your own note-taking style so that your notes make sense to you when you review them later. Think of your notes as an outline.

- Use headings and subheadings.
- List items 1, 2, 3, etc.
- Use a phrase or word, rather than a sentence.
- Note examples with a one-word reminder.
- Develop your own abbreviations (e.g., INS for insurance; PIF for patient information form).
- Don't spend time rewriting your notes to make them look better. As long as you can read them and they make sense to you, that's what is important.

Watch for signals. Good note-taking depends on your ability to listen actively in class. Listen and watch for signals that will help you select the main ideas. For example, the instructor may

- repeat a point several times
- speak loudly to emphasize
- write on the board or put on an overhead
- distribute a handout
- say things such as: "There are three reasons for this...." or "The most important thing to remember is...."

Review your notes that same day, when the class is still fresh in your mind. Add important points you might have missed, if necessary. Recalling material that day signals to the brain that this material must be stored for future use.

A good test of effective note-taking is: Could you summarize the lecture to someone who wasn't there, using your own words? If you can, you've done a good job of taking notes.

WRITING ESSAYS

When instructors assign an essay writing exercise, many students panic. Writing is often not a student's strong point. The best tip about writing an essay is not to leave it to the last minute! As soon as the instructor assigns the essay topic, think about it, start forming ideas in your mind, and begin your research.

Most essay writing assignments in this course are relatively short—typically 250 to 500 words. This should not be too daunting for most students. The next page looks at an example essay topic and some ideas on how to "flesh it out."

Let's say the instructor assigned a 350- to 400-word essay on health insurance reform or the importance of HIPAA compliance. Think about the topic, remembering what you've read and what the instructor has said in his or her lectures. Then, begin your research. Log on to the Internet and get some ideas. *Do not* copy any information you find; just use it as a source and then form your own ideas and opinions around it. The following steps can help guide you through the essay writing process:

- Decide on your topic (or use the topic assigned by the instructor).
- Prepare an outline or diagram of your ideas.
- Form a thesis statement.

NOTE: A **thesis statement** tells the reader what the essay is about, and what point you, the author, will be making. A thesis statement has two parts:

- The first part states the topic; for example:
  - Insurance reform …
  - HIPAA compliance …
- The second part states the point of the essay; for example:
  - … is taking a toll on the American middle class.
  - … is crucial in today's medical practices.

Once a thesis statement is formed, begin writing your essay:

- Write the introduction.
- Write the body:
  - Write the main points.
  - Write the sub points.
  - Elaborate on the sub points.
- Write the conclusion.
- Proofread, edit, and add the finishing touches (e.g., name, date).

The essay illustrated in Box 1 demonstrates the principles of writing a basic essay. The different parts of the essay have been labeled. The thesis statement is in bold, the topic sentences are in italics, and each main point is underlined. When you write your own essay, you will probably not need to identify the different parts of the essay unless your instructor asks you to do so. They are marked in this example so that you can more easily identify them.

Box 1: Sample Essay

THE NEW REVOLUTION IN HEALTHCARE: ELECTRONIC MEDICAL RECORDS

Electronic medical records (EMRs) have been around in one form or another for a long time, but **recent advances in technology and continued efforts to streamline and improve the healthcare system have brought EMRs to the center stage of the current healthcare debate**. Many "experts" have suggested ways that computerized databases can improve the care of patients and reduce costs at all levels of the healthcare system.

There are many benefits of EMRs. For instance, a recent EMR system installed at Icon Medical Center allows patient records to be viewed anytime from anywhere in the complex. Records can be accessed concurrently by hospital staff and physicians in adjacent office buildings. *Greater coordinated care has been achieved by interfacing the EMR system with hospital clinical applications.* This has resulted in a more complete care assessment and reduced critical errors. Compliance with HIPAA and other government regulations has also been improved.

There is a downside to EMRs. *The risk of breaching patient confidentiality and medico-legal concerns head the top of the list of disadvantages.* Another disadvantage is the cost and time expended to convert existing paper records to an electronic system.

There will be a need for more uniform national standards for data entry and security if EMRs are to become the norm. *If an EMR system is to provide a comprehensive solution for today's practice environment, it must accomplish multiple functions.* These functions include streamlining workflow efficiency, improving adherence to treatment standards, providing detailed financial practice analysis, enhancing patient education and interaction, and optimizing compliance with regulatory and managed care guidelines.

NOTE: When you use Times New Roman Font, 12 point size, 1" margins, double-spaced text, and a title, a one-page essay is approximately 325 to 350 words, depending on paragraphing. To count the number of words in your essay, if using Microsoft Word, click on "Tools," then on "Word Count." In WordPerfect, click on "File," "Properties," and "Information."

PREPARING FOR TESTS

There are three stages of test preparation:

- *Long-term*—from the beginning of school to the test
- *Short-term*—the time leading up to the test when study and review become crucial (often the week or so before)
- *Immediate*—the day or night before

Long-Term Preparation

From day one, keep the final exam or test in mind, asking yourself, "What do I need to know?" Some useful strategies include the following:

- Looking at the objectives stated in the course outlines
- Reviewing regularly
- Looking at old tests/exams if available

Try to understand the material, rather than just memorizing it.

Short-Term Preparation

Use these strategies as you begin your test-studying in earnest:

- Organizing your information
- Combining related information to help you understand it
- Practicing "active study" techniques (e.g., paraphrasing your notes [saying them in your own words])
- Pacing and scheduling your study
- Using memory aids such as mnemonics and/or acronyms (e.g., PIF for patient information form) to aid recall of hard-to-remember lists and terms. An example of a typical mnemonic that allows someone to remember the musical bass clef is **G**ood **B**oys **D**o **F**ine **A**lways (g-b-d-f-a).

Immediate Preparation

By the time you get to the day or night immediately before your test, your study technique should be review (as opposed to relearning). Keep these guidelines in mind as you refresh your knowledge:

- Get enough sleep.
- Eat properly.
- Take breaks, relax, and exercise.
- Focus your attention.
- Keep a positive attitude.

Cramming

Cramming is not learning; rather, it is short-term remembering. However, when time is short, you may occasionally have to cram. If that is the case, do the following:

- Make choices—don't attempt to remember everything.
- Turn what you're studying into questions.
- Recite.
- Relax; takes some long, deep breaths (being nervous and upset will not help).

Before You Begin

- **Preview the test before you answer anything**. This gets you thinking about the material. Make sure to note the point value of each question. This will give you some ideas on how to budget your time.
- **Do a "mind dump."** Using what you remember from your study sessions, make notes of anything you think you might forget. Write down things that you used in learning the material that might help you remember. Outline your answers to discussion questions.
- **Quickly calculate how much time you should allow for each section** according to the point value. (You don't want to spend 30 minutes on an essay question that counts only 5 points.)

Taking the Test

- **Read the directions**. (Can more than one answer be correct? Are you penalized for guessing?) Never assume that you know what the directions say.
- **Answer the easy questions first**. This will give you the confidence and momentum to get through the rest of the test, because you are sure these answers are correct.
- **Go back to the difficult questions**. While looking over the test and doing the easy questions, your subconscious mind will have been working on the answers to the harder ones. Also, later items on the test might give you useful or needed information for earlier items.
- **Answer all questions** (unless you are penalized for wrong answers).
- **Ask the instructor to explain any items that are not clear**. Do not ask for the answer, but phrase your question in a way that shows the instructor that you have the information but are not sure what the question is asking.
- **Try to answer the questions from the instructor's point of view**. Try to remember what the instructor emphasized and believed was important.

- **Use the margin to explain why you chose the answer** if the question does not seem clear or if the answer seems ambiguous.
- **Circle key words in difficult questions**. This will force you to focus on the central point.
- **Express difficult questions in your own words**. Rephrasing can make it clear to you, but be sure you don't change the meaning of the question.
- **Use all of the time allotted for the test**. If you have extra time, cover up your answers and actually rework the question.

How to Use the Student CD

The following section will introduce and briefly walk you through the two software elements located on the CD bound into this Workbook. After inserting the CD into your computer and opening the icon, you will see the start screen with these four options:

- Electronic Forms
- Guided Completion
- Instructions
- Quit

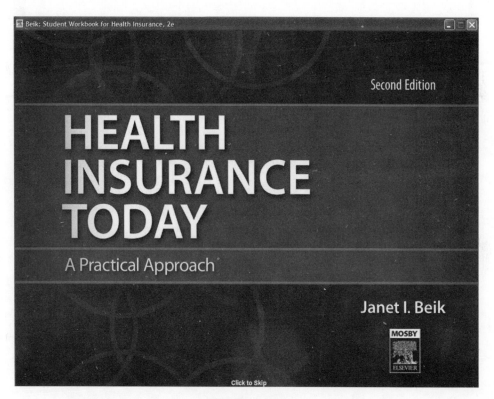

CD Start Screen

The Electronic Forms tab takes you to a file with the Electronic Forms. The Guided Completion tab starts the Guided Completion software. The Instructions tab presents further, more specific instructions about the software. The Quit tab takes you back to your desktop.

ELECTRONIC FORMS

The Electronic Forms are the most basic and versatile software option. Quite simply, the Electronic Forms are documents designed to look like select forms used throughout this Workbook with an option to print and turn in to your instructor for an assignment. There are two different blank Electronic Forms for use throughout the Workbook:

- CMS-1500
- A ledger card

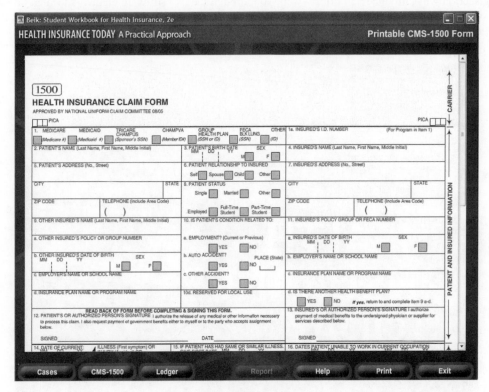

Electronic Forms

GUIDED COMPLETION

The Guided Completion element walks the user through a CMS-1500 form one block at a time. This feature matches with select, generally introductory CMS-1500 claim form completion exercises throughout the Workbook. You are able to enter the information block-by-block, and if you need assistance, there will be a section help button to give you a hint. Upon completing the claim, you can print out a copy of the completed claim form.

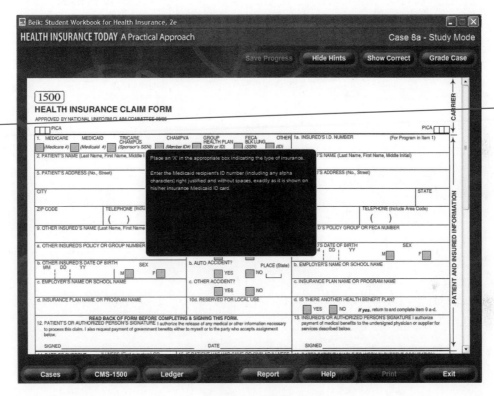

Guided Completion

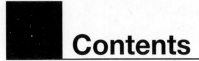

Contents

Student Workbook

Health Insurance Today: A Practical Approach

1 Medical Insurance: Where Did It Come From?

Chapter 1 of the textbook, *Health Insurance Today: A Practical Approach,* provides a brief history and background of medical insurance, how it got started, and its transformation into what we know today as modern health insurance. It is important to know this information to have a complete understanding of the topic.

These accompanying workbook activities are intended to enhance the student's knowledge and understanding of the material included in Chapter 1. Students should follow the instructor's directions for completing each section. A checklist and a student evaluation are included at the end of the chapter exercises to help the student assess his or her comprehension of the material covered in the corresponding chapter.

WORKBOOK CHAPTER OBJECTIVES

After completing the workbook activities for Chapter 1, the student should be able to:
- Define the terms used in the chapter.
- Answer the review questions to within the evaluation criteria set by the instructor.
- Evaluate and provide rational opinions regarding the critical thinking issues.
- Use individual or group thinking techniques to reach valid conclusions on problem-solving issues/scenarios.
- Complete assigned projects or participate in class discussions as directed by the instructor.
- Achieve the required proficiency on all performance objectives.
- Perform Internet exploration/searches as assigned.
- Do the enrichment activities as assigned.

DEFINING CHAPTER TERMS

Using the computer (or typewriter), students should key an accurate definition for each of the chapter terms listed. These definitions should be in the students' own words. When finished, students should compare their definitions with those listed in the glossary at the back of the textbook, correcting any inaccuracies.

Consolidated Omnibus Budget Reconciliation Act (COBRA)
cost sharing
deductible
entity/entities
fee-for-service
group plan
health insurance
Health Insurance Portability and Accountability Act (HIPAA)
Health Maintenance Organization (HMO) Act
indemnify

indemnity insurance
indigent
insurance
insured
insurer
managed healthcare
medical insurance
policy
preexisting conditions
premium
preventive medicine

ASSESSMENT

The following activities/exercises are intended to present a variety of learning opportunities for mastering the information presented in the text and to prepare the student for on-the-job performance. The instructor will tailor these activities/exercises to meet the specific needs and time requirements of the course.

Review tests help the instructor measure the extent to which the student has learned the chapter material. Before attempting to complete the test, the student should review the chapter.

1

Multiple Choice

Directions: In the questions/statements presented, choose the response that **best** answers/completes the stem by circling the letter that precedes it.

1. Financial protection against loss or harm typically is referred to as:
   a. An event
   b. Insurance
   c. A premium
   d. Preventive medicine

2. Health insurance narrows down "undesired events" to:
   a. Illnesses
   b. Injuries
   c. Preventive medicine
   d. a and b

3. Keeping a person well or detecting and treating an emerging illness in its early stages is referred to as:
   a. Outpatient care
   b. Preventive medicine
   c. Emergency medicine
   d. Individualized treatment

4. The beginnings of modern health insurance occurred in 1850 in:
   a. Italy
   b. Russia
   c. England
   d. Germany

5. Health insurance was "born" in the United States in 1929 with a plan that later became known as:
   a. Medicare
   b. Blue Cross
   c. Managed care
   d. National healthcare

6. Blue Cross and Blue Shield plans traditionally established premiums wherein everybody in the community paid the same premium, called:
   a. A premium set
   b. Standard rating
   c. Community rating
   d. Equalizing premium rating

7. A profound change in form from one stage to the next in the life history of an organism is referred to scientifically as:
   a. Change
   b. Mutation
   c. Adulteration
   d. Metamorphosis

2

8. HMOs were first recognized in the United States in the:
    a. 1850s
    b. 1920s
    c. 1970s
    d. 1990s

9. A type of insurance that provides comprehensive major medical benefits and allows insured individuals to choose any provider when seeking medical care is called:
    a. A fee-for-service plan
    b. Managed care
    c. Indemnity insurance
    d. a and c

10. Many individuals employed full-time (or for a specific number of hours per week) are eligible for:
    a. A group insurance plan
    b. An individual (or private) plan
    c. Premium-free healthcare coverage
    d. Preventive healthcare only

11. When certain illnesses or injuries exist before the effective date of an insurance policy and are not covered by the policy, these conditions are commonly referred to as:
    a. Riders
    b. Latent clauses
    c. Uncovered situations
    d. Preexisting conditions

12. If an insurance company thinks an applicant presents too much of a risk, he or she will be put into a category referred to as a(n):
    a. High-risk pool
    b. Uninsurable group
    c. "Watch dog" category
    d. Risk assessment cluster

13. To get around the problem of individuals with preexisting conditions being afraid to change jobs for fear of losing healthcare coverage, Congress introduced:
    a. Blue Cross and Blue Shield
    b. Medicare
    c. Medicaid
    d. HIPAA

14. Experts believe that increasing healthcare costs are due to:
    a. The "graying of America"
    b. Advances in medical technology
    c. More demand for healthcare
    d. All of the above

15. Any health plan that attempts to control or coordinate the use of healthcare to contain expenditures, improve quality, or both falls under the category of:

a. Managed healthcare

b. A fee-for-service plan

c. An indemnity plan

d. All of the above

True/False

Directions: Place a "T" in the blank preceding the statement if it is true; place an "F" if it is false.

_____ 1. Medical insurance and health insurance are interchangeable terms.

_____ 2. Medical insurance narrows down the "undesirable events" to illnesses and injuries.

_____ 3. Health insurance in the United States began shortly after the turn of the 19th century when physicians agreed to provide certain services to Texans for a very nominal fee.

_____ 4. Politics has never played a role in the growth and change of health insurance.

_____ 5. There are a dozen major sources from which people can gain access to health insurance.

_____ 6. People in the middle of the wage spectrum are often the ones who have the most difficult time acquiring health insurance.

_____ 7. Advances in medical technology have tended to keep healthcare costs down.

_____ 8. People buy health insurance to protect themselves from financial loss or ruin.

_____ 9. COBRA and HIPAA were enacted by Congress in the same year—1996.

_____ 10. The two basic categories of health insurance plans are indemnity (fee-for-service) and managed care.

Fill-in-the-Blank

Directions: Insert the word(s) in the following sentences that **best** completes the statement.

1. The word "insurance" comes from the Latin word _____.

2. The beginnings of modern health insurance occurred in _____ (country) in _____ (year).

3. The name of the Massachusetts company that first offered medical expense coverage similar to today's health insurance is _____.

4. In 1929, Justin Kimball, a Baylor University professor in Dallas, introduced a plan that evolved into _____.

5. The Blue Shield plan got its start in the _____ (geographical area of United States).

6. _____ and _____ are the federal healthcare programs that began during President Johnson's term in 1965.

7. A(n) _____ is a plan that provides healthcare from specific physicians and hospitals who contract with that plan.

8. The "traditional" or "standard" type of healthcare plan is called a(n) _____ plan or _____-_____-_____ plan.

9. An insurance policy that covers several individuals, often sharing common professions, is called a(n) _____ policy.

10. Certain illnesses or injuries that exist before an effective date of an insurance policy are commonly referred to as _____ _____.

4

CRITICAL THINKING ACTIVITIES

A. Think about the term "preventive medicine." How can practicing preventive medicine help curb the rising cost of healthcare?

B. The section "Access to Health Insurance" lists three groups that are typically without healthcare coverage. List these three groups, and explain this phenomenon.

C. Why and how does "media intervention" affect healthcare costs?

PROBLEM-SOLVING/GROUP ACTIVITY

Your instructor will separate the class into groups. Each group will be assigned a particular decade or time period from the PBS website chart. Research the particular decade(s) your group has been assigned, and prepare a short presentation on the important developments and acts of that time period.

PROJECTS/DISCUSSION TOPICS

A. Research and be prepared to discuss the theory of cost containment in healthcare. Zero in on federal and individual states' specific methods of keeping healthcare costs under control.

B. Prepare for (or lead) a class discussion on one of the following key medical insurance issues:
   1. How people get medical insurance
   2. Access to medical insurance
   3. Why healthcare costs so much
   4. Reasons for health insurance

CASE STUDY

Margaret and Jeremy Tinsman were, so they thought, in the prime of their life. Margaret was a homemaker, and Jeremy was a successful used car salesman. Both were covered under a group healthcare plan through Jeremy's employer. At 53, Jeremy had a debilitating stroke, which left him completely paralyzed on his left side and unable to speak. Subsequently, Jeremy had to quit his job. What options are open to Margaret and Jeremy as far as health insurance is concerned? What role, if any, does HIPAA play in this scenario?

INTERNET EXPLORATION

A. Browse the World Wide Web to learn more about the major factors that are contributing to the increased costs of healthcare insurance.

B. Using the Internet, find out how "group insurance plans" differ from "individual/private" plans.

```
┌─────────────────────────────────────┐
│                                     │
│                                     │
│         REFERENCE NOTEBOOK          │
│             FOR THE                 │
│      HEALTH INSURANCE PROFESSIONAL  │
│                                     │
│                                     │
│                                     │
│                                     │
│                                     │
│                                     │
│                                     │
│                                     │
│                                     │
│           Property of (Student's Name) │
│                   (Complete Date)   │
│                                     │
│                                     │
│                                     │
└─────────────────────────────────────┘
```

Fig. 1-1 Sample cover sheet.

APPLICATION EXERCISES

Create a Health Insurance Professional's Notebook.

1. Supplies needed:
   a. black, 3-ring, 1-inch binder
   b. prepunched, color-coded, tabbed dividers
   c. self-adhesive labels for dividers

2. Create a title page for notebook (Fig. 1-1).

3. Prepare six individual labels as follows:
   a. COMMERCIAL/BCBS
   b. MEDICAID
   c. MEDICARE
   d. TRICARE/CHAMPVA
   e. WORKERS' COMP
   f. MISCELLANEOUS CARRIERS

4. Place labels on tabbed dividers and insert into notebook.

6

Chapter Check List

Student name: _____

Chapter completion date: _____

1.	Record	Your start time and date: _____
2.	Read	The assigned chapter in the text
3.	View	PowerPoint slides (if available)
4.	Complete	Exercises in the Workbook as assigned
5.	Compare	Your answers to the answers posted on the bulletin board/website/handout
6.	Correct	Your answers
7.	Complete	All tests and required activities
8.	Read	Assigned readings (if any)
9.	Complete	Chapter performance objectives (competencies), if any
10.	Evaluate	Chapter performance and submit to your instructor
11.	Record	Your ending time and date: _____
12.	Move on	Begin next chapter as assigned

Student name: _____

Chapter completion date: _____

Evaluate your classroom performance. Complete the self-evaluation, and submit it to your instructor. When your instructor returns this form to you, compare your self-evaluation with the evaluation completed by your instructor.

Skill	Student Self-Evaluation			Instructor Evaluation		
	Good	Average	Poor	Good	Average	Poor
Attendance/punctuality						
Personal appearance						
Applies effort						
Is self-motivated						
Is courteous						
Has positive attitude						
Completes assignments in timely manner						
Works well with others						

Student's initials: _____

Date: _____

Points Possible: _____

Points Awarded: _____

Chapter Grade: _____

Instructor's initials: _____

Date: _____

2 Tools of the Trade: A Career as a Health (Medical) Insurance Professional

Chapter 2 addresses what "tools" the student needs to succeed in a career as a health insurance professional. These tools include skills and interests applicable to the world of health insurance. Although job duties and responsibilities differ from one facility to another, certain core skills are the same across the field. Additionally, students should realize that the term "health insurance professional" encompasses diverse specialties in which credentialing is possible, heightening their career success and potential further. Students are encouraged to explore the Internet to "zero in" on the particular specialty of interest.

WORKBOOK CHAPTER OBJECTIVES

After completing the workbook activities for Chapter 2, the student should be able to:
- Define the terms used in the chapter.
- Answer the review questions to within the evaluation criteria set by the instructor.
- Use "critical thinking" skills to evaluate, make decisions, and communicate his or her viewpoint clearly and accurately for the scenarios presented.
- Demonstrate college entry-level "core" skills in five of the six areas listed in the text.
- Identify and discuss job duties and responsibilities of various specialties under the umbrella of "health insurance professional."
- Explore career prospects.
- Investigate certification possibilities.

DEFINING CHAPTER TERMS

Using the computer (or typewriter), students should key an accurate definition for each of the chapter terms listed. These definitions should be in the students' own words. When finished, students should compare their definitions with those listed in the glossary at the back of the textbook, correcting any inaccuracies.

application
autonomy
certification
CMS-1500 claim form
communication
comprehension
diligence

initiative
integrity
objectivity
paraphrase
prioritize
professional ethics

ASSESSMENT

Multiple Choice
Directions: In the questions/statements presented, choose the response that **best** answers/completes the stem by circling the letter that precedes it.

1. The nationally recognized title for a health insurance professional is:
    a. Nationally certified health insurance professional (NCHIP)
    b. Health Insurance Professional of America (HIPA)
    c. Academy of Health Insurance Professionals (AHIP)
    d. There is no nationally recognized title or acronym for this broad specialty

2. To increase the potential for success, candidates entering the health insurance field should possess which of the following college entry-level skills?
   a. Reading and comprehension
   b. Basic business math
   c. English and grammar
   d. All of the above

3. Typical program length in community colleges and technical schools for a career as a health insurance professional can range from:
   a. 2-4 months
   b. 6-8 months
   c. 1-2 years
   d. 2-4 years

4. The concept that learning will not stop when individuals graduate from a college or career program, but that they will continue to learn for the rest of their life is called:
   a. Career identity
   b. Job dedication
   c. Lifelong learning
   d. Permanent commitment

5. The process of organizing daily responsibilities by the order of their importance is called:
   a. Organizing
   b. Prioritizing
   c. Multitasking
   d. Categorizing

6. Self-discipline, possessing a positive attitude, and diligence are examples of:
   a. Desirable personality traits
   b. Qualities of character
   c. Behavioral characteristics
   d. All of the above

7. Writing down important facts from lectures and readings *in your own words* is called:
   a. Paraphrasing
   b. Active listening
   c. Paying attention to detail
   d. Two-way communication

8. Possessing the ability to work without direct supervision and the ability to make decisions without being subject to approval by or undue influence from another individual is called:
   a. Freedom from restraint
   b. A workplace "right"
   c. Endorsement
   d. Autonomy

9. The growth of certain types of medical facilities has increased greatly the demand for employees with a solid background in coding and excellent computer skills. These are:

 a. Outpatient clinics

 b. Inpatient hospitals

 c. Ambulatory care facilities

 d. Both a and c

10. As an alternative to working in a medical office, health insurance professionals have the option of working *independently* from:

 a. Computer "cafes"

 b. Home-based offices

 c. Contract associations

 d. Health information networks

11. Graduates of a health insurance professional program can enhance their career through:

 a. Autonomy

 b. Certification

 c. Preauthorization

 d. Computerization

12. The standard insurance form used by all government and most commercial insurance payers is the:

 a. CMS-1400

 b. CMS-1500

 c. HIPAA Standard Form

 d. There is no "standard" form

True/False

Directions: Place a "T" in the blank preceding the statement if it is true; place an "F" if it is false.

_____ 1. To succeed as a health insurance professional, an individual should possess specific college entry-level skills in several areas.

_____ 2. All learning institutions offer programs where students can receive extensive hands-on training and practice in medical insurance billing and coding.

_____ 3. Length for a typical health insurance professional program varies from several months to several years.

_____ 4. A 4-year degree is not offered in any medical field except nursing.

_____ 5. Preparation is a crucial key for success in any career.

_____ 6. "Lifelong learning" means that learning does not stop when an individual completes college or a career program.

_____ 7. Autonomy—doing things on your own without supervision—is frowned on in medical facilities.

_____ 8. A career as a health insurance professional offers the individual a variety of tasks and responsibilities.

_____ 9. The career prospects of a health insurance professional are limited to physicians' offices.

_____ 10. HIPAA has limited the amount of jobs available in healthcare because of its encouragement of computer-to-computer claim filing.

_____ 11. One of the biggest rewards of a career in the healthcare field is the knowledge that you are helping people.

_____ 12. There is no nationally recognized certification specifically referred to as a "health insurance professional."

Short Answer

Note: If space provided is inadequate, use a separate piece of blank paper.

1. List the six college entry-level skills that candidates should possess to maximize success as a health insurance professional.

_____

_____

_____

_____

_____

_____

2. Explain why each of the following "core" courses are typically included in a health insurance professional program.

   Anatomy and Physiology: _____

   Medical Terminology: _____

   Keyboarding: _____

   Microsoft Word: _____

   Business English: _____

   Medical Office Administrative Skills: _____

3. List at least five types of facilities that offer a graduate of a health insurance professional or billing and coding program opportunities for entry-level employment.

_____

_____

_____

_____

_____

4. In addition to the essential classroom skills, individuals experienced in working as health insurance professionals suggest that candidates for this field also should possess certain job skills. Choose three of these "on-the-job" skills listed in the text and write a short paragraph explaining why this skill is important to a health insurance professional. (Use a blank sheet of paper to complete this assignment.)

_____

_____

_____

CRITICAL THINKING ACTIVITIES

A. Fig. 2-1 shows an article that appeared in a recent newspaper, which contains a mixture of facts and opinions. Read the article, and then label the bracketed areas as "fact" or "opinion." When you have finished, make up a title representing the main idea of the article.

Exercise

The following are excerpts from an article that appeared recently in *The Hawkeye* that contains a mixture of facts and opinions. Read the article, and then label the bracketed areas as fact or opinion. When you have finished, make up a heading to show the main idea of the article.

_____

Health care in America is fast becoming a matter of stock prices, CEOs' salaries, cost savings, and cutbacks–not new cancer therapies, breakthrough drugs, or new help for intractable diseases. Its heroes and role models aren't the white-coated scientists who discover new cures but the suits who put together the big deals; not the physicians who save lives but the corporate honchos who cut healthcare jobs and find innovative ways to deny treatment.

Millions of Americans will be pushed into managed-care organizations of various types in the next few years. Many of them will be vulnerable to a pattern of abuses that is emerging as health-care becomes just another business opportunity for investors and executives, and doctors are being told, in essence, to put up and shut up.

To get away with curtailing high-tech and expensive care, some HMOs force physicians to sign agreements that contain "gag" orders forbidding them to tell patients about treatments or referrals to specialists the HMO will not provide, even though they might be successful. The American Medical Association calls gag orders "unethical" and "harmful to patients."

Some emerging remedies are worrisome. For example, state legislatures are hurrying to pass laws to give more protection to HMO patients. Two states have made gag rules illegal, and several others are considering such laws. Many states now require HMOs to pay for two days of hospital care for mothers after childbirth, instead of pushing them out in half that time.

But this process is a slow and difficult way to assure patients will get the necessary care they used to take for granted. And it's troubling that there seems to be a need for legislators to intervene in what should be private, professional relationships between patient and doctor.

Fig. 2-1 Critical Thinking Exercise.

PROBLEM-SOLVING/COLLABORATIVE (GROUP) ACTIVITIES

Your instructor will assign groups and give instructions for oral presentation(s) or discussion(s) on one or more of the following topics:

- Employment prospects for the healthcare professional are increasing.
- Alternative career prospects exist for the healthcare professional other than working in physicians' offices or clinics.
- The recent HIPAA laws have created new job opportunities for health insurance professionals.
- Personal and professional rewards can be gained from a career as a health insurance professional.

PROJECTS/DISCUSSION TOPICS

A. Select someone you know who is working in a health career. Prepare a list of 10 questions to ask this person regarding his or her job. Interview this individual, using the question list as a guide. Develop a short, 3- to 5-minute oral presentation explaining this individual's role in healthcare and any other information you were able to gather from the interview.

B. In anticipation of completing your education as a health insurance professional, generate a list of career opportunities available in your area for which you would be qualified. Outline the skills and traits you will need for each and the approximate beginning wages.

CASE STUDY

You are having lunch with Carrie Phillips, a long-time friend, and you inform her that you have enrolled in a college program to pursue a career in healthcare. She is excited for you and informs you that she also is interested in this field, but because of obligations that keep her house-bound, she cannot spend time away from home attending classes. As a favor to your friend, and for your own information, investigate what *distance learning* opportunities are available in the medical billing and insurance field. Prepare a short report of your findings to tell Carrie the next time you have lunch.

INTERNET EXPLORATION

A. Log on to the World Wide Web and find out what career certifications are available in the various specialties associated with a health insurance professional.

B. Using search words such as "health career opportunities in (your state)," search the Internet for information on what is currently available for a health insurance professional. Note any specific requirements for the positions available.

C. As an alternative to "B," zero in on your specific area of interest in healthcare, and search the Web for job opportunities either in your area or elsewhere in the United States if you are considering or are willing to relocate. Also note the various wage scales different areas of the United States offer.

PERFORMANCE OBJECTIVES

The **Secretary's Commission on Achieving Necessary Skills (SCANS)** states that a "high-performance" workplace requires workers who have a solid foundation in *basic literacy and computational skills*, in *thinking skills* necessary to put knowledge to work, and in *personal qualities* that make workers dedicated and trustworthy. In Chapter 1, you completed a performance objective for four of the five basic skills—reading, writing, listening, and speaking. Now, your instructor will administer the performance objective you will be taking to determine competency in the "thinking skills" category, which include the following:

- Creative thinking—generates new ideas
- Decision making—specifies goals and constraints, generates alternatives, considers risks, and evaluates and chooses best alternative
- Problem solving—recognizes problems, and devises and implements plan of action
- Seeing things in the mind's eye—organizes and processes symbols, pictures, graphs, objects, and other information
- Knowing how to learn—uses efficient learning techniques to acquire and apply new knowledge and skills
- Reasoning—discovers a rule or principle underlying the relationship between two or more objects, and applies it when solving a problem

Performance Objective 2-1—Thinking Skills

Conditions: Student will develop a 250-word written composition using the following topic as the subject: "Modern Healthcare Is a Team Effort."

Instructions: In your essay, discuss what you think this means and how you believe you will fit into a "high-performance" workplace. After doing a self-evaluation and some serious introspection, discuss some of your personal attributes that might have to be modified to perform effectively in a team setting, indicate what you would change about yourself, and how you would go about making these changes. Use the six thinking skills outlined previously in developing your essay. Compositions must be keyed and double-spaced using 1-inch margins all around, Times New Roman font, 12 point. Proofread your document before submission. Remember, using spell check does not catch all errors. Pay close attention to grammar and punctuation rules using reference manuals available.

Supplies/Equipment: Internet-ready computer/printer/textbook and reference material

Time Allowed: To be determined by instructor

Accuracy Needed to Pass: 70%

Procedural Steps	Points Earned	Comments
Evaluator: Note time began: _____		
Carefully read and study the applicable documents.		
1. Student adequately defined the topic and gave reasons why he or she would or would not fit into a "high-performance" workplace. (10)		
2. Student listed and discussed necessary modifications/changes in personal attributes. (20)		
3. Student discussed how these modifications would be accomplished. (20)		
4. Essay shows evidence that the student used all or most of the six "thinking skills." (20)		
5. Student used proper sentence structure, English grammar, and correct punctuation/ spacing in essay using rules from reference materials. (15)		
6. Proofread/edit essay. (10)		
7. Ensure essay is properly identified according to instructions/print a hard copy. (5)		
Optional: May deduct points for taking more time than allowed.		

Total Points = 100

Student's Score: _____

Evaluator: _____

Comments: _____

_____

_____

15

APPLICATION EXERCISES

Reference Notebook Assignment

Using the Table of Contents in the textbook as a reference, and Fig. 2-2 as a guide, create a table of contents for your reference notebook. Save this table of contents as an electronic file to add additional information as the course progresses. For now, page numbers will be blank.

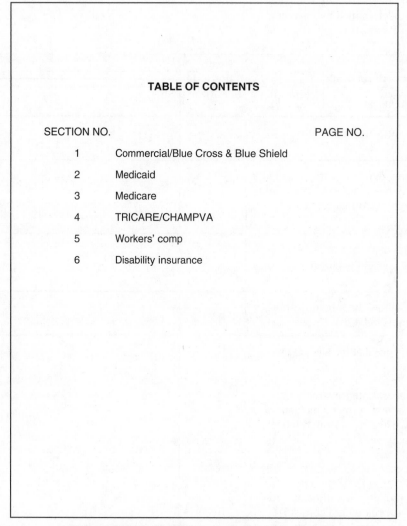

Fig. 2-2 Example of reference notebook table of contents.

SELF-EVALUATION

Chapter Check List

Student name: _____

Chapter completion date: _____

1.	Record	Your start time and date: _____
2.	Read	The assigned chapter in the text
3.	View	PowerPoint slides (if available)
4.	Complete	Exercises in the Workbook as assigned
5.	Compare	Your answers with the answers posted on the bulleting board/website/handout
6.	Correct	Your answers
7.	Complete	All tests and required activities
8.	Read	Assigned readings (if any)
9.	Complete	Chapter performance objectives (competencies), if any
10.	Evaluate	Chapter performance and submit to your instructor
11.	Record	Your ending time and date: _____
12.	Move on	Begin next chapter as assigned

Student name: _____

Chapter completion date: _____

Evaluate your classroom performance. Complete the self-evaluation, and submit it to your instructor. When your instructor returns this form to you, compare your self-evaluation with the evaluation completed by your instructor.

Skill	Student Self-Evaluation			Instructor Evaluation		
	Good	Average	Poor	Good	Average	Poor
Attendance/punctuality						
Personal appearance						
Applies effort						
Is self-motivated						
Is courteous						
Has positive attitude						
Completes assignments in timely manner						
Works well with others						

Student's initials: _____

Date: _____

Instructor's initials: _____

Date: _____

Points Possible: _____

Points Awarded: _____

Chapter Grade: _____

3 The Legal and Ethical Side of Medical Insurance

Chapter 3 addresses the legal and ethical issues regarding the protection of the rights of patients, the healthcare provider, and the entire healthcare team. When patients visit a medical facility, healthcare professionals (and patients) are governed by basic guidelines. Some of these guidelines are of a legal nature, such as those set by governmental licensing agencies and state and federal law, whereas others are ethical, such as those imposed by professional organizations that define appropriate conduct.

Legal and ethical issues that the health insurance professional is exposed to on a daily basis have taken on new meaning with the advent of the federal HIPAA privacy rule, especially the important aspect of patient confidentiality. Students should be able to understand lawful and ethical medical conduct, and apply this conduct to the workplace to promote practice policies and goals. In addition, students need to understand the relationship between law and ethics, and foster a deeper consideration of legal and ethical issues and issues of quality of care, patient safety, and prevention of medical errors. These workbook activities are intended to enhance the material presented in the text and help the student attain the above-mentioned workplace goals.

WORKBOOK CHAPTER OBJECTIVES

After completing the workbook activities for Chapter 3, the student should be able to:
- Define the terms used in the chapter.
- Answer the review questions to within the evaluation criteria set by the instructor.
- Evaluate and provide rational opinions regarding critical thinking issues.
- Analyze data, make decisions, and communicate his or her beliefs (either individually or collaboratively) clearly and accurately regarding certain legal or ethical issues.
- Complete assigned exercises, and actively participate in group discussions.
- Achieve the stated competency level in all performance objectives.
- Do all applications exercises to required accuracy.
- Conduct a self-evaluation on classroom performance.

DEFINING CHAPTER TERMS

Using the computer (or typewriter), students should key an accurate definition for each of the chapter terms listed. These definitions should be in the students' own words. When finished, students should compare their definitions with those listed in the glossary in the back of the textbook, correcting any inaccuracies.

abandoning
abuse
acceptance
accountability
ancillary
binds
breach of confidentiality
competency
confidentiality
consideration
durable power of attorney
emancipated minor
ethics
etiquette
first party (party of the first part)
fraud

implied contract
implied promises
incidental disclosure
litigious
medical ethics
medical etiquette
medical record (health record)
negligence
offer
portability
privacy
privacy statement
respondeat superior
second party (party of the second part)
subpoena *duces tecum*
third party (party of the third part)

Multiple Choice

Directions: In the questions/statements presented, choose the response that **best** answers/completes the stem by circling the letter that precedes it.

1. The practice of medicine is:
   a. A business
   b. Always profitable
   c. Supported by tax dollars
   d. Is often considered a charity

2. The primary goal(s) of the health insurance professional is(are):
   a. To complete and submit insurance claims
   b. To conduct billing and collection procedures
   c. To generate as much money for the practice as is legally and ethically possible
   d. All of the above

3. A breach of medical care can result in:
   a. A denied claim
   b. A malpractice lawsuit
   c. Cancellation of an insurance policy
   d. The health insurance professional losing his or her license

4. Loosely translated, the Latin term *respondeat superior* means:
   a. The physician is always the boss
   b. Failure to exercise a reasonable degree of care
   c. The physician must respond to all legal accusations
   d. The employer is ultimately responsible for employee actions

5. Failure to exercise a reasonable degree of care is referred to as:
   a. Negligence
   b. *Respondeat superior*
   c. Omission by default
   d. Employer liability

6. A health insurance policy and the relationship between a healthcare provider and a patient are considered:
   a. Dual agreements
   b. Legal contracts
   c. Faultless covenants
   d. All of the above

7. In terms of contract law, when an individual completes an application for health insurance, he or she is:
   a. Making an offer
   b. Completing an acceptance
   c. Submitting a consideration
   d. Proving competency

8. When the insurance company agrees to grant health insurance coverage to an individual, this is called:
   a. Making an offer
   b. Completing an acceptance
   c. Submitting a consideration
   d. Proving competency

9. The binding force in any contract that gives it legal status—the *thing of value* that each party gives to the other—is the:
   a. Offer
   b. Acceptance
   c. Consideration
   d. Legal object

10. For a contract to be enforceable, it must be:
    a. Legal
    b. In writing
    c. At least 48 hours old
    d. All of the above

11. The parties to a legal contractual agreement must be:
    a. Emancipated
    b. At least 21 years old
    c. Mentally competent
    d. A citizen of the United States

12. Minors who are married or living separate and apart from their parents and not receiving any financial support from them are:
    a. Uninsurable
    b. Illegal minors
    c. Emancipated minors
    d. Unable to enter into a contract

13. The contract between a healthcare provider and a patient is referred to as a(n):
    a. Overt contract
    b. Implied contract
    c. Contract by default
    d. Representative contract

14. Ceasing to provide care to a patient without following prudent steps is a breach of the physician/patient contract, referred to as:
    a. Disclosure
    b. Negligence
    c. Abandonment
    d. Infringement

15. The act that regulates disclosure of confidential information is the:
    a. Fraud and Abuse Act
    b. Federal Privacy Act of 1974
    c. Federal False Claim Amendments Act of 1986
    d. Federal Omnibus Budget Reconciliation Act of 1980 (OBRA)

Chapter **3** **The Legal and Ethical Side of Medical Insurance**

16. The act allowing current or former employees or dependents younger than age 65 to become eligible for Medicare because of end-stage renal disease is the:

    a. Federal Privacy Act of 1974

    b. Federal False Claim Amendments Act of 1986

    c. Consolidated Omnibus Budget Reconciliation Act of 1986 (COBRA)

    d. Federal Omnibus Budget Reconciliation Act of 1987 (OBRA)

17. Standards of human conduct—sometimes called morals—of a particular group or culture are commonly known as:

    a. Mores

    b. Ethics

    c. Etiquette

    d. Conventions

18. Following the rules and conventions governing correct or polite behavior in society is called:

    a. Mores

    b. Ethics

    c. Etiquette

    d. Conventions

19. A clinical, scientific, administrative, and legal documentation of facts containing information relating to a patient's care and treatment is called a:

    a. Contract

    b. Health record

    c. Consultation report

    d. History and physical

20. A health record is considered privileged communication; information in it should not be disclosed without a patient's:

    a. Approval

    b. Knowledge

    c. Implied consent

    d. Written consent

21. If additional information needs to be added to a patient's record, it should be in the form of a(n):

    a. Appropriate addendum

    b. Separate typewritten page

    c. Computer-generated document

    d. Penciled note in the margin of the history and physical

22. Adequate and complete documentation helps to:

    a. Determine the level of service

    b. Establish medical necessity

    c. Justify the fee(s) charged

    d. All of the above

23. Lack of proper documentation often results in:

    a. Denied claims

    b. Reduced claim payments

    c. Patients losing their healthcare benefits

    d. a and b are correct

24. HIPAA's objective stating that employees cannot be denied health insurance coverage when moving from one group health plan to another is called:

    a. Insurance portability

    b. Preexisting conditions

    c. Unfair competition

    d. Covered expenses

25. If two people who know each other meet inadvertently in a physician's reception area, HIPAA refers to this exposure as:

    a. Defendable circumstances

    b. Incidental disclosure

    c. Unavoidable contact

    d. Accidental events

26. Timeliness, according to the Joint Commission, is within _____ hours of the encounter.

    a. 6

    b. 12

    c. 24

    d. 48

27. Situations that do not come under the umbrella of patient confidentiality include:

    a. Communicable diseases

    b. Abuse of a child (or an adult)

    c. Wounds inflicted by firearms

    d. All of the above

28. A signed release of information may not be required when:

    a. The patient is a Medicaid recipient

    b. The patient is a Medicare recipient

    c. The patient is being treated as a result of an on-the-job injury

    d. a and c are correct

29. A legal document that requires an individual to appear in court with a piece of evidence that can be used or inspected by the court is called a(n):

    a. Judgment

    b. Arrest warrant

    c. Small claims suit

    d. Subpoena *duces tecum*

30. What results when confidential information is disclosed to a third party without patient consent or court order?

    a. A malpractice lawsuit

    b. Subpoena *duces tecum*

    c. A breach of confidentiality

    d. All of the above

Chapter **3** **The Legal and Ethical Side of Medical Insurance**

True/False

Directions: Place a "T" in the blank preceding the statement if it is true; place an "F" if it is false.

_____ 1. The health insurance professional should be knowledgeable in the area of medical law and liability.

_____ 2. Medical laws regulating insurance are the same from state to state.

_____ 3. Direct and indirect patient contact involves ethical and legal responsibility.

_____ 4. The health insurance professional can be a party to legal action in the event of error or omission.

_____ 5. In contract law, the promise to pay the premium is the "consideration" of the individual seeking health insurance coverage.

_____ 6. All states require that all types of insurance policies be filed with, and approved by, the state regulatory authorities before the policy may be sold.

_____ 7. A contract between an insurance company and the insured party cannot be terminated.

_____ 8. A patient can terminate the contract with the physician simply by paying all incurred charges and not returning to the practice.

_____ 9. The healthcare provider can terminate the physician/patient contract by simply discharging the patient.

_____ 10. If the physician wants to withdraw from a particular case, he or she must notify the patient by a letter sent by certified mail with a return receipt.

_____ 11. An insurance company often is referred to as the third party to a contract.

_____ 12. Laws are universal rules to be observed by everyone, but different cultures follow different moral and ethical codes.

_____ 13. A medical (health) record is considered a legal document.

_____ 14. Records are the property of the healthcare provider and must be preserved as long as the patient is alive.

_____ 15. Timely, accurate, and complete documentation is crucial to good patient care.

_____ 16. All patient record documentation must be performed by the physician.

_____ 17. Appropriate documentation serves as the basis for the defense of malpractice claims and lawsuits.

_____ 18. HIPAA's impact is felt only in medical facilities.

_____ 19. One significant change HIPAA has made for businesses is that health records must be kept separate from routine personnel records.

_____ 20. It now is commonly accepted that patients are the legal owners of their medical records.

_____ 21. How long medical records are kept and how they are stored and disposed of varies from practice to practice and state to state.

_____ 22. Every healthcare organization and provider must guarantee confidentiality and privacy of the healthcare information they collect, maintain, use, and transmit electronically.

_____ 23. A written release of information is not necessary to process an insurance claim for a patient's financial benefit.

_____ 24. There are never any exceptions to patient confidentiality.

_____ 25. In health insurance, fraud and abuse are technically the same thing.

Short Answer

Note: If space provided is inadequate, use a separate piece of blank paper.

1. Explain in your own words what is meant by a "litigious" society.

   _____

   _____

2. List and explain each of the five elements of a legal contract.

   _____

   _____

   _____

   _____

   _____

3. Explain the contractual relationship between the healthcare provider and the patient.

   _____

4. Under what circumstances and how might a healthcare provider terminate a contract between the provider and a patient?

   _____

5. How do medical ethics differ from medical etiquette?

   _____

6. List HIPAA's four primary objectives.

   _____

   _____

   _____

   _____

7. List and discuss the seven steps a medical practice must undertake to become HIPAA compliant.

   _____

   _____

   _____

   _____

   _____

   _____

   _____

CRITICAL THINKING ACTIVITIES

A. You receive a telephone call from an attorney asking for information on Eric Downs, a patient who was treated in your office recently for injuries resulting from an automobile accident. How would you handle this phone call?

B. Write a paragraph detailing how an implied contract is created between a healthcare provider and a patient. Explain why this type of contract is binding, and what must transpire for it to be "set aside."

PROBLEM-SOLVING/COLLABORATIVE (GROUP) ACTIVITIES

A. Medical ethics is a current area of concern for practitioners and consumers. The textbook lists several debatable topics on ethical issues, such as

- Birth control
- Abortion
- Experimentation
- Prolongation of life
- Quality of life
- Withholding care
- Euthanasia
- Who makes the medical decisions
- Who has the knowledge and the right to make these decisions

Your instructor will assign teams to discuss or debate one or more of these issues. Choose a topic of interest, and be prepared to discuss the pro or con side of the issue.

B. At Broadmoor Medical Clinic, the staff takes turns manning the telephone during the noon lunch break. Today, it is your turn. Patient Sally Albright phones and requests a refill on her prescription for captopril (high blood pressure medicine). List all the information you should get from Sally.

C. Assume that Sally's healthcare provider has authorized a prescription refill: captopril, 25 mg, 1 by mouth in a.m., #100 × 2 refills. Additionally, the physician has told you that Sally needs to come in for a weekly blood pressure check. Should Sally's telephone call, the resulting prescription refill, and the physician's request of weekly blood pressure checks be documented in her health record? If so, illustrate an appropriate method of documentation.

PROJECTS/DISCUSSION TOPICS

A. **Individual or Group:** The textbook lists several exceptions to confidentiality. List these, and explain in your own words why you think they should, or should not, be exceptions.

B. **Individual:** Research a current article regarding healthcare fraud and abuse. Prepare a 1-page (200-word) essay or a 2- to 3-minute oral presentation summarizing the information.

CASE STUDIES

A. Brent Underwood, a health insurance professional in the Beach Front Medical Clinic, is convinced by Bertha Parker, a 60-year-old patient of the clinic, that she is a "financial hardship" case. Brent tells Ms. Parker that he will send in a claim to her insurance company and "write off" any balance that they do not pay. Determine if Brent is within his legal rights as a health insurance professional to do this for Bertha. If not, decide if his actions constitute fraud or abuse.

B. Mary Larson visits Dr. Jacob Astor, her obstetrician, for a suspected pregnancy. Dr. Astor performs an examination, determines she is pregnant, and asks you, one of his versatile healthcare professionals, to arrange for an ultrasound. The office is very busy, so you inform Mary that you will schedule the procedure later and call her with the appointment date and time. Later that day, you telephone Mary's residence, and her husband answers the telephone. You inform him of the appointment time that has been set up for Mary's ultrasound. Is this a breach of confidentiality? Why or why not?

C. You are employed as a health insurance professional for Dr. Gail Lorber, a family practice physician. Dr. Ian Sutton telephones from the State University Epidemiology laboratory. He informs you that he is doing a clinical study on infectious diseases and is requesting a list of all patients who have been treated for hepatitis A, B, and C in the last 5 years. Do you need to procure a written release from each patient to give this information to Dr. Sutton? Why or why not?

INTERNET EXPLORATION

A. **Preventing Fraud and Abuse:** Using search words such as "preventing healthcare fraud and abuse," research the Internet and find some good websites that discuss this topic. Generate a list of at least five ways a health insurance professional can help to curb this growing problem.

B. **Criminal versus Civil Law:** Conduct research on the Internet to determine the difference between criminal law and civil (tort) law. Make your findings detailed and specific.

C. **"The 4 Ds of Negligence":** Research the Internet, determine what the "4 Ds" of negligence are, and briefly explain each. To enhance your definitions, give an example for further explanation.

Chapter **3** **The Legal and Ethical Side of Medical Insurance**

Performance Objective 3-1—Documenting Information Accurately

Conditions: Student will read the following case study, after which he or she will generate an entry in the patient's health record that illustrates the fundamentals of accurate documentation.

Instructions: In the following case study, determine the important information that requires documentation in the patient's health record. Using your computer, key a "chart note" illustrating proper and adequate documentation.

Case Study: Helen Arbuckle telephones the office at 9:45 AM on 04/06/XX and informs you that she was in the office a week ago. At that time, Dr. Herschell prescribed Xanax for her anxiety episodes. She was instructed by Dr. Herschell to take the medication as he prescribed and let him know in 1 week how she was doing. If she felt her condition had not improved significantly, she was to schedule another appointment as soon as there was an opening. She has not noticed any improvement and wants to schedule another appointment as soon as possible, which you do.

Supplies/Equipment: Computer/printer/notes/textbook/reference materials

Time Allowed: _____

Accuracy Needed to Pass: 90%

Procedural Steps	Points Earned	Comments
Evaluator: Note time began: _____		
Student read the case study in the instructions given.		
1. Student correctly generated the proper heading for the "chart note" (keyed patient's name and date at the top of the document). (10)		
2. Student accurately recorded the required information from Mrs. Arbuckle's telephone call. (50)		
3. Student affixed the proper signature/identification to the chart note. (5)		
4. Student proofread/edited/printed hard copy. (10)		
Optional: May deduct points for taking more time than allowed.		

Total Points = 75

Student's Score: _____

Evaluator: _____

Comments: _____

_____

_____

_____

_____

Performance Objective 3-2—Identifying, Documenting, and Reporting Abuse and Fraud

Conditions: Student will research and generate an outline to present at a "staff meeting" for creating a policy for identifying, documenting, and reporting abuse and fraud in the medical office.

Instructions: The policy outline should include, but not be limited to, the following:

- A general definition of fraud and abuse
- Purpose of the policy
- Reasons for the policy
- Examples of fraud and abuse that frequently occur in medical facilities
- Methods used to discourage fraud and abuse
- How to gather evidence
- Responsibilities of team members
- Mandatory reporters
- Names of individuals/firms to report incidents to

Key and generate a hard copy of your outline using your computer and printer. Use 1-inch margins all around, Times New Roman Font, 12 point. Double-space outline entries. Identify your document according to instructions. *Cite your references.*

Supplies/Equipment: Internet-ready computer/printer/notes/textbook/references materials

Time Allowed: 50 minutes

Accuracy Needed to Pass: 70%

Procedural Steps	Points Earned	Comments
Evaluator: Note time began: _____		
1. Student generated document in acceptable outline form for presentation at "staff meeting." (10)		
2. Document included the required number of "relevant" topics listed in "logical" order. (25)		
3. Student followed specific formatting guidelines as noted in the instructions. (10)		
4. Student properly cited references. (10)		
5. Student proofread/edited/printed hard copy. (10)		
6. Student affixed proper identification to document. (5)		
Optional: May deduct points for taking more time than allowed.		

Total Points = 70

Student's Score: _____

Evaluator: _____

Comments: _____

_____

_____

_____

APPLICATION EXERCISES

Reference Notebook Assignment

Prepare a section in your notebook for filing information on specific laws and regulations in your state that govern insurance. Include pertinent telephone and fax numbers, websites, and addresses for contacting agencies that can help you with insurance questions.

SELF-EVALUATION

Chapter Check List

Student name: _____

Chapter completion date: _____

1.	Record	Your start time and date: _____
2.	Read	The assigned chapter in the text
3.	View	PowerPoint slides (if available)
4.	Complete	Exercises in Workbook as assigned
5.	Compare	Your answers with the answers posted on the bulletin board/website/handout
6.	Correct	Your answers
7.	Complete	All tests and required activities
8.	Read	Assigned readings (if any)
9.	Complete	Chapter performance objectives (competencies), if any
10.	Evaluate	Your personal performance and submit it to your instructor
11.	Record	Your ending time and date: _____
12.	Move on	Begin next chapter as assigned

PERFORMANCE EVALUATION

Student name: _____

Chapter completion date: _____

Evaluate your classroom performance. Complete the self-evaluation, and submit it to your instructor. When your instructor returns this form to you, compare your self-evaluation with the evaluation completed by your instructor.

Skill	Student Self-Evaluation			Instructor Evaluation		
	Good	Average	Poor	Good	Average	Poor
Attendance/punctuality						
Personal appearance						
Applies effort						
Is self-motivated						
Is courteous						
Has positive attitude						
Completes assignments in timely manner						
Works well with others						

Student's initials: _____

Date: _____

Instructor's initials: _____

Date: _____

Points Possible: _____

Points Awarded: _____

Chapter Grade: _____

Chapter **3** **The Legal and Ethical Side of Medical Insurance**

4 Types and Sources of Health Insurance

Chapter 4 introduces the student to different types of health insurance, sources of health insurance, and terms common to third-party carriers. The types and sources of health insurance were discussed in this chapter, and the major carriers are addressed in more depth later on in the textbook. There are basically two types of health insurance: indemnity, often referred to as fee-for-service, and managed care. The following workbook exercises have been developed to reinforce the concepts and materials in Chapter 4.

WORKBOOK CHAPTER OBJECTIVES

After completing the workbook activities for Chapter 4, the student should be able to:
- Define the terms used in the chapter.
- Answer the review questions to within the evaluation criteria set by the instructor.
- Use critical thinking skills to evaluate, make decisions, and communicate his or her viewpoint clearly and accurately.
- Redefine and use collaborative learning skills.
- Research the Internet successfully for up-to-date information on relevant topics.
- Perform basic mathematical computations.
- Apply learning experiences to applicable circumstances.

DEFINING CHAPTER TERMS

Using the computer (or typewriter), students should key an accurate definition for each of the chapter terms listed. These definitions should be in the students' own words. When finished, students should compare their definitions with those listed in the glossary at the back of the textbook, correcting any inaccuracies.

balance billing
birthday rule
cafeteria plan
CHAMPVA
CMS-1500 form
coinsurance
comprehensive plan
Consolidated Omnibus Budget Reconciliation Act
   (COBRA)
coordination of benefits (COB)
deductible
disability insurance
enrollees
exclusions
flexible spending account (FSA)
group contract
indemnity (fee-for-service)
insured

maintenance of benefits (MOB)
managed care
Medicaid
medical savings account (MSA)
medically necessary
Medicare
Medicare supplement plans
Medigap
nonparticipating provider (nonPAR)
out-of-pocket maximum
participating provider (PAR)
policyholder
preexisting condition
premium
Social Security Disability Insurance (SSDI)
TRICARE
usual, customary, and reasonable (UCR)
workers' compensation

33

Multiple Choice

Directions: In the questions/statements presented, choose the response that **best** answers/completes the stem by circling the letter that precedes it.

1. The two basic types of health insurance are:
   a. Major medical and comprehensive
   b. Indemnity and fee-for-service
   c. Indemnity and managed care
   d. Commercial and federal

2. Which of the following is not a way that these two types of plans differ in their basic approach to paying healthcare benefits?
   a. Choice of providers
   b. Choice of premium types
   c. Out-of-pocket costs for covered services
   d. How bills are paid

3. With an indemnity policy, patients:
   a. Can choose any provider they want
   b. Can change physicians at any time
   c. Pay a monthly "premium"
   d. Pay no yearly deductible
   e. a, b, and c

4. The value of a provider's service is based on specific historical data, referred to as:
   a. The usual, customary, and reasonable (UCR) fee
   b. Medically necessary charge
   c. Average provider fee
   d. Geographical data fee

5. The universal form used to submit claims to third-party payers is the:
   a. CMS-1100
   b. HCFA-1000
   c. CMS-1500
   d. There is no universal form

6. The type of insurance that tells patients what physicians they can see and monitors enrollees' medications and treatments so that costs remain as low as possible is:
   a. Indemnity
   b. Comprehensive
   c. Managed care
   d. Major medical

7. An insurance contract with a company or other groups of common interest wherein all employees are insured under a single policy is referred to as a(n):
   a. Indemnity policy
   b. Group policy
   c. Mutual benefits policy
   d. Common policy

8. The kind of policy purchased by a self-employed individual or one who works for a company that does not offer a group policy is a(n):

    a. Individual policy

    b. Group policy

    c. Mutual benefits policy

    d. Common policy

9. The federal health insurance program that provides benefits to individuals age 65 or older and individuals younger than 65 with certain disabilities is called:

    a. Medicare

    b. Medicaid

    c. Disability insurance

    d. TRICARE/CHAMPVA

10. The name of the federal entitlement program that covers certain categories of low-income individuals and certain disabled individuals is called:

    a. Medicare

    b. Medicaid

    c. Disability insurance

    d. TRICARE/CHAMPVA

11. Insurance that pays workers who are injured or disabled on the job or experience job-related illnesses is called:

    a. Workers' compensation

    b. Medicare

    c. Medicaid

    d. TRICARE/CHAMPVA

12. The type of plan available to self-employed individuals that works in conjunction with special low-cost, high-deductible health insurance is called a(n):

    a. Self-employed savings account (SESA)

    b. Flexible spending account (FSA)

    c. Medical savings account (MSA)

    d. Investment retirement account (IRA)

True/False

Directions: Place a "T" in the blank preceding the statement if it is true; place an "F" if it is false.

_____ 1.   Fee-for-service and indemnity insurance are the same.

_____ 2.   The portion of the medical fee that the patient is responsible for is called coinsurance.

_____ 3.   All third-party insurers have the same UCR rates.

_____ 4.   To receive maximum payment, healthcare providers must use the CMS-1500 form for all claims.

_____ 5.   All managed care plans allow patients to choose any healthcare provider they want.

_____ 6.   Under no circumstances will an insurance policy cover services rendered for "preexisting conditions."

_____ 7.   Managed care is medical care that is provided by a corporation established under state and federal laws.

_____ 8.   Individual health insurance policies historically have higher premiums than employer group policies.

_____ 9.   Medicaid is a joint federal-state health program that is run by the individual states.

_____ 10.   Medicare is the military's comprehensive healthcare program.

_____ 11. SSDI is an insurance program administered by HIPAA for individuals who are unable to work.

_____ 12. Workers' compensation laws are designed to ensure injured or disabled employees are provided with monetary awards, eliminating the need for litigation.

Matching

Directions: Insert the letter of the definition that correctly corresponds to the terms listed.

_____ 1. COBRA

_____ 2. indemnity insurance

_____ 3. FSA

_____ 4. preexisting condition

_____ 5. coinsurance

_____ 6. MSA

_____ 7. nonparticipating provider (nonPAR)

_____ 8. premium

_____ 9. deductible

_____ 10. UCR

a. The amount the insured must pay before insurance coverage begins

b. The part of a provider's charge that the insurance carrier will allow as covered expenses

c. The portion of the fee (often a percentage) that the insured must pay

d. A provider who is under no contractual agreement with the insurance carrier to accept reimbursement as payment in full

e. A special tax shelter set up for the purpose of paying medical bills

f. An IRS Section 125 cafeteria plan

g. Traditional healthcare in which patients can choose any provider they want (including specialists) and change physicians at any time

h. Illnesses or injuries that occurred before the start of a health insurance contract

i. A law that provides continuation of group health coverage when an individual leaves his or her place of employment

j. A periodic fee that is paid to an insurer for healthcare coverage

CRITICAL THINKING ACTIVITIES

A. You have learned that the CMS-1500 is a "universal" form for submitting health insurance claims to most third-party payers. What advantages and disadvantages can you think of for having a universal form?

B. Compare and contrast an MSA with an FSA.

C. Write a "news event" on a current health insurance topic. This should be a paragraph of at least 150 words, and it should explain the "event" thoroughly enough for your peers to understand.

D. Express your opinion (pro or con) of "managed care" in one to two paragraphs.

E. In a 2004 ABC News poll, it was found that "62 percent of the population said that they would favor a system of universal health insurance financed by the government, paid for by the tax payers, as opposed to the system we now have, the employer-based system where many people are uninsured." What is your opinion on this subject?

Key your answer according to established essay formatting rules and print a hard copy.

PROBLEM-SOLVING/COLLABORATIVE THINKING ACTIVITIES

A. Imagine you are married with two minor children. Your spouse comes home from work and announces that his or her employer has offered a choice of health insurance policies. One is an indemnity plan with a $250 yearly deductible and an 80/20 copayment. The other is a managed care plan (HMO) requiring only a $25 per encounter payment.

   1. Do you have enough information for making an educated choice?

   2. If so, which plan would you choose and why?

   3. If not, what further information do you need before you can make a decision?

PROJECTS/DISCUSSION TOPICS

Choose one of the following topics and, according to your instructor's guidelines, prepare an outline for an oral discussion:

1. What does it mean not to have health insurance?
2. The costs versus the benefits of health insurance
3. Consolidated Omnibus Budget Reconciliation Act (COBRA)
4. Health insurance in other countries (e.g., Canada, Great Britain)
5. Compare and contrast participating (PAR) and nonPAR providers.

CASE STUDIES

A. Sally and Joe Barnes have three children, ages 12, 8, and 5. Sally has a 60% teaching contract with the Oak Crest County School System, and Joe works full-time for Amex Auto Sales. Both have a group policy through their employer. Sally's date of birth is 08/17/64, and Joe's is 03/10/65. Which policy is primary for their children?

B. Dr. Maxwell Stark is a PAR provider with Blue Cross and Blue Shield; Dr. Forrest Wilson is nonPAR with the same insurer. Both providers are specialists in gastroenterology. Both physicians charge $1000 for a colonoscopy. Blue Cross and Blue Shield allows $700 as its UCR fee for this procedure. Assuming each provider has a patient who undergoes a colonoscopy, each patient has satisfied his or her yearly deductible, and each has paid the same amount of coinsurance (20% of the "allowable" charge—$140), how much can Dr. Stark bill his colonoscopy patient? How much can Dr. Wilson bill his patient?

INTERNET EXPLORATION

Research and analyze long-term care insurance. Compose a list of advantages and disadvantages of this type of health insurance. Imagine you are having a discussion with your 62-year-old aunt. What would you tell her about long-term care insurance?

The remaining basic foundation skill is mathematics. Individuals seeking entry-level positions should be able to "perform basic computations and approach practical problems by choosing appropriately from a variety of mathematical techniques."

Performance Objective 4-1—Math Skills

Conditions: Student will read the following math problem and choose an appropriate method to arrive at the correct answer (must show your work).

Supplies/Equipment: Calculator, pencil, sheet of plain paper, (allowed) reference materials

Time Allowed: 15 minutes

Accuracy Needed to Pass: 100%

Problem: You are employed as a health insurance professional by Bright Horizons Medical Center. You note that your supply of CMS-1500 forms is getting low, and it's time to reorder. According to the catalog, these forms can be ordered two ways: a case containing 250 forms priced at $0.20 each, or a case of 1500 (quantity) forms priced at $195 per 1000. Which is the more economical method for purchasing these forms?

Procedural Steps	Points Earned	Comments
Evaluator: Note time began: _____		
1. Carefully read the problem.		
2. Using an appropriate mathematical technique, calculate the correct answer.		
3. Insert your answer in the blank provided. (10)		
4. Show your calculations, and make sure the method you used to arrive at the solution is accurate. (10)		
Optional: May deduct points for taking more time than allowed.		

Total Points = 20

Student's Score: _____

Evaluator: _____

Comments: _____

_____

_____

_____

_____

Health Insurance Professional's Notebook

If your instructor has chosen this project for you to complete, you now should have the following items generated for your notebook:

- A cover page
- Six tabbed and labeled dividers
- A Table of Contents (not final)

Now, create a cover sheet for each of the six main sections (Fig. 4-1). After these documents have been created, insert them in your notebook behind the tabbed dividers.

MEDICAID

TABLE OF CONTENTS

   I.   Federal regulations

   II.   State regulations for _____ (insert your state here)

   III.   Eligibility chart/table

   IV.   Sample forms

   V.   Sample identification card(s)

   VI.   Current fiscal intermediary name/address/phone

   VII.   Guidelines for completing the CMS-1500

   VIII.   CMS-1500 template

(List other pertinent topics.)

Fig. 4-1 Sample section cover sheet.

Chapter Check List

Student name: _____

Chapter completion date: _____

1.	Record	Your start time and date: _____
2.	Read	The assigned chapter in the text
3.	View	PowerPoint slides (if available)
4.	Complete	Exercises in Workbook as assigned
5.	Compare	Your answers with the answers posted on the bulletin board/website/handout
6.	Correct	Your answers
7.	Complete	All tests and required activities
8.	Read	Assigned readings (if any)
9.	Complete	Chapter performance objectives (competencies), if any
10.	Evaluate	Your personal performance and submit it to your instructor
11.	Record	Your ending time and date: _____
12.	Move on	Begin next chapter as assigned

PERFORMANCE EVALUATION

Student name: _____

Chapter completion date: _____

Evaluate your classroom performance. Complete the self-evaluation, and submit it to your instructor. When your instructor returns this form to you, compare your self-evaluation with the evaluation completed by your instructor.

Skill	Student Self-Evaluation			Instructor Evaluation		
	Good	Average	Poor	Good	Average	Poor
Attendance/punctuality						
Personal appearance						
Applies effort						
Is self-motivated						
Is courteous						
Has positive attitude						
Completes assignments in timely manner						
Works well with others						

Student's initials: _____

Date: _____

Instructor's initials: _____

Date: _____

Points Possible: _____

Points Awarded: _____

Chapter Grade: _____

5 The "Universal" Claim Form: CMS-1500

Chapter 5 introduces the student to the CMS-1500—the "universal" claim form used by all government and most third-party payers. Although most medical facilities now submit claims electronically, or are in the process of doing so, it is important for students to understand the basic structure and function of the paper form. It is important that students know where the information comes from that applies to each of the 33 blocks of the CMS-1500 form. After students learn the fundamentals of the paper claims, they should be able to understand better how electronic claims are generated. The following workbook exercises familiarize students further with the CMS-1500 claim form and guide them through the multistage process of collecting and "abstracting" the necessary information from various documents to complete and submit a "clean" claim.

WORKBOOK CHAPTER OBJECTIVES

After completing the workbook activities for Chapter 5, the student should be able to:
- Define the terms used in the chapter.
- Answer the review questions to within the evaluation criteria set by the instructor.
- Analyze hypothetical situations, applying logical concepts for rational decision making to health insurance scenarios.
- Apply reasoning and problem-solving skills (individually or in a group) to arrive at practical solutions to common health insurance issues.
- Conduct Internet research to learn more about selected topics.
- Abstract information from healthcare documents for the purpose of accurate claims completion.
- Collect information and documents for inclusion in the Health Insurance Professional's Notebook.
- Perform self-evaluation on successful content mastery for Chapter 5.

DEFINING CHAPTER TERMS

Using the computer (or typewriter), students should key an accurate definition for each of the chapter terms listed. These definitions should be in the students' own words. When finished, students should compare their definitions with those listed in the glossary at the back of the textbook, correcting any inaccuracies.

abstract
ASCII (American Standard Code for Information Interchange)
assign benefits
beneficiary
claims clearinghouse
clean claims
CMS-1500 (form)
demographic information

encounter form
mono-spaced fonts
OCR scannable
optical character recognition (OCR)
patient ledger card
release of information
small provider
waiver

43

Multiple Choice

Directions: In the questions/statements presented, choose the response that **best** answers/completes the stem, and circle the letter that precedes it.

1. A major innovation that made the process of health insurance claims submission simpler was the development of:
   a. HIPAA
   b. A universal form
   c. The American Medical Association
   d. Optical character recognition (OCR) scanners

2. The front side of the CMS-1500 claim form is printed in:
   a. All italics
   b. Two languages
   c. OCR scannable red ink
   d. Times New Roman, 12-point font

3. The most common *format* used for *text files* in computers and on the Internet is:
   a. OCR
   b. ASCII
   c. Universal 100
   d. Times New Roman

4. OCR formatting rules specify:
   a. All entries in uppercase
   b. No punctuation
   c. MM/DD/YYYY birth date format
   d. All of the above

5. A "small provider" of services is one with less than:
   a. 5 full-time equivalent employees
   b. 15 full-time equivalent employees
   c. 20 full-time equivalent employees
   d. 25 full-time equivalent employees

6. The patient information form is considered a legal document and should be updated no less often than:
   a. Once a month
   b. Once a year
   c. Every 2 years
   d. Every 5 years

7. A patient's name, address, Social Security number, and employment data are commonly referred to as:
   a. Viable data
   b. Pertinent facts
   c. Transient statistics
   d. Demographic information

8. An individual covered under Medicare is referred to as a(n):
   a. Enrollee
   b. Beneficiary
   c. Recipient
   d. Covered entity

9. An insurance policy that covers an individual, his or her spouse, and eligible dependents is referred to as a(n):
   a. Dual plan
   b. Family plan
   c. Multiple plan
   d. Individual plan

10. A multipurpose form used by most medical practices for billing is called a(n):
    a. Superbill
    b. Encounter form
    c. Routing form
    d. All of the above

11. In noncomputerized practices, patient charges and payments can be tracked manually on a(n):
    a. Encounter form
    b. CMS-1500 form
    c. Patient ledger card
    d. Patient information form

12. The CMS-1500 claim form has _____ separate blocks.
    a. 24
    b. 28
    c. 30
    d. 33

13. After the health insurance professional has completed the claim form, it should be:
    a. Proofread
    b. Mailed to the patient
    c. Mailed to the insurance carrier
    d. Submitted to the provider for signature

14. An example of a method for manual claims follow-up is using an:
    a. Insurance log
    b. Encounter form
    c. Insurance register
    d. a and c are correct

15. A company that receives claims, consolidates them, and transmits them in batches to third-party payers is called a:
    a. Third-party payer
    b. Clearinghouse
    c. Claims consolidator
    d. Covered entity

True/False

Directions: Read the following sentences. If it is true, place a "T" in the blank preceding the number. If it is false, place an "F" in the blank, and then rewrite the sentence in the space provided beneath so that it reads true. The first one is done for you as an example.

_F_   1.   The American Medical Association is responsible for creating the universal claim form known as the CMS-1500.

The Health Care Financing Administration is responsible for creating the universal claim form known as the CMS-1500.

_____

_____ 2.   The CMS-1500 form (originally known as the HCFA-1500) was developed for the purpose of submitting Medicare claims.

_____

_____ 3.   The federal government has passed a law mandating that the universal claim form be used for all third-party payers.

_____

_____ 4.   The CMS-1500 form is in two parts. The top portion is for the physician/supplier information, and the bottom portion for the patient/insured information.

_____

_____ 5.   The CMS-1500 form is composed of 33 blocks.

_____

_____ 6.   Because the CMS-1500 is a "universal" form, every major payer has exactly the same guidelines for completing each block.

_____

_____ 7.   The use of OCR formatting guidelines is preferred, but not mandatory, when completing the CMS-1500 claim form.

_____

_____ 8.   Correct OCR guidelines require the use of the MM DD YY format for all dates.

_____

_____ 9.   The health insurance professional's most important responsibility is to obtain the maximum amount of reimbursement in the minimal amount of time that the patient's health record would support.

_____

_____ 10.   The HIPAA Administrative Simplification Compliance Act (ASCA) prohibits the Department of Health and Human Services (HHS) from paying all claims that are not submitted electronically, without exception.

_____

_____ 11. The patient information form lists demographic and insurance information.

_____

_____ 12. The health insurance professional must obtain written permission from the patient to release healthcare information to any person or business entity except the patient's insurance carrier.

_____

Short Answer/Fill-in-the-Blanks

1. Name the two major sections of the CMS-1500 claim form.

   _____

   _____

2. List the situations when a space is required instead of the usual punctuation or symbols in OCR formatting.

   _____

   _____

   _____

   _____

3. When the health insurance professional has completed the claim form, it is crucial that the form is thoroughly examined for _____ and _____.

4. What is the health insurance professional's most important task?

   _____

5. Who uses the paper CMS-1500 form?

   _____

6. ASCA prohibits HHS from paying Medicare claims that are not submitted electronically, unless the Secretary grants a(n) _____ for this requirement.

7. Define a "small provider."

   _____

8. List three reasons why healthcare facilities use a patient information form.

   _____

   _____

   _____

9. Explain the rationale for making a photocopy of both sides of a patient's insurance ID card.

_____

10. What is the significance of a patient "assigning benefits"?

_____

11. Define a medical record.

_____

12. List six things a complete medical record should provide.

_____

_____

_____

_____

_____

_____

13. List at least six types of information typically found on an encounter form.

_____

_____

_____

_____

_____

_____

14. List at least five reasons why a claim might be rejected.

_____

_____

_____

_____

_____

48

15. What are three advantages of electronic claims filing?

_____

_____

_____

CRITICAL THINKING ACTIVITIES

A. You are employed as a health insurance professional in a family practice facility. Eloise Grafton, the office supervisor, asks you to generate a document for the Office Procedures Manual explaining the steps involved in the insurance claims and billing process. Begin with the patient's arrival at the office through the checkout process at the reception area when the encounter is concluded. Include a diagram or a flow chart to enhance understanding.

B. Write a paragraph explaining the purpose and function of the **encounter form.** Be specific and thorough. Use examples as necessary.

PROBLEM-SOLVING/COLLABORATIVE (GROUP) ACTIVITIES

A. Your instructor will give you two blank patient information forms. Along with a partner, role-play health insurance professional and patient. When you play the part of the "patient," complete the patient information form using your own personal information, or create a fictitious character. Then ask your partner, the "health insurance professional," to check the form for omissions or errors. Reverse roles and repeat the procedure.

B. Carefully examine the completed claim form (Adam Rogers) in Fig. 5-1. Highlight or circle any shaded blocks that contain errors. Then, in Table 5-1, insert a "C" in Column 2 if the information in the block is correct; insert an "I" if it is incorrect. Lastly, illustrate how the information should be entered correctly in Column 3.

1500

HEALTH INSURANCE CLAIM FORM

APPROVED BYNATIONALUNIFORMCLAIMCOMMITTEE 08/05

PICA — PICA — CARRIER

1. MEDICARE (Medicare #) ☐ MEDICAID (Medicaid #) ☐ TRICARE CHAMPUS (Sponsor's SSN) ☐ CHAMPVA (Member ID#) ☐ GROUP HEALTH PLAN (SSN or ID) ☒ FECA BLK LUNG (SSN) ☐ OTHER (ID) ☐

1a. INSURED'S I.D. NUMBER (For Program in Item 1): XQS123456789

2. PATIENT'S NAME (Last Name, First Name, Middle Initial): ROGERS ADAM L

3. PATIENT'S BIRTH DATE MM DD YY: 10 21 54 — SEX M ☒ F ☐

4. INSURED'S NAME (Last Name, First Name, Middle Initial): SAME

5. PATIENT'S ADDRESS (No., Street): 1500 WEST 50TH ST

6. PATIENT RELATIONSHIP TO INSURED: Self ☒ Spouse ☐ Child ☐ Other ☐

7. INSURED'S ADDRESS (No., Street):

CITY: MILTON — STATE: XY

8. PATIENT STATUS: Single ☒ Married ☐ Other ☐ — Employed ☐ Full-Time Student ☐ Part-Time Student ☐

CITY — STATE

ZIP CODE — TELEPHONE (Include Area Code) ( )

ZIP CODE — TELEPHONE (Include Area Code) ( )

9. OTHER INSURED'S NAME (Last Name, First Name, Middle Initial)

10. IS PATIENT'S CONDITION RELATED TO:

11. INSURED'S POLICY GROUP OR FECA NUMBER

a. OTHER INSURED'S POLICY OR GROUP NUMBER

a. EMPLOYMENT? (Current or Previous) ☐ YES ☐ NO

a. INSURED'S DATE OF BIRTH MM DD YY — SEX M ☐ F ☐

b. OTHER INSURED'S DATE OF BIRTH MM DD YY — SEX M ☐ F ☐

b. AUTO ACCIDENT? ☐ YES ☐ NO — PLACE (State)

b. EMPLOYER'S NAME OR SCHOOL NAME: RARITAN HYDRAULICS

c. EMPLOYER'S NAME OR SCHOOL NAME

c. OTHER ACCIDENT? ☐ YES ☐ NO

c. INSURANCE PLAN NAME OR PROGRAM NAME

d. INSURANCE PLAN NAME OR PROGRAM NAME

10d. RESERVED FOR LOCAL USE

d. IS THERE ANOTHER HEALTH BENEFIT PLAN? ☐ YES ☐ NO *If yes,* return to and complete item 9 a-d.

READ BACK OF FORM BEFORE COMPLETING & SIGNING THIS FORM.

12. PATIENT'S OR AUTHORIZED PERSON'S SIGNATURE I authorize the release of any medical or other information necessary to process this claim. I also request payment of government benefits either to myself or to the party who accepts assignment below.

SIGNED *Adam L Rogers* DATE 9/10/XX

13. INSURED'S OR AUTHORIZED PERSON'S SIGNATURE I authorize payment of medical benefits to the undersigned physician or supplier for services described below.

SIGNED

PATIENT AND INSURED INFORMATION

14. DATE OF CURRENT: ILLNESS (First symptom) OR INJURY (Accident) OR PREGNANCY(LMP) MM DD YY: 09 10 20XX

15. IF PATIENT HAS HAD SAME OR SIMILAR ILLNESS. GIVE FIRST DATE MM DD YY

16. DATES PATIENT UNABLE TO WORK IN CURRENT OCCUPATION FROM MM DD YY TO MM DD YY

17. NAME OF REFERRING PROVIDER OR OTHER SOURCE: HORNER WILLIAMS MD

17a. 655432112

17b. NPI 231314800

18. HOSPITALIZATION DATES RELATED TO CURRENT SERVICES FROM MM DD YY TO MM DD YY

19. RESERVED FOR LOCAL USE

20. OUTSIDE LAB? ☐ YES ☐ NO — $ CHARGES

21. DIAGNOSIS OR NATURE OF ILLNESS OR INJURY (Relate Items 1, 2, 3 or 4 to Item 24E by Line)

1. 892 . 0

2. ___ . ___

3. ___ . ___

4. ___ . ___

22. MEDICAID RESUBMISSION CODE — ORIGINAL REF. NO.

23. PRIOR AUTHORIZATION NUMBER

	24. A. DATE(S) OF SERVICE From MM DD YY	To MM DD YY	B. PLACE OF SERVICE	C. EMG	D. PROCEDURES, SERVICES, OR SUPPLIES (Explain Unusual Circumstances) CPT/HCPCS	MODIFIER	E. DIAGNOSIS POINTER	F. $ CHARGES	G. DAYS OR UNITS	H. EPSDT Family Plan	I. ID. QUAL.	J. RENDERING PROVIDER ID. #
1	09 10 XX	09 10 XX	11		99202		1	60 00	1		NPI	0020202 / 231314800
2	09 10 XX	09 10 XX	11		90703		1	20 00	1		NPI	0020202 / 231314800
3											NPI	
4											NPI	
5											NPI	
6											NPI	

25. FEDERAL TAX I.D. NUMBER: 42 1898989 — SSN ☐ EIN ☒

26. PATIENT'S ACCOUNT NO.

27. ACCEPT ASSIGNMENT? (For govt. claims, see back) ☒ YES ☐ NO

28. TOTAL CHARGE $ 80 00

29. AMOUNT PAID $

30. BALANCE DUE $

31. SIGNATURE OF PHYSICIAN OR SUPPLIER INCLUDING DEGREES OR CREDENTIALS (I certify that the statements on the reverse apply to this bill and are made a part thereof.)
HORNER WILLIAMS MD
Horner Williams MD 09/14/20XX
SIGNED DATE

32. SERVICE FACILITY LOCATION INFORMATION
BROADMOOR MEDICAL CLINIC
4353 PINE RIDGE DRIVE
MILTON XY 12345-0001
a. X100XX1000 b.

33. BILLING PROVIDER INFO & PH # ( )
BROADMOOR MEDICAL CLINIC
4353 PINE RIDGE DRIVE
MILTON XY 12345-0001
a. X100XX1000 b.

PHYSICIAN OR SUPPLIER INFORMATION

NUCC Instruction Manual available at: www.nucc.org — APPROVED OMB-0938-0999 FORM CMS-1500 (08/05)

Fig. 5-1 CMS-1500 form for Adam Rogers.

Table 5-1 Table of Corrections		
Block No.	C/I	Corrected Information
2		
3		
5		
10		
11d		
17		
17a		
24b		
24g		
25		
32b		
33		
33a		
33b*		
*After May 23, 2007, Block 33b is not to be reported.		

C. Study the insurance ID card in Fig. 5-2. Answer the following questions with regard to the information on the card.

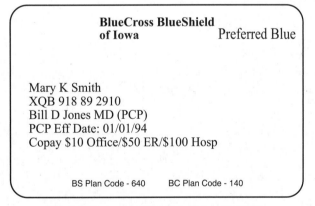

**BlueCross BlueShield
of Iowa**   Preferred Blue

Mary K Smith
XQB 918 89 2910
Bill D Jones MD (PCP)
PCP Eff Date: 01/01/94
Copay $10 Office/$50 ER/$100 Hosp

BS Plan Code - 640   BC Plan Code - 140

Fig. 5-2 Insurance ID card for Mary K. Smith.

1. In whose name is this insurance policy written?
2. What identification code should be entered in Block 1a of the CMS-1500 form?
3. What is the name of the insured's primary care physician?
4. When was this primary care physician assigned to the insured?
5. Explain what the numbers mean in the last line of the card: **Copay $10 Office/$50 ER/$100 Hosp**

Chapter **5** The "Universal" Claim Form: CMS-1500

Your instructor will assign one or more of the following topics:

A. Discuss the pros and cons of filing claims electronically.

B. Create a table comparing/contrasting direct claims filing versus using a claims clearinghouse. Include advantages and disadvantages of both methods.

C. Study the OCR formatting guidelines in the text, and then generate a list outlining the "do's" and "don'ts" for your Health Insurance Professional Notebook.

D. Fig. 5-3 illustrates the back of an insurance ID card. Discuss the function and importance of each line of information on this ID card.

SOUTHEAST IOWA SCHOOLS
HEALTH CARE PLAN

You, the insured, or someone acting on your behalf must call for certification of coverage for the below named services:

• prior to all scheduled inpatient hospital admissions, skilled nursing facility and mental health facility admissions;

• within 24 hours of an inpatient obstetrical admission;

• within 48 hours of an emergency inpatient admission (72 hours for holidays and weekends);

THE NUMBER TO CALL IS 1-800-373-1020. (Phones are answered 24 hours a day, seven days a week.)

ADDITIONAL PROVISIONS: A maternity evaluation form must be submitted to EBS by the sixth month of pregnancy. Contact EBS at (800) 373-1327 or (319) 752-3200.

This Plan now has a PREFERRED PROVIDER NETWORK. Non-preferred providers may bill you for charges in excess of Usual, Reasonable, and Customary fees. Contact EBS for a Preferred Provider listing.

Fig. 5-3 Back side of an insurance ID card.

CASE STUDIES

A. Using the information on Mary K. Smith's patient information form (Fig. 5-4) and her insurance ID card (see Fig. 5-2), complete Blocks 1 through 13 in the top half of the CMS-1500 claim form (Fig. 5-5), or use the electronic form in the Student Software CD.

B. Using the information in the encounter form (Mary K. Smith) shown in Fig. 5-6, complete the bottom half of the CMS-1500 claim form (Fig. 5-7), or use the electronic form in the Student Software. Use the following information:

Provider Block	
Broadmoor Medical Clinic	Clinic EIN # 42-1898989
4353 Pine Ridge Drive	Dr. R. L. Jones NPI 1234567890
Milton, XY 12345-0001	Dr. Marilou Lucerno NPI 2907511822
Clinic NPI # X100XX1000	Date claims 1 day after examination
Telephone: 555-656-7890	

PATIENT INFORMATION SHEET

Today's date: 6/12/XX

HEAD OF HOUSEHOLD

Head of household: Mary K. Smith

Social Security #: 918-89-2910

Sex: F Date of birth: 7/24/68

Address: 409 Oak St.

City, St: Milton, XY Zip: 12345

Home phone #: 555-765-1234

Occupation: Waitress

Employer's name: Grover's Pizza

Employer's address: 1516 Main St.

Employer's City, St: Milton, XY Zip: 12345

Employer's phone #: 555-766-4321

PATIENT INFORMATION

Patient's legal name: Mary K. Smith

Nickname: — Relationship to head of household: same

Date of birth _____ Age ____ Sex ____ Marital Status: S

Employer name ____ **SAME AS ABOVE**

Employer address ____

Social Security ____

Employer phone # ____

Worker's Compensation Carrier (If applicable): -N/A

City, St: ____ Zip ____

Referring Physician: none

Allergies ____

EMERGENCY INFORMATION

Other contact not living with you: Betty Keyes

Home phone# ____ Work phone# ____

Address: Rt 63 Box 112 City: Milton St: XY Zip: 12345

Patient relationship to other contact: daughter

If patient is a child, parent name: N/A

INSURANCE INFORMATION

Primary insurance: BlueCross/BlueShield Subscriber: Mary K. Smith

ID #: XQB 918-89-2910 Relationship to subscriber: self

Secondary insurance: none Subscriber ____

ID # ____ Relationship to subscriber ____

OTHER FAMILY MEMBERS:

Name: Darrell P. Beckett Date of birth: 2/21/90

Name: Cathy M. Beckett Date of birth: 4/6/95

Name ____ Date of birth: ____

Name ____ Date of birth: ____

I understand that it is my responsibility that any incurred charges are paid.

To the extent necessary to determine liability for payment to obtain reimbursement, process claim forms, I authorize the release of any medical information necessary to process claims.

I hereby assign all medical and/or surgical benefits, to include major medical benefits to which I am entitled, including Medicare, private insurance, and other health plans to Family Medicine of Mt. Pleasant, P.C.

This assignment will remain in effect until revoked by me in writing, a photocopy of this assignment is to be considered as valid as an original. I hereby authorize said assignee to release all information necessary to secure the payment.

Signed: Mary K. Smith Date: 6/12/04

If patient is a minor, parent or guardian signature.

Fig. 5-4 Patient information sheet for Mary K. Smith.

HEALTH INSURANCE CLAIM FORM

APPROVED BY NATIONAL UNIFORM CLAIM COMMITTEE 08/05

☐☐ PICA

							PICA ☐☐

CARRIER

1. MEDICARE MEDICAID TRICARE CHAMPUS CHAMPVA GROUP HEALTH PLAN FECA BLK LUNG OTHER	1a. INSURED'S I.D. NUMBER (For Program in Item 1)
☐ (Medicare #) ☐ (Medicaid #) ☐ (Sponsor's SSN) ☐ (Member ID#) ☐ (SSN or ID) ☐ (SSN) ☐ (ID)	

2. PATIENT'S NAME (Last Name, First Name, Middle Initial)	3. PATIENT'S BIRTH DATE MM DD YY SEX M ☐ F ☐	4. INSURED'S NAME (Last Name, First Name, Middle Initial)

5. PATIENT'S ADDRESS (No., Street)	6. PATIENT RELATIONSHIP TO INSURED Self ☐ Spouse ☐ Child ☐ Other ☐	7. INSURED'S ADDRESS (No., Street)

CITY	STATE	8. PATIENT STATUS Single ☐ Married ☐ Other ☐	CITY	STATE

ZIP CODE	TELEPHONE (Include Area Code) ( )	Employed ☐ Full-Time Student ☐ Part-Time Student ☐	ZIP CODE	TELEPHONE (Include Area Code) ( )

9. OTHER INSURED'S NAME (Last Name, First Name, Middle Initial)	10. IS PATIENT'S CONDITION RELATED TO:	11. INSURED'S POLICY GROUP OR FECA NUMBER

a. OTHER INSURED'S POLICY OR GROUP NUMBER	a. EMPLOYMENT? (Current or Previous) ☐ YES ☐ NO	a. INSURED'S DATE OF BIRTH MM DD YY SEX M ☐ F ☐

b. OTHER INSURED'S DATE OF BIRTH MM DD YY SEX M ☐ F ☐	b. AUTO ACCIDENT? PLACE (State) ☐ YES ☐ NO	b. EMPLOYER'S NAME OR SCHOOL NAME

c. EMPLOYER'S NAME OR SCHOOL NAME	c. OTHER ACCIDENT? ☐ YES ☐ NO	c. INSURANCE PLAN NAME OR PROGRAM NAME

d. INSURANCE PLAN NAME OR PROGRAM NAME	10d. RESERVED FOR LOCAL USE	d. IS THERE ANOTHER HEALTH BENEFIT PLAN? ☐ YES ☐ NO *If yes*, return to and complete item 9 a-d.

PATIENT AND INSURED INFORMATION

READ BACK OF FORM BEFORE COMPLETING & SIGNING THIS FORM.

12. PATIENT'S OR AUTHORIZED PERSON'S SIGNATURE I authorize the release of any medical or other information necessary to process this claim. I also request payment of government benefits either to myself or to the party who accepts assignment below.	13. INSURED'S OR AUTHORIZED PERSON'S SIGNATURE I authorize payment of medical benefits to the undersigned physician or supplier for services described below.
SIGNED _____ DATE _____	SIGNED _____

Fig. 5-5 Top half of CMS-1500 form (for Mary K. Smith).

BROADMOOR MEDICAL CLINIC

DATE OF SERVICE 6/12/XX

PATIENT ID#: 918892910

CHIEF COMPLAINT: Annual exam

PATIENT NAME: Mary K. Smith

CONFIDENTIAL: X

PROVIDER NAME: R.L. Jones, M.D.
NPI 1234567890

BILLED VISIT? X

Office Vs, New/Est	Code
99201	99211
99202	99212
99203	99213
99204	99214
99205	99215

Telephone Calls	Code
Intermediate	99372
Complex/Lengthy	99373

Prev Medicine, New	Code
5-11 yo	99383
12-17 yo	99384
✓ 18-39 yo 130.00	99385

Prev Medicine, Est.	Code
5-10 yo	99393
12-17 yo	99394
18-39 yo	99395

Counseling/Risk Fx	Code
Individual:	
15 min	99401
30 min	99402
45 min	99403
60 min	99404
Group:	
30 min	99411
60 min	99412
Health Risk Assess:	
Administer	99420

AdminVaccine	Code
Administer one:	99471
Admin, ea add'l:	90472
Admin, oral, one:	90473
Admin, oral, ea add'l:	90474

AdminTher Injection	Code
Therapeutic inj	90782
IM antibiotic	90788

Drugs Administered IM/SC	Code
Tetracycline 250 mg	J0120
Ampicillin Na 500 mg	J0290
Rocephin 250 mg	J0696
Depo-Provera 150 mg	J1055
Benadryl to 50 mg	J1200
Erythrocin 500 mg	J1364
Gentamicin to 80 mg	J1580
Wycillan 600,000 U	J2510
Pen G 600,000 U	J2540
Streptomy to 1 Gm	J3000

Vaccine(s)	Code
Adenovirus	90476
BCG/Tb	90585
Cholera	90724
Diptheria	90719
DT	90702
DTaP	90700
DTaP-HepB-IPV	90723
DTaP-HIB	90721
DTP	90701
DTP-HIB	90720
Flu, 3+ yo	90658
Hep A, 2ds	90633
Hep B 2ds	90743
Hep B 3ds	90744
Hep B adult	90746
Hep B/HIB	90748
Hib/HbOC, 4 ds	90645
Hib/PRP-D, boost	90646
Hib/PRP-OMP, 3 ds	90647
Hib/PRP-T, 4 ds	90648
IPV	90713
Measles	90705
Meningococcal	90733
MMR	90707
MMRV	90710
MR	90708
Mumps	90704
OPV	90712
Pneumococcal	90732
Rotavirus, live, oral	90680
Rubella	90706
Td	90718
Tetanus Tox	90703
Typhoid (AKD)	90693
Typhoid (ViCPS)	90691
Typhoid (H-P)	90692
Varicella	90716

Team Conference	Code
Pt not pres, 30 min	99361
Pt not pres, 60 min	99362

Respiratory SystemTx	Code
Peak flow	94200
Nebulizer demo	94664
Repeat neb Tx	94640-76
Pulse oximetry	94760

Inhaled Drugs	Code
Albuterol/0.5 mg	J7618

ScreeningTests	Code
Vision	99173
Hearing (air only)	92551

Allergy Injections	Code
Single inj (OV incl)	95115
2+ inj (OV incl)	95117

Health/Behavior Assess	Code
Initial, ea 15 min	96150
Re-assess	96151
Indiv int'vent/15"	96152
Group/15 min	96153
Family/15 min	96154
Fam w/o pt/15 min	96155

Education	Code
Group	99078
Supplies	99071

Surgical Procedures	Code
I & D:	
abscess	10060
foreign body	10120
Debridement:	
10% body surf	11000
ea add'l 10%	11000
Biopsy:	
lesion, skin	11100
ea add'l lesion	11001
Repair Wound:	
Trunk, ext, scalp, neck:	
2.5 cm or <	12001
Face, ears, nose, lips	
eyelids 2.5 cm or <	12011
Tx dehiscence	12020
Burns:	
1st deg, local	16000
Destruction lesion:	
Flat warts, up to 14	17110
Common warts, 1st	17000
ea add'l wart, 2-14	17003
Penis	54050
Vulva	56501
Removal foreign body:	
Eye, external	65205
Nose	30300
Skin	Office Vs
Removal ear wax	69210
Strain/Sprain	Office Vs

Laboratory:	Code
Venipuncture	36415

CLIAWaivedTests	Code
Glucometer	82962
Hematocrit	85014QW
Hemoglobin	85018QW
Mononucleosis	86308QW
Rapid strep test	87880QW
Urine dipstick	81002
Urine pregnancy	81025

CLIA Phys Perf Micro	Code
Wet mount-any	Q0111
KOH prep	Q0112
✓ UA dip, non-auto, w/micro	81000 15.00
UA dip, auto, w/micro	81001

CLIA Intermediate	Code
✓ CBC 15.00	85025
Chlamydia culture	87110
GC culture	87081
Lead	83655
Sickle cell screen	85660
TB intradermal	86580
Throat culture	87070
Urine culture	87086

CLIA Complex	Code
HIV	86703
✓ PAP smear, thin prep	88144 25.00
VDRL	86592

Diagnosis(es):

1. V 70.0
2.
3.
4.

Signature of provider:

Bill Jones, MD

Return to clinic: 1 year

Fig. 5-6 Encounter form (for Mary K. Smith).

55

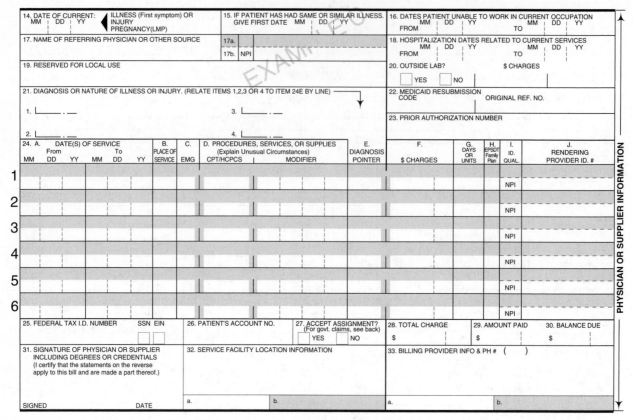

Fig. 5-7 Bottom half of CMS-1500 form (for Mary K. Smith).

INTERNET EXPLORATION

A. Research the Internet and locate a specific example of a HIPAA-compliant authorization form for use or disclosure of protected health information (PHI).

B. Your office manager has informed you that the practice is considering electronic claims submission. She has asked you to do some research to find the names of two or three clearinghouses and compare what they have to offer, specifically considering services offered, software and equipment needed, and corresponding costs. Research the Internet using "claims clearinghouse" as your search word, and create a memo to your office manager providing him or her with at least two clearinghouse companies to show a comparison of services provided by the company, their costs, and required equipment/software.

Performance Objective 5-1—Patient Ledger Card

Conditions: Student will create a ledger card for a new patient using the information abstracted from the patient information form and the insurance ID card for Adam Rogers.

Supplies/Equipment: Electronic form/typewriter/pen; patient information form (Fig. 5-8), insurance ID card (Fig. 5-9), blank ledger card (Fig. 5-10) or the electronic ledger card in the Student Software CD.

Time Allowed: 20 minutes

Accuracy Needed to Pass: 90%

Procedural Steps	Points Earned	Comments
Evaluator: Note time began:_____		
1. Carefully read and study the applicable documents.		
2. Type the patient's correct name and address in the appropriate position. (10)		
3. Type the insurance information in the upper, left-hand corner of the ledger card (ensure none of the information falls within the address block). (20)		
4. Type the amount of coinsurance the patient must pay for each office visit in the upper right-hand corner. (5)		
5. Type the number to call for preadmission certification below the coinsurance amount. (5)		
Optional: May deduct points for taking more time than allowed.		

Total Points = 40

Student's Score: _____

Evaluator: _____

Comments: _____

_____

_____

_____

_____

PATIENT INFORMATION SHEET

Today's date: _9/10/XX_

HEAD OF HOUSEHOLD

Head of household: _patient_

Social Security #: _123-45-6789_

Sex: _M_ Date of birth: _10/21/54_

Address: _400 Maple Av_

City, St: _Milton, XY_ Zip: _12345_

Home phone #: _SSS-800-2222_

Occupation: _night watchman_

Employer's name: _Raritan Hydraulics_

Employer's address: _1500W. 60th St._

Employer's City, St: _Milton, XY_ Zip: _12345_

Employer's phone #: _SSS-800-3210_

PATIENT INFORMATION

Patient's legal name: _Adam L. Rogers_ Nickname _____ Relationship to head of household: _self_

Date of birth: _12/21/54_ Age _____ Sex: _M_ Marital Status: _S_

Employer name: _Raritan Hydraulics_ Social Security #: _123-45-6789_

Employer address: _1500W. 60th St._ Employer phone #: _SSS-800-6611_

City, St: _Milton, XY_ Zip: _12345_ Worker's Compensation Carrier (If applicable): _NA_

Referring Physician: _____ Allergies: _NONE_

EMERGENCY INFORMATION

Other contact not living with you: _Phillip Rogers_ Home phone#: _SSS-800-2104_ Work phone#: _SSS-800-3210_

Address: _2925 Sunnylawn_ City: _Milton_ St: _XY_ Zip: _12345_

Patient relationship to other contact: _son_ If patient is a child, parent name: _____

INSURANCE INFORMATION

Primary insurance: _BlueCross & BlueShield_ Subscriber: _patient_ _Adam L. Rogers_

ID #: _XQS 123456789_ Relationship to subscriber: _self_

Secondary insurance: _____ Subscriber: _____

ID #: _____ Relationship to subscriber: _____

OTHER FAMILY MEMBERS:

Name _____ Date of birth: _____

Name _____ Date of birth: _____

Name _____ Date of birth: _____

Name _____ Date of birth: _____

I understand that it is my responsibility that any incurred charges are paid.

To the extent necessary to determine liability for payment to obtain reimbursement, process claim forms, I authorize the release of any medical information necessary to process claims.

I hereby assign all medical and/or surgical benefits, to include major medical benefits to whichI am entitled, including Medicare, private insurance, and other health plans to Family Medicine of Mt. Pleasant, P.C.

This assignment will remain in effect until revoked by me in writing, a photocopy of this assignment is to be considered as valid as an original. I hereby authorize said assignee to release all information necessary to secure the payment.

Signed _Adam L. Rogers_ Date _9/10/04_

If patient is a minor, parent or guardian signature.

Fig. 5-8 Patient information sheet (for Adam Rogers).

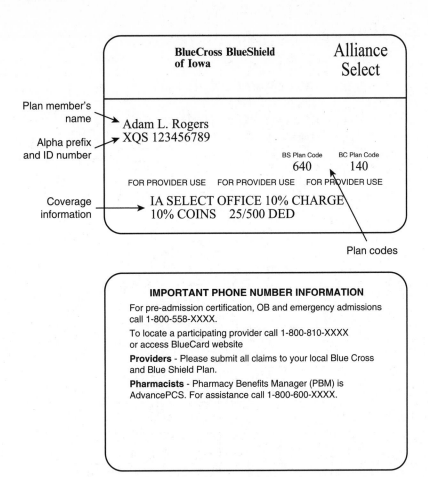

Plan member's name

Alpha prefix and ID number

Coverage information

Plan codes

Fig. 5-9 Front and back of ID card for Adam Rogers.

STATEMENT

BROADMOOR MEDICAL CLINIC
4353 Pine Ridge Drive
Milton, XY 12345-0001
Telephone: 555-656-7890

| DATE | PROFESSIONAL SERVICE DESCRIPTION | CHARGE | | CREDITS | | | | CURRENT BALANCE | |
				PAYMENTS		ADJUSTMENTS			

Due and payable within 10 days. Pay last amount in balance column ⇧

Fig. 5-10 Blank ledger card.

Performance Objective 5-2—Patient Ledger Card

Conditions: Using the ledger card (paper or electronic) created in Performance Objective 5-1, student will enter the procedures and charges abstracted from the encounter form for Adam Rogers.

Supplies/Equipment: Pen, patient encounter form (Fig. 5-11)

Time Allowed: 20 minutes

Accuracy Needed to Pass: 100%

Procedural Steps	Points Earned	Comments
Evaluator: Note time began: _____		
1. Carefully read and study the applicable documents.		
2. Enter the correct date. (5)		
3. Enter the descriptions for the professional services rendered along with the applicable codes. (20)		
4. Post the corresponding charges for each service rendered. (10)		
5. Post the amount of coinsurance collected on this date from the patient. (5)		
6. Enter the current balance in the proper column. (10)		
Optional: May deduct points for taking more time than allowed.		

Total Points = 50

Student's Score: _____

Evaluator: _____

Comments: _____

_____

_____

_____

_____

BROADMOOR MEDICAL CLINIC

DATE OF SERVICE 9/10/04

PATIENT ID#: 123456789

CHIEF COMPLAINT: Stepped on a nail

PATIENT NAME: Adam L. Rogers

CONFIDENTIAL: _____

PROVIDER NAME: Horner Williams

BILLED VISIT? yes

NPI 2313141800

Office Vs, New/Est	Code		Code
99201		99211	
99202 60.00		99212	
99203		99213	
99204		99214	
99205		99215	

Telephone Calls	Code
Brief	99371
Intermediate	99372
Complex/Lengthy	99373

Prev Medicine, New	Code
5-11 yo	99383
12-17 yo	99384
18-39 yo	99385

Prev Medicine, Est.	Code
5-10 yo	99393
12-17 yo	99394
18-39 yo	99395

Counseling/Risk Fx	Code
Individual:	
15 min	99401
30 min	99402
45 min	99403
60 min	99404
Group:	
30 min	99411
60 min	99412
Health Risk Assess:	
Administer	99420

AdminVaccine	Code
Administer one:	99471
Admin, ea add'l:	90472
Admin, oral, one:	90473
Admin, oral, ea add'l:	90474

AdminTher Injection	Code
Therapeutic inj	90782
IM antibiotic	90788

Drugs Administered IM/SC	Code
Tetracycline 250 mg	J0120
Ampicillin Na 500 mg	J0290
Rocephin 250 mg	J0696
Depo-Provera 150 mg	J1055
Benadryl to 50 mg	J1200
Erythrocin 500 mg	J1364
Gentamicin to 80 mg	J1580
Wycillan 600,000 U	J2510
Pen G 600,000 U	J2540
Streptomy to 1 Gm	J3000

Vaccine(s)	Code
Adenovirus	90476
BCG/Tb	90585
Cholera	90724
Diptheria	90719
DT	90702
DTaP	90700
DTaP-HepB-IPV	90723
DTaP-HIB	90721
DTP	90701
DTP-HIB	90720
Flu, 3+ yo	90658
Hep A, 2ds	90633
Hep B 2ds	90743
Hep B 3ds	90744
Hep B adult	90746
Hep B/HIB	90748
Hib/HbOC, 4 ds	90645
Hib/PRP-D, boost	90646
Hib/PRP-OMP, 3 ds	90647
Hib/PRP-T, 4 ds	90648
IPV	90713
Measles	90705
Meningococcal	90733
MMR	90707
MMRV	90710
MR	90708
Mumps	90704
OPV	90712
Pneumococcal	90732
Rotavirus, live, oral	90680
Rubella	90706
Td	90718
Tetanus Tox 20.00	90703
Typhoid (AKD)	90693
Typhoid (ViCPS)	90691
Typhoid (H-P)	90692
Varicella	90716

Team Conference	Code
Pt not pres, 30 min	99361
Pt not pres, 60 min	99362

Respiratory SystemTx	Code
Peak flow	94200
Nebulizer demo	94664
Repeat neb Tx	94640-76
Pulse oximetry	94760

Inhaled Drugs	Code
Albuterol/0.5 mg	J7618

ScreeningTests	Code
Vision	99173
Hearing (air only)	92551

Allergy Injections	Code
Single inj (OV incl)	95115
2+ inj (OV incl)	95117

Health/Behavior Assess	Code
Initial, ea 15 min	96150
Re-assess	96151
Indiv int'vent/15"	96152
Group/15 min	96153
Family/15 min	96154
Fam w/o pt/15 min	96155

Education	Code
Group	99078
Supplies	99071

Surgical Procedures	Code
I & D:	
abscess	10060
foreign body	10120
Debridement:	
10% body surf	11000
ea add'l 10%	11000
Biopsy:	
lesion, skin	11100
ea add'l lesion	11001
Repair Wound:	
Trunk, ext, scalp, neck:	
2.5 cm or <	12001
Face, ears, nose, lips	
eyelids 2.5 cm or <	12011
Tx dehiscence	12020
Burns:	
1st deg, local	16000
Destruction lesion:	
Flat warts, up to 14	17110
Common warts, 1st	17000
ea add'l wart, 2-14	17003
Penis	54050
Vulva	56501
Removal foreign body:	
Eye, external	65205
Nose	30300
Skin	Office Vs
Removal ear wax	69210
Strain/Sprain	Office Vs

Laboratory:	Code
Venipuncture	36415

CLIAWaivedTests	Code
Glucometer	82962
Hematocrit	85014QW
Hemoglobin	85018QW
Mononucleosis	86308QW
Rapid strep test	87880QW
Urine dipstick	81002
Urine pregnancy	81025

CLIA Phys Perf Micro	Code
Wet mount-any	Q0111
KOH prep	Q0112
UA dip, non-auto, w/micro	81000
UA dip, auto, w/micro	81001

CLIA Intermediate	Code
CBC	85025
Chlamydia culture	87110
GC culture	87081
Lead	83655
Sickle cell screen	85660
TB intradermal	86580
Throat culture	87070
Urine culture	87086

CLIA Complex	Code
HIV	86703
PAP smear, thin prep	88144
VDRL	86592

Diagnosis(es):

1. 892.0
2.
3.
4.

Signature of provider:

Horner Williams, MD

Return to clinic: PRN

Fig. 5-11 Encounter form (for Adam Rogers).

Health Insurance Professional's Notebook

A. Collect at least one each of the following documents from a local medical office or clinic. Label the various parts as to what information the area typically contains.

- Patient information form
- Insurance ID card (front and back)
- Ledger card
- Encounter form
- CMS-1500 claim form

B. Create a section in your Health Insurance Professional's Notebook under the title "Sample Documents," and file the documents collected in "A" in this section. This notebook is for your own personal use after you become employed, so include as much information as necessary on these documents so that they can be a valuable reference tool on the job.

Chapter Check List

Student name: _____

Chapter completion date: _____

1.	Record	Your start time and date: _____
2.	Read	The assigned chapter in the text
3.	View	PowerPoint slides (if available)
4.	Complete	Exercises in the Workbook as assigned
5.	Compare	Your answers with the answers posted on the bulletin board/website/handout
6.	Correct	Your answers
7.	Complete	All tests and required activities
8.	Read	Assigned readings (if any)
9.	Complete	Chapter performance objectives (competencies), if any
10.	Evaluate	Chapter performance and submit to your instructor
11.	Record	Your ending time and date: _____
12.	Move on	Begin next chapter as assigned

Student name: _____

Chapter completion date: _____

Evaluate your classroom performance. Complete the self-evaluation, and submit it to your instructor. When your instructor returns this form to you, compare your self-evaluation with the evaluation completed by your instructor.

Skill	Student Self-Evaluation			Instructor Evaluation		
	Good	Average	Poor	Good	Average	Poor
Attendance/punctuality						
Personal appearance						
Applies effort						
Is self-motivated						
Is courteous						
Has positive attitude						
Completes assignments in timely manner						
Works well with others						

Student's initials: _____

Date: _____

Instructor's initials: _____

Date: _____

Points Possible: _____

Points Awarded: _____

Chapter Grade: _____

6 Traditional Fee-for-Service/Private Plans

Chapter 6 takes an in-depth look at commercial insurance, specifically traditional fee-for-service (FFS) (indemnity) and private plans. The core of Chapter 6 zeros in on one of the best-known third-party payers in the United States: Blue Cross and Blue Shield. The author has elected to include Blue Cross and Blue Shield under the broad umbrella of commercial insurance because it no longer operates as a national entity, but as separate regional organizations. In this workbook chapter, numerous opportunities are presented to explore the national Blue Cross and Blue Shield Association and the regional company that serves the area in which the student resides.

WORKBOOK CHAPTER OBJECTIVES

After completing the workbook activities for Chapter 6, the student should be able to:
* Define the terms used in the chapter.
* Answer the review questions to within the evaluation criteria set by the instructor.
* Analyze, apply, and evaluate information given in "real-world" situations, applying logical concepts for rational decision making to current health insurance issues.
* Apply systematic processes that focus on analyzing situations (including decision-making steps) to arrive at reasonable solutions in problem-solving scenarios and case studies.
* Conduct Internet research to become more knowledgeable about the best-known healthcare insurer in the United States, Blue Cross and Blue Shield.
* Abstract applicable information from healthcare documents necessary for completion of various forms used in healthcare billing and the claims process.
* Generate information and documents for inclusion in the student's personal Health Insurance Professional's Notebook.
* Create appropriate correspondence to a patient explaining professional fees.
* Perform self-evaluation on successful content mastery of Chapter 6.

DEFINING CHAPTER TERMS

Using the computer (or typewriter), students should key an accurate definition for each of the chapter terms listed. These definitions should be in the students' own words. When finished, students should compare their definitions with those listed in the glossary at the back of the textbook, correcting any inaccuracies.

administrative services organization (ASO)
autonomy
basic health insurance
BlueCard Program
BlueCard Worldwide
Blue Cross and Blue Shield Federal Employee Program (FEP)
carve out
coinsurance
commercial health insurance
comprehensive insurance
covered expenses
deductible
Employee Retirement Income Security Act of 1974 (ERISA)
explanation of benefits (EOB)
Federal Employees Health Benefits (FEHB) Program
fee-for-service (FFS)/indemnity plan
fiscal intermediary
group insurance

Healthcare Service Plans
health insurance policy premium
health maintenance organization (HMO)
insurance cap
lifetime maximum cap
major medical insurance
managed care plan
Medicare supplement plans
nonforfeitable interest
participating provider (PAR)
point-of-service (POS) plan
policyholder
preferred provider organization (PPO)
reasonable and customary fee
self-insured/self-insurance
single or specialty service plans
stop loss insurance
supplemental coverage
third-party administrator (TPA)
third-party payer

Multiple Choice

Directions: In the questions/statements presented, choose the response that **best** answers/completes the stem, and circle the letter that precedes it.

1. The type of health insurance that offers the most choices of providers, in which patients can choose any provider they want and can change providers at any time is a(n):
   a. Managed care plan
   b. Indemnity plan
   c. FFS plan
   d. b or c

2. An example of a third-party payer is:
   a. A commercial insurance company
   b. Blue Cross and Blue Shield
   c. Medicare/Medicaid
   d. All of the above

3. Group insurance typically is:
   a. The most expensive kind
   b. Paid entirely by the employer
   c. A contract between an insurance company and an employer
   d. Mandated by the federal government

4. The type of insurance that comprises a group of providers who share the financial risk of the plan or who have an incentive to deliver cost-effective, but quality, service is a(n):
   a. Managed care plan
   b. Indemnity plan
   c. FFS plan
   d. b or c

5. The best type of healthcare plan is a(n):
   a. HMO
   b. Indemnity plan
   c. PPO
   d. No one type is universally best

6. Most FFS plans include the patient paying a:
   a. Periodic payment (premium)
   b. Yearly deductible
   c. Per-visit coinsurance
   d. All of the above

7. The typical levels of coverage in an FFS plan include:
   a. Basic/major medical/comprehensive
   b. Basic/preventive care/planned care
   c. Outpatient/inpatient/emergency
   d. Auto/workers' comp/long-term care

8. With FFS insurance, which of the following is typically true?
   a. Only employers can offer it through a group policy
   b. The higher the deductible, the lower the premium
   c. All healthcare expenses count toward the yearly deductible
   d. After the yearly deductible is met, the policy covers 100% of services

9. The amount of money the policyholder has to pay out-of-pocket for any one incident or in any 1 year is limited by:
   a. Yearly deductible
   b. Per-visit coinsurance
   c. Insurance cap
   d. Periodic premium

10. When the fee charged by a provider falls within the parameters of the fee commonly charged for that particular service within a specific geographic area, it is said to be:
    a. Medically necessary
    b. A participating fee
    c. Reasonable and customary
    d. Medicare approved

11. A provider who signs a contractual arrangement with a third-party insurance contractor and agrees to accept the amount paid by the carrier as payment in full is referred to as a:
    a. Participating provider (PAR)
    b. Nonparticipating provider (nonPAR)
    c. Primary care provider (PCP)
    d. Principal attending physician (PAP)

12. The government health insurance program that provides coverage for its own civilian employees is called:
    a. Medicare
    b. Medicaid
    c. Federal Employees Health Benefits (FEHB) Program
    d. Blue Cross and Blue Shield

13. When the employer—not an insurance company—is responsible for the cost of its employees' medical services, the employer has a:
    a. Workers' compensation program
    b. Third-party group plan
    c. Self-insured program
    d. Disability benefits plan

14. The federal law designed to protect the rights of beneficiaries of employee benefit plans offered by employers and that sets minimum standards for pension plans in private industry is called:
    a. Social Security
    b. Workers' compensation
    c. Employee Retirement Income Security Act (ERISA)
    d. Consolidated Omnibus Budget Reconciliation Act (COBRA)

15. A person or organization that processes claims and performs other contractual administrative services is commonly referred to as a:
   a. Third-party administrator (TPA)
   b. Management commissioner (MC)
   c. Fiscal intermediary
   d. Third-party payer

True/False

Directions: Place a "T" in the blank preceding the statement if it is true; place an "F" if it is false.

_____ 1. With managed healthcare, patients can choose any physician they want and can change physicians any time.

_____ 2. A third-party payer is any organization that provides payment for specified coverages provided under a health plan.

_____ 3. Group insurance is generally more expensive because it covers more individuals.

_____ 4. Traditional FFS insurance is gradually becoming less popular than managed care.

_____ 5. With FFS insurance, the policyholder controls the choice of physician and facility.

_____ 6. FFS plans all have the same deductible amount.

_____ 7. "Reasonable and customary" is a term used to refer to the commonly charged or prevailing fees for health services within a geographic area.

_____ 8. Commercial health insurance is standard in price and the kinds of benefits that the policy covers.

_____ 9. Most organizations that are self-insured are large entities, which can draw from hundreds or thousands of enrollees.

_____ 10. Stop-loss insurance is protection from the devastating effect of exorbitant medical claims.

_____ 11. Blue Cross policies cover inpatient hospital care; Blue Shield covers physicians' services.

_____ 12. Blue Cross and Blue Shield offers only indemnity (FFS) plans.

_____ 13. If an individual belongs to a BlueCard PPO, the initials PPO appear inside a blue globe.

_____ 14. Blue Cross and Blue Shield organizations are no longer governed at a national level, and each has its own specific guidelines for completing the CMS-1500 claim form.

_____ 15. It is important to consult all patient insurance plans for their specific guidelines to avoid claim delays and rejections.

_____ 16. Normally, when husband and wife are covered under separate policies, primary coverage follows the patient.

_____ 17. An explanation of benefits (EOB) is a document prepared by the carrier that gives details of how the claim was adjudicated.

_____ 18. The time limit for filing claims is the same for all third-party payers—1 year.

_____ 19. Filing CMS-1500 paper claims for commercial carriers is much the same as with all other carriers.

_____ 20. HIPAA mandates that all commercial claims be submitted electronically.

Short Answer/Fill-in-the-Blank

1. Name four basic types of plans.

   _____

   _____

   _____

   _____

2. List three out-of-pocket costs that are standard for patients to pay with FFS plans.

   _____

   _____

   _____

3. List four functions commonly performed by TPAs and administrative services organizations.

   _____

   _____

   _____

   _____

4. Explain what a "carve out" is and give an example.

   _____

5. Explain (in your own words) the difference between a PAR and a nonPAR provider.

   _____

6. What is a fiscal intermediary, and what functions does it perform?

   _____

7. Explain what is meant by "timely filing" as it relates to claims.

   _____

8. Timely filing for Blue Cross and Blue Shield claims is _____ days.

Chapter **6** **Traditional Fee-for-Service/Private Plans**

A. You are working as a health insurance professional at Silverstone Mental Health Clinic. Patient Philippe Sanchez comes in for an appointment with Dr. Gerald T. Field, a psychiatrist. This is Mr. Sanchez's first visit to the clinic. Fig. 6-1 shows Mr. Sanchez's completed patient information form. There are two insurance companies listed, with Sunset Assurance, a family policy in his wife's name, listed first. The second one is a single policy in the patient's name. Mr. Sanchez explains that the family policy is in Maria's name through her employer, but it does not cover treatment for mental health. "Send my bill to the packing plant," he states. "They will take care of it." Further questions only confuse Mr. Sanchez, and it is apparent that he knows little about the two policies. How can you, the health insurance professional, determine the following?

- Which carrier is actually primary?
- Do both policies cover mental health treatment?
- Should you send a claim to both third-party payers?
- Where would you find out more information about the coverage of the American Indemnity policy and the Sunset Assurance policy?

Registration Data

1. Your Name   **Sanchez Philippe M**   Sex ☒ Male ☐ Female   Date of Birth **06/16/1969**
   (Last)   (First)   (Middle)

2. Social Security #: **111-22-3333**   Marital Status: S ⓜ D Se W

3. Address: **811 46th St.**   4. **SSS-621-876S**
   (Street)   (Phone)
   Wilton   **X Y**   **12345**
   (City)   (State)   (Zip)

5. Employer: **Southwest Packers Inc**   Occupation: **Inspector**
   Employer Address: **Hwy 409 West, Wilton**   **SSS-621-S432**
   (Work Phone)
   Spouse: **Maria**   Employer: **Wilton Comm. Schools** Occupation: **Teacher Aide**
   Employer Address: **1667 Parkway, Wilton**   **SSS-621-8864**
   (Work Phone)

6.

Other Household Members	Date of Birth	Relationship
Emilio	05/03/1995	Son
Rita	01/24/1998	daughter
	/ /	
	/ /	
	/ /	

7. Medical Insurance Information

	Ins. Company Name	Policy No.	Policy Holder	Sgl.	Fmly.	Primary	Sec.
(1)	Sunset Assurance	001-445678	Maria	☐	☒	☐	☐
(2)	American Indemnity	04691IFML	Philippe	☒	☐	☐	☐
( )				☐	☐	☐	☐

Type of Coverage

8. Person to Contact in an Emergency **Maria**   Relationship to you **wife**
   DOB 03/18/1972
   Their Work Phone **SSS-621-8864**   Their Home Phone **SSS-621-876S**

9. Party with primary responsibility for payment: ☒ Self   ☐ Other
   Name _____   Relationship to you _____
   Address _____   Home Phone _____

For Office Use Only

Date Completed _____   Account No. _____   Patient No. _____

Household Status   ☐ Head of Household

☐ Spouse   ☐ Child   ☐ Other: _____

Head of Household Name _____

Fig. 6-1 Registration data sheet for Philippe Sanchez.

B. Eloise Stout comes to the orthopedic clinic (where you work) for treatment of a Colles' fracture. She informs you that she lives out of state and is here on vacation visiting her daughter. Fig. 6-2 shows a facsimile of her insurance ID card. From the information on the ID card, answer the following questions:

- What Blue Cross and Blue Shield plan does the patient have?
- What does the alpha prefix signify?
- If a "suitcase logo" appeared in the upper right-hand corner of this card (as it normally does with this specific program), what would it indicate?
- Will the patient be able to receive the same benefits as she would at home?
- What form will you use to submit the claim?
- Where will you send the completed claim?

Note: You may have to go to a website for some answers. Use "Blue Card Program" as search words.

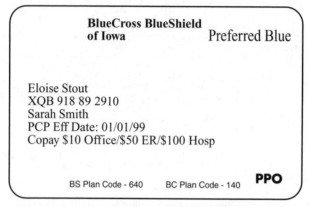

Fig. 6-2 Sample of a Blue Cross and Blue Shield ID card.

Note: Blue Cross and Blue Shield's address is 2604 West 32nd, Des Moines, IA 52230.

C. Many health insurance professional students have difficulty understanding the differences between Blue Cross and Blue Shield's Federal Employee Program (FEP) and the FEHB Program. Write a critical thinking paragraph briefly explaining each program and highlight the differences.

D. Following are two patient scenarios. Using the criteria given, calculate the total amount each patient will have to pay out-of-pocket, including the coinsurance and deductible. Assume in both cases that Blue Cross and Blue Shield's usual, customary, and reasonable fee for this procedure is $4250, and none of the yearly deductible has been met.

Patient No. 1

Steven Barnes	**Provider is PAR**
Cholecystectomy	Charge: $5000
Deductible: $500	Coinsurance 80/20
Total patient responsibility	

Patient No. 2

Sylvia Manley	Provider is nonPAR
Hysterectomy	Charge: $5000
Deductible: $250	Coinsurance 90/10
Total patient responsibility	

Illustrate on the portions of the following ledger cards how these charges and payments would be posted. The amount in the current balance column should reflect the total out-of-pocket amount the patient owes.

Note: When posting services/payments, make sure you include the date the insurance claim was submitted (1 day after service) and the date the claim was paid (3/13/20XX).

Patient No. 1 (Steven Barnes)

Date of Service	Procedure/Service	Amount Charged	Amount Paid	Adjustments	Current Balance
02/13/20XX	Cholecystectomy	5000.00			5000.00

Patient No. 2 (Sylvia Manley)

Date of Service	Procedure/Service	Amount Charged	Amount Paid	Adjustments	Current Balance
02/13/20XX	Hysterectomy	5000.00			5000.00

PROJECTS/DISCUSSION TOPICS

A. Research and prepare for an in-class discussion on the process involved in a commercial insurer (e.g., Blue Cross) becoming a fiscal intermediary.

B. Research the Blue Cross and Blue Shield carrier in your state/area. Prepare a presentation or create a bulletin board display depicting the various plans, options, and programs your local Blue Cross and Blue Shield organization offers health insurance consumers in your community (**hint:** go to **http://www.bcbs.com** and enter your Zip Code).

C. There are several topics listed under "Featured Programs" on the Blue Cross and Blue Shield Association home page. Choose one of these topics, read the entire item, and write a critical thinking paragraph focusing on the main points of the article.

CASE STUDIES

A. Review the Patient Information Form for Philippe Sanchez (see Fig. 6-1). Assume you have contacted American Indemnity and learned that they are primary and will accept claims submitted on the universal form (CMS-1500). Complete the top portion of the claim form (Fig. 6-3), or use the electronic file in the Student Software CD, using the information from his registration data. (American Indemnity's address is 2345 West Palm Avenue, Petaluma, CA, 99001.) (Patient has an up-to-date release of information and assignment of benefits on file.)

1500

HEALTH INSURANCE CLAIM FORM

APPROVED BY NATIONAL UNIFORM CLAIM COMMITTEE 08/05

PICA | PICA | CARRIER

1. MEDICARE (Medicare #) ☐ MEDICAID (Medicaid #) ☐ TRICARE CHAMPUS (Sponsor's SSN) ☐ CHAMPVA (Member ID#) ☐ GROUP HEALTH PLAN (SSN or ID) ☐ FECA BLK LUNG (SSN) ☐ OTHER (ID) ☐ | 1a. INSURED'S I.D. NUMBER (For Program in Item 1)

2. PATIENT'S NAME (Last Name, First Name, Middle Initial) | 3. PATIENT'S BIRTH DATE MM DD YY SEX M ☐ F ☐ | 4. INSURED'S NAME (Last Name, First Name, Middle Initial)

5. PATIENT'S ADDRESS (No., Street) | 6. PATIENT RELATIONSHIP TO INSURED Self ☐ Spouse ☐ Child ☐ Other ☐ | 7. INSURED'S ADDRESS (No., Street)

CITY STATE | 8. PATIENT STATUS Single ☐ Married ☐ Other ☐ | CITY STATE

ZIP CODE TELEPHONE (Include Area Code) ( ) | Employed ☐ Full-Time Student ☐ Part-Time Student ☐ | ZIP CODE TELEPHONE (Include Area Code) ( )

9. OTHER INSURED'S NAME (Last Name, First Name, Middle Initial) | 10. IS PATIENT'S CONDITION RELATED TO: | 11. INSURED'S POLICY GROUP OR FECA NUMBER

a. OTHER INSURED'S POLICY OR GROUP NUMBER | a. EMPLOYMENT? (Current or Previous) ☐ YES ☐ NO | a. INSURED'S DATE OF BIRTH MM DD YY SEX M ☐ F ☐

b. OTHER INSURED'S DATE OF BIRTH MM DD YY SEX M ☐ F ☐ | b. AUTO ACCIDENT? ☐ YES ☐ NO PLACE (State) | b. EMPLOYER'S NAME OR SCHOOL NAME

c. EMPLOYER'S NAME OR SCHOOL NAME | c. OTHER ACCIDENT? ☐ YES ☐ NO | c. INSURANCE PLAN NAME OR PROGRAM NAME

d. INSURANCE PLAN NAME OR PROGRAM NAME | 10d. RESERVED FOR LOCAL USE | d. IS THERE ANOTHER HEALTH BENEFIT PLAN? ☐ YES ☐ NO *If yes*, return to and complete item 9 a-d.

READ BACK OF FORM BEFORE COMPLETING & SIGNING THIS FORM.

12. PATIENT'S OR AUTHORIZED PERSON'S SIGNATURE I authorize the release of any medical or other information necessary to process this claim. I also request payment of government benefits either to myself or to the party who accepts assignment below.

SIGNED ________ DATE ________

13. INSURED'S OR AUTHORIZED PERSON'S SIGNATURE I authorize payment of medical benefits to the undersigned physician or supplier for services described below.

SIGNED ________

PATIENT AND INSURED INFORMATION

Fig. 6-3 Top half of CMS-1500 form (for Philippe Sanchez).

B. The encounter form in Fig. 6-4 documents procedures, services, and a diagnosis for Susan Martin, a 9-year-old girl. Fig. 6-5 shows her completed patient information sheet. Using these two documents, complete the following tasks:

1. Complete the patient ledger card in Fig. 6-6, or the electronic file, for this patient.

2. Using the information on the encounter form (see Fig. 6-4) and the completed ledger card (see Fig. 6-6), complete the bottom half (provider/supplier section) of the claim form in Fig. 6-7, or use the electronic file.

BROADMOOR MEDICAL CLINIC

ACCT. #: 02 201	DATE OF SERVICE: 12/04/20XX	CATEGORY:	DIAGNOSIS: 787.0/780.6

PATIENT'S NAME: Martin, Susan A.

CPT	✔	DESCRIPTION	FEE	CPT	✔	DESCRIPTION	FEE	CPT	✔	DESCRIPTION	FEE
OFFICE VISIT - NEW PATIENT				**IMMUNIZATIONS**				**INJECTIONS (CONT'D.)**			
99201		Focused		90701		DtaP		J3410		Vistaril	
99202		Expanded		90632		Hep A (Adult)		J3420		Vitamin B12	
99203		Detailed		90633		Hep A (Ped)		J2000		Xylocaine	
99204		Comprehensive		90744		Hep B (Ped)		**PROCEDURES**			
99205		Complex		90746		Hep B (Adult)		46600		Anoscopy	
OFFICE VISIT - ESTABLISHED PATIENT				90737		Hib		92551		Audio Screening	
99211		Minimal		90657		Influenza		11730		Avulsion Nail, Partial or	
99212	✔	Focused	80.00	90707		MMR				Complete, Single	
99213		Expanded		90732		Pneumococcal		11200		Rem. of Skin Tags up to 15	
99214		Detailed		90718		Td		11201		Each Additional 10	
				90703		Tetanus Toxoid		10060		I & D Simple Abscess	
				90716		Varicella		10120		Removal FB Skin	
PHYSICAL EXAM - NEW PATIENT								11740		I & D Subung. Hematoma	
99381		Age Under 1 Year		**INJECTIONS**				58310		IUD Removal	
99382		Age 1 - 4 Years		J1200		Benadryl up to 50 mg		94010		Spirometry	
99383		Age 5 - 11 Years		J0540		Bicillin up to 1,200,000 mg		A4570		Splint	
99384		Age 12 - 17 Years		J0690		Cefazolin Sodium 250 mg		99173		Vision Screening	
99385		Age 18 - 39 Years		J0704		Celestone		**LABORATORY**			
99386		Age 40 - 64 Years		J0780		Compazine		82270		Blood Occult	
99387		Age 65+ Years		J1100		Decadron		85680		TB Intradermal	
				J0970		Delestrogen		81000		Urine Dip Stick	
PHYSICAL EXAM - ESTABLISHED PATIENT				J1050		Depo Provera		84703		Serum Pregnancy Test	
99391		Age Under 1 Year		J1510		Gamma Globulin		87082		Strep Screen	
99392		Age 1 - 4 Years		J3301		Kenalog					
99393		Age 5 - 11 Years		J1940		Kasix		36415		Venipuncture	
99394		Age 12 - 17 Years		J2550		Phenergan		99000		Handling	
99395		Age 18 - 39 Years		J3490		Rocephin					
99396		Age 40 - 64 Years		J1070		Testosterone		**MISCELLANEOUS**			
99397		Age 65+ Years		J3250		Tigan					
				J1885		Torodol					

ICD-9 ☐ DIAGNOSIS

CARDIOLOGY
794.31 ☐ Abn Ekg
786.50 ☐ Chest Pain, Nos
780.4 ☐ Dizziness And Giddiness
787.1 ☐ Heartburn
272.0 ☐ Hypercholesterolem
272.4 ☐ Hyperlipidemia Nec/Nos
401.1 ☐ Hypertension Benign
401.9 ☐ Hypertension Nos
401.0 ☐ Hypertension, Malig.
785.1 ☐ Palpitations

ENDOCRINE
250.01 ☐ IDDM Controlled
250.03 ☐ IDDM Uncontrolled
250.02 ☐ NIDDM Uncontrolled
250.00 ☐ NIDDM Controlled
251.2 ☐ Hypoglycemia
244.9 ☐ Hypothyroidism
242.90 ☐ Hyperthyroidism

EAR, NOSE, THROAT
386.30 ☐ Labyrinthitis Nos
382.9 ☐ Otitis Media, Ac./Chr.
462. ☐ Pharyngitis Acute
477.9 ☐ Rhinitis, Allergic
461.9 ☐ Sinusitis, Ac Nos
473.9 ☐ Sinusitis, Chronic
528.0 ☐ Stomatitis
034.0 ☐ Strep Throat

388.30 ☐ Tinnitus Nos
463. ☐ Tonsillitis, Acute
474.0 ☐ Tonsillitis, Chronic

FEMALE / GYNECOLOGY
795.0 ☐ Abn Pap Smear-Cervix
793.8 ☐ Abn Findings-Breast
626.0 ☐ Amenorrhea
611.72 ☐ Breast Mass/Lump
616.0 ☐ Cervicitis
V25.09 ☐ Contracep. Mgmt.
625.3 ☐ Dysmenorrhea
626.4 ☐ Menstruation, Irreg.
625.2 ☐ Menstruation, Excessive
614.9 ☐ Pelvic Inflam Dis
V22.2 ☐ Preg State, Incidential
616.10 ☐ Vaginitis

PHYSICAL EXAM
V20.1 ☐ Well Child
V72.84 ☐ Pre-Op Exam

GASTRO-INTESTINAL
789.06 ☐ Abnormal Pain, Epigastric
794.3 ☐ Abn. Liver Function Study
578.1 ☐ Blood in Stool
564.0 ☐ Constipation
787.91 ☐ Diarrhea
562.11 ☐ Diverticulitis
530.81 ☐ Esophageal Reflux
535.5 ☐ Gastritis/Duodenitis Nos
455.6 ☐ Hemorrhoids

787.0 ☒ Nausea And Vomiting
533.90 ☐ Peptic Ulcer Nos
569.3 ☐ Rectal Bleeding

GENITO-URINARY
585. ☐ Chronic Renal Failure
595.0 ☐ Cystitis Acute
788.1 ☐ Dysuria
599.7 ☐ Hematuria
601.0 ☐ Prostatitis Acute
599.0 ☐ UTI

HEMATOLOGY
790.6 ☐ Abn Blood Chemistry Nec
285.9 ☐ Anemia Nos
280.1 ☐ Anemia, Iron Def

INFECTIOUS
616.3 ☐ Abcess: Bartholin Gland
682.9 ☐ Abcess: Skin
780.6 ☒ Fever: Unkn. Origin

IMMUNOLOGY - ALLERGIES
995.3 ☐ Allergic Reaction Nos
477.0 ☐ Allergy, Hay Fever
042. ☐ Human ImmunoVirus Dis.

ORTHOPEDICS
716.90 ☐ Arthritis Unspec.
724.5 ☐ Backache Nos
727.3 ☐ Bursitis Nec
354.0 ☐ Carpal Tunnel Syndrome
719.40 ☐ Joint Pain-Unspec.
729.1 ☐ Myalgia And Myositis Nos.

733.00 ☐ Osteoporosis
845.00 ☐ Sprain: Ankle
847.2 ☐ Sprain: Back
847.0 ☐ Sprain: Cervical
840.9 ☐ Sprain: Shoulder
729.81 ☐ Swelling of Limb
726.00 ☐ Tendonitis

NEUROLOGY
784.0 ☐ Headache
346.9 ☐ Migraine Nos
724.3 ☐ Sciatica
307.81 ☐ Tension Headache
780.4 ☐ Vertigo

OPHTHALMOLOGY
373.00 ☐ Blepharitis Nos
372.30 ☐ Conjunctivitis
918.1 ☐ Corneal Abrasion

PULMONARY / RESPIRATORY
493.9 ☐ Asthma Nos
466.0 ☐ Bronchitis Acute
490. ☐ Bronchitis Nos
486. ☐ Pneumonia
786.2 ☐ Cough
786.0 ☐ Dyspnea/Resp Abn
487. ☐ Influenza
786.52 ☐ Painful Respiration
786.09 ☐ SOB
465.9 ☐ URI
079.9 ☐ Viral Syndrome

PSYCH / MENTAL HEALTH
303.9 ☐ Alcoholism
300.00 ☐ Anxiety State Nos
300.00 ☐ Depression

SKIN / DERMATOLOGIC
706.1 ☐ Acne Nec
691. ☐ Dermatitis, Atopic
692. ☐ Dermatitis, Contact
110.1 ☐ Dermatophytosis, Nail
691.0 ☐ Diaper Rash
054.9 ☐ Herpes Simplex Nos
053.9 ☐ Herpes Zoster Nos
054.19 ☐ Herpes Genital Nec
684. ☐ Impetigo
703.0 ☐ Ingrowing Nail
215.9 ☐ Nevus
110.1 ☐ Onychomycosis
696.1 ☐ Psoriasis
706.2 ☐ Sebaceous Cyst
708.8 ☐ Urticaria Nec
078.1 ☐ Warts, Viral

OTHER - MISC.
780.7 ☐ Malaise and Fatigue
780.2 ☐ Syncope

WRITE - IN

INSTRUCTIONS: fluids & rest / OTC acetominophen for fever / No Rx at this time	RETURN APPOINTMENT: ___ Days ___ Weeks ___ Months ☒ PRN ___ 15 ___ 30 ___ 45	PAID ☐ CASH ☐ CHECK ☐ CR. CD.	PREV. BAL. 146.50
			TODAY'S FEE 80.00
			AMT. REC'D. 10.00

Fig. 6-4 Encounter form (for Susan Martin).

PATIENT INFORMATION SHEET

Today's date: 12/04/20XX

HEAD OF HOUSEHOLD

Head of household: Anna P. Costello

Social Security # 333-00-1111

Sex: F   Date of birth 4/2/76

Address: 603 Maplelawn

City, St: Wilton, XY   Zip 12345

Home phone # 555-621-1111

Occupation: seamstress

Employer's name: Apex Mattress Factory

Employer's address: North Ft. Gaslight Rd.

Employer's City, St: Wilton, XY   Zip 12345

Employer's phone # 555-621-2330

PATIENT INFORMATION

Patient's legal name: Susan Ann Martin   Nickname _____   Relationship to head of household: daughter

Date of birth 6/1/19XX   Age 9   Sex F   Marital Status _____

Employer name: student   Social Security # 911-999-0000

Employer address _____   Employer phone # _____

City, St: _____   Zip _____   Worker's Compensation Carrier (If applicable) _____

Referring Physician _____   Allergies penicillin

EMERGENCY INFORMATION

Other contact not living with you: Patsy Evans   Home phone# 555-654-3210   Work phone# _____

Address 26 Fox Ct., #152   City Wilton   St XY   Zip 12345

Patient relationship to other contact: grandmother   If patient is a child, parent name: Anna Costello

INSURANCE INFORMATION

Primary insurance BCBS   Subscriber Anna Costello

ID # XYZ911999000   Relationship to subscriber daughter

Secondary insurance: _____   Subscriber _____

ID # _____   Relationship to subscriber _____

OTHER FAMILY MEMBERS:

Name _____   Date of birth: _____

Name _____   Date of birth: _____

Name _____   Date of birth: _____

Name _____   Date of birth: _____

I understand that it is my responsibility that any incurred charges are paid.

To the extent necessary to determine liability for payment to obtain reimbursement, process claim forms, I authorize the release of any medical information necessary to process claims.

I here by assign all medical and/or surgical benefits, to include major medical benefits to which I am entitled, including Medicare, private insurance, and other health plans to Family Medicine of Mt. Pleasant, P.C.

This assignment will remain in effect until revoked by me in writing, a photocopy of this assignment is to be considered as valid as an original. I hereby authorize said assignee to release all information necessary to secure the payment.

Signed Anna P. Costello   Date 12/04/20XX

If patient is a minor, parent or guardian signature.

Fig. 6-5 Patient information sheet (for Susan Martin).

STATEMENT

BROADMOOR MEDICAL CLINIC
4353 Pine Ridge Drive
Milton, XY 12345-0001
Telephone: 555-656-7890

DATE	PROFESSIONAL SERVICE DESCRIPTION	CHARGE		CREDITS				CURRENT BALANCE	
				PAYMENTS		ADJUSTMENTS			

Due and payable within 10 days.   **Pay last amount in balance column** ⇧

Fig. 6-6 Blank patient ledger card (for Susan Martin).

Fig. 6-7 Bottom half of CMS-1500 form (for Susan Martin).

C. Let's assume that in Case Study A, Mr. Sanchez's mental health treatment is covered under both of the policies he listed on his new patient registration form. You have determined that Maria's family policy through Wilton Community Schools is primary. Explain the procedure for filing dual claims when the patient is covered under a secondary policy.

Broadmoor Medical Clinic	Clinic EIN # 42-1898989
4353 Pine Ridge Drive	Dr. R.G. Jones NPI 1234567890
Milton, XY 12345-0001	Dr. Marilou Lucero NPI 2907511822
Clinic NPI X100XX1000	Group # GRW0000
Telephone: 555-656-7890	Date claim 1 day after examination

D. Examine the EOB form shown in Fig. 6-8, then match each column number with the correct written explanation by placing the correct column number in the blank space preceding the written explanation.

_____ Amount applied to coinsurance

_____ Amount patient is responsible for paying

_____ Amount the provider charged for each service

_____ Amount(s) applied to copay, deductible, or not covered

_____ Balance the insurer will apply to benefits

_____ Coordination of benefits adjustment

_____ Date(s) patient received services

_____ Description of services rendered

_____ Fee adjustment

_____ Percentage of coverage

_____ Total amount paid by insurance plan

EXPLANATION OF BENEFITS

(This is NOT a bill)

July 1, 2002

Group number:	0000123
Member:	Jane M Sample
Member's ID:	123456789 02
Claim number:	8000000001
Provider:	Smith, Robert
Payment Reference ID:	2002062510100013

1	2	3	4	5	6	7	8	9	10	11
Service/ product description	Dates you received service/product (m/d/y to m/d/y)	Charges billed by provider	Minus provider's fee adjustment	Minus your copay (C), deductible (D) or amount not covered (*)	Total amount eligible for benefits	%	Minus your co-insurance amount	Plus or (minus) coordination of benefits adjustment	Total paid by your plan	Amount you're responsible for
OFFICE VISIT	06/15/02 06/15/02	75.00	12.00	15.00 C	48.00	100%			48.00	15.00
LAB	06/15/02 06/15/02	89.12	15.36	50.00 D	23.76	100%			23.76	50.00
X-RAY	06/15/02 06/15/02	100.00	20.00		80.00	80%	16.00		64.00	16.00
SURGERY	06/15/02 06/15/02	50.00		50.00 575	0.00	0%			0.00	$0.00
Totals		**$314.12**	**$47.38**	**$115.00**	**$151.76**		**$16.00**		**$135.76**	**$131.00**

Your 2002 medical deductible satisfied so far: $100.00
Your 2002 family medical deductible satisfied so far: $300.00

Amount we paid your provider: **$135.76**

Amount you're responsible for: **$131.00**

* Message Codes:

575   This procedure is considered cosmetic. Your plan does not cover cosmetic services.

Fig. 6-8 Explanation of benefits form.

A. Blue Cross and Blue Shield is one of the most popular insurers in the United States. Log on to their website (**http://www.bcbs.com**) and research the available information to answer the following questions:

1. Who should the health insurance professional contact when there is a billing question?
2. List the various types of coverage Blue Cross and Blue Shield offers its enrollees.
3. Blue Cross and Blue Shield has _____ member companies and covers approximately _____ (number) of people.
4. What is "Blueworks"?
5. What type of coverage would you likely purchase if you were traveling outside of the United States?
6. To submit a claim for medical care overseas, you complete a(n) _____ and send it to the _____.

B. Search the Blue Cross and Blue Shield Association website, and locate the current guidelines for completing the new CMS-1500 form in your particular area.

C. Log on to the Blue Cross and Blue Shield website. Under "Media Resources," there is an informational item titled "Guidelines for the Role of Participating Physicians in Health Plans." Read and study this article and be prepared for an in-class discussion.
http://www.bcbs.com/bluefinder

D. Using search words "PAR versus nonPAR providers," search the Internet for advantages and disadvantages of each. Then prepare for a debate/in-class discussion on this topic.

E. Log on to **http://www.bcbs.com** and click on "Blueworks." Surf the topics under the caption "What the Blues Are Doing Now." Do any of these items relate to your state? If so, research the topic(s) and prepare a 3- to 5-minute oral presentation to the class highlighting new Blue Cross and Blue Shield programs/initiatives to improve healthcare. If your state is not among the topics listed, choose one that you find of particular interest to present.
http://www.bcbs.com/blueworks/index.html

Performance Objective 6-1—Patient Case Study 6-1

Conditions: Complete an encounter form and ledger card using the information on the documents in Case Study 6-1.

Supplies/Equipment: Ledger form (paper or electronic)/pen; patient information form (Fig. 6-9), ID card (Fig. 6-10), encounter form (Fig. 6-11), ledger card (Fig. 6-12)

Time Allowed: 20 minutes

Accuracy Needed to Pass: 100%

Procedural Steps	Points Earned	Comments
Evaluator: Note time began: _____		
Carefully read and study the applicable documents.		
Encounter Form 1. Calculate the total charge of all services checked, and enter the amount under "TODAY'S FEE." (10)		
2. Still using the encounter form and assuming the patient paid the coinsurance, calculate the amount paid, and enter it under "AMT. REC'D." (10)		
Ledger Card 3. Complete the ledger card by listing each procedure/service separately. Post today's payment, and calculate the balance due. (30)		
Optional: May deduct points for taking more time than allowed.		

Total Points = 50

Student's Score: _____

Evaluator: _____

Comments: _____

_____

_____

_____

_____

Registration Data

1. Your Name _Ebers_ _Karen_ _S_ Sex ☐ Male Date of Birth _07/28/2002_
   (Last) (First) (Middle) ☒ Female

2. Social Security #: _222-99-0000_ Marital Status: Ⓢ M D Se W

3. Address: _14276 Valley View Lane_ 4. _SSS-756-1234_
   (Street) (Phone)
   Hopkins, _XY_ _98765_
   (City) (State) (Zip)

5. Employer: _Sunrise Care Center (mother)_ Occupation: _dietician_
   Employer Address: _189 West Elm St._ _SSS-786-3321_
   Hopkins, XZ 98765 (Work Phone)
   Spouse: _N/A_ Employer: _____ Occupation: _____
   Employer Address: _____ (Work Phone)

6.
Other Household Members	Date of Birth	Relationship
Tricia Lambert	03/18/72	mother
Adam Ebers	11/04/99	brother
	/ /	
	/ /	
	/ /	

7. Medical Insurance Information

	Ins. Company Name	Policy No.	Policy Holder	Sgl.	Type of Coverage Fmly.	Primary	Sec.
( )	BCBS	XYZSII-11-0022	mother	☐	☒	☐	☐
( )				☐	☐	☐	☐
( )				☐	☐	☐	☐

8. Person to Contact in an Emergency _Tricia Lambert_ Relationship to you _mother_
   Their Work Phone _756-3321_ Their Home Phone _756-1234_

9. Party with primary responsibility for payment: ☐ Self ☒ Other
   Name _Tricia Lambert_ Relationship to you _mother_
   Address _(see above)_ Home Phone _____

For Office Use Only

Date Completed _____ Account No. _____ Patient No. _____

Household Status ☐ Head of Household

☐ Spouse ☐ Child ☐ Other: _____

Head of Household Name _____

Fig. 6-9 Registration data sheet (for Karen Ebers).

Chapter **6** **Traditional Fee-for-Service/Private Plans**

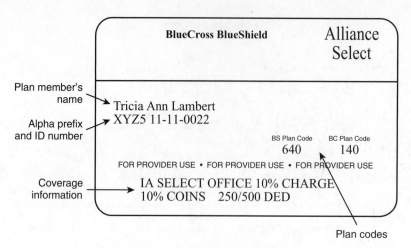

Plan member's name →

Alpha prefix and ID number →

Coverage information →

BlueCross BlueShield

Alliance
Select

Tricia Ann Lambert
XYZ5 11-11-0022

BS Plan Code   BC Plan Code
640   140

FOR PROVIDER USE • FOR PROVIDER USE • FOR PROVIDER USE

IA SELECT OFFICE 10% CHARGE
10% COINS   250/500 DED

Plan codes

Fig. 6-10 ID card (for Tricia Ann Lambert).

BROADMOOR MEDICAL CLINIC

ACCT. #: 11122	DATE OF SERVICE: 10-07-20XX	CATEGORY:	DIAGNOSIS: V 20.1
PATIENT'S NAME: Ebers, Karen S.		HEALTHCARE PROVIDER: Dr. Marilou Lucero	

CPT	✔	DESCRIPTION	FEE	CPT	✔	DESCRIPTION	FEE	CPT	✔	DESCRIPTION	FEE
OFFICE VISIT - NEW PATIENT				**IMMUNIZATIONS**				**INJECTIONS (CONT'D.)**			
99201		Focused		90701		DtaP		J3410		Vistaril	
99202		Expanded		90632		Hep A (Adult)		J3420		Vitamin B12	
99203		Detailed		90633		Hep A (Ped)		J2000		Xylocaine	
99204		Comprehensive		90744		Hep B (Ped)		**PROCEDURES**			
99205		Complex		90746		Hep B (Adult)		46600		Anoscopy	
OFFICE VISIT - ESTABLISHED PATIENT				90737		Hib		92551	✔	Audio Screening	35.00
99211		Minimal		90657		Influenza		11730		Avulsion Nail, Partial or	
99212		Focused		90707		MMR				Complete, Single	
99213		Expanded		90732		Pneumococcal		11200		Rem. of Skin Tags up to 15	
99214		Detailed		90718		Td		11201		Each Additional 10	
99215		Comprehensive		90703	✔	Tetanus Toxoid	20.00	10060		I & D Simple Abscess	
				90716		Varicella		10120		Removal FB Skin	
PHYSICAL EXAM - NEW PATIENT								11740		I & D Subung. Hematoma	
99381		Age Under 1 Year		**INJECTIONS**				58310		IUD Removal	
99382		Age 1 - 4 Years		J1200		Benadryl up to 50 mg		94010		Spirometry	
99383	✔	Age 5 - 11 Years	125.00	J0540		Bicillin up to 1,200,000 mg		A4570		Splint	
99384		Age 12 - 17 Years		J0690		Cefazolin Sodium 250 mg		99173	✔	Vision Screening	40.00
99385		Age 18 - 39 Years		J0704		Celestone		**LABORATORY**			
99386		Age 40 - 64 Years		J0780		Compazine		82270		Blood Occult	
99387		Age 65+ Years		J1100		Decadron		85680		TB Intradermal	
				J0970		Delestrogen		81000		Urine Dip Stick	
PHYSICAL EXAM - ESTABLISHED PATIENT				J1050		Depo Provera		84703		Serum Pregnancy Test	
99391		Age Under 1 Year		J1510		Gamma Globulin		87082		Strep Screen	
99392		Age 1 - 4 Years		J3301		Kenalog					
99393		Age 5 - 11 Years		J1940		Lasix		36415		Venipuncture	
99394		Age 12 - 17 Years		J2550		Phenergan		99000		Handling	
99395		Age 18 - 39 Years		J3490		Rocephin					
99396		Age 40 - 64 Years		J1070		Testosterone		**MISCELLANEOUS**			
99397		Age 65+ Years		J3250		Tigan					
				J1885		Torodol					

ICD-9 ☐ DIAGNOSIS				
CARDIOLOGY	388.30 ☐ Tinnitus Nos	787.0 ☐ Nausea And Vomiting	733.00 ☐ Osteoporosis	**PSYCH / MENTAL HEALTH**
794.31 ☐ Abn Ekg	463. ☐ Tonsillitis, Acute	533.90 ☐ Peptic Ulcer Nos	845.00 ☐ Sprain: Ankle	303.9 ☐ Alcoholism
786.50 ☐ Chest Pain, Nos	474.0 ☐ Tonsillitis, Chronic	569.3 ☐ Rectal Bleeding	847.2 ☐ Sprain: Back	300.00 ☐ Anxiety State Nos
780.4 ☐ Dizziness And Giddiness	**FEMALE / GYNECOLOGY**	**GENITO-URINARY**	847.0 ☐ Sprain: Cervical	300.00 ☐ Depression
787.1 ☐ Heartburn	795.0 ☐ Abn Pap Smear-Cervix	585. ☐ Chronic Renal Failure	840.9 ☐ Sprain: Shoulder	**SKIN / DERMATOLOGIC**
272.0 ☐ Hypercholesterolem	793.8 ☐ Abn Findings-Breast	595.0 ☐ Cystitis Acute	729.81 ☐ Swelling of Limb	706.1 ☐ Acne Nec
272.4 ☐ Hyperlipidemia Nec/Nos	626.0 ☐ Amenorrhea	788.1 ☐ Dysuria	726.00 ☐ Tendonitis	691. ☐ Dermatitis, Atopic
401.1 ☐ Hyptertension Benign	611.72 ☐ Breast Mass/Lump	599.7 ☐ Hematuria	**NEUROLOGY**	692. ☐ Dermatitis, Contact
401.9 ☐ Hypertension Nos	616.0 ☐ Cervicitis	601.0 ☐ Prostatitis Acute	784.0 ☐ Headache	110.1 ☐ Dermatophytosis, Nail
401.0 ☐ Hypertension, Malig.	V25.09 ☐ Contracept. Mgmt.	599.0 ☐ UTI	346.9 ☐ Migraine Nos	691.0 ☐ Diaper Rash
785.1 ☐ Palpitations	625.3 ☐ Dysmenorrhea	**HEMATOLOGY**	724.3 ☐ Sciatica	054.9 ☐ Herpes Simplex Nos
ENDOCRINE	626.4 ☐ Menstruation, Irreg.	790.6 ☐ Abn Blood Chemistry Nec	307.81 ☐ Tension Headache	053.9 ☐ Herpes Zoster Nos
250.01 ☐ IDDM Controlled	625.2 ☐ Menstruation, Excessive	285.9 ☐ Anemia Nos	780.4 ☐ Vertigo	054.10 ☐ Herpes Genital Nec
250.03 ☐ IDDM Uncontrolled	614.9 ☐ Pelvic Inflam Dis	280.1 ☐ Anemia, Iron Def	**OPHTHALMOLOGY**	684. ☐ Impetigo
250.02 ☐ NIDDM Uncontrolled	V22.2 ☐ Preg State, Incidental	**INFECTIOUS**	373.00 ☐ Blepharitis Nos	703.0 ☐ Ingrowing Nail
250.00 ☐ NIDDM Controlled	616.10 ☐ Vaginitis	616.3 ☐ Abcess: Bartholin Gland	372.30 ☐ Conjunctivitis	215.9 ☐ Nevus
251.2 ☐ Hypoglycemia	**PHYSICAL EXAM**	682.9 ☐ Abcess: Skin	918.1 ☐ Corneal Abrasion	110.1 ☐ Onychomycosis
244.9 ☐ Hypothyroidism	V20.1 ☑ Well Child	780.6 ☐ Fever: Unkn. Origin	**PULMONARY / RESPIRATORY**	696.1 ☐ Psoriasis
242.90 ☐ Hyperthyroidism	V72.84 ☐ Pre-Op Exam	**IMMUNOLOGY - ALLERGIES**	493.9 ☐ Asthma Nos	706.2 ☐ Sebaceous Cyst
EAR, NOSE, THROAT	**GASTRO-INTESTINAL**	995.3 ☐ Allergic Reaction Nos	466.0 ☐ Bronchitis Acute	708.8 ☐ Urticaria Nec
386.30 ☐ Labyrinthitis Nos	789.06 ☐ Abnormal Pain, Epigastric	477.0 ☐ Allergy, Hay Fever	490. ☐ Bronchitis Nos	078.1 ☐ Warts, Viral
382.9 ☐ Otitis Media, Ac./Chr.	794.3 ☐ Abn. Liver Function Study	042. ☐ Human ImmunoVirus Dis.	486. ☐ Pneumonia	**OTHER - MISC.**
462. ☐ Pharyngitis Acute	578.1 ☐ Blood in Stool	**ORTHOPEDICS**	786.2 ☐ Cough	780.7 ☐ Malaise and Fatigue
477.9 ☐ Rhinitis, Allergic	564.0 ☐ Constipation	716.90 ☐ Arthritis Unspec.	786.0 ☐ Dyspnea/Resp Abn	780.2 ☐ Syncope
461.9 ☐ Sinusitis, Ac Nos	787.91 ☐ Diarrhea	724.5 ☐ Backache Nos	487. ☐ Influenza	**WRITE - IN**
473.9 ☐ Sinusitis, Chronic	562.11 ☐ Diverticulitis	727.3 ☐ Bursitis Nec	786.52 ☐ Painful Respiration	
528.0 ☐ Stomatitis	530.81 ☐ Esophageal Reflux	354.0 ☐ Carpal Tunnel Syndrome	786.09 ☐ S O B	
034.0 ☐ Strep Throat	535.5 ☐ Gastritis/Duodenitis Nos	719.40 ☐ Joint Pain-Unspec.	465.9 ☐ URI	
	455.6 ☐ Hemorrhoids	729.1 ☐ Myalgia And Myositis Nos.	079.9 ☐ Viral Syndrome	

INSTRUCTIONS:	RETURN APPOINTMENT: 1 year	PAID	PREV. BAL. — 0 —
	___ Days ___ Weeks ___ Months (PRN)	☐ CASH ☐ CHECK	TODAY'S FEE
	___ 15 ___ 30 ___ 45	☐ CR. CD.	AMT. REC'D.

Fig. 6-11 Encounter form (for Karen Ebers).

BCBS XYZ 511110022
$250; 90/10 10% COINS
A/C #11122

STATEMENT

BROADMOOR MEDICAL CLINIC
4353 Pine Ridge Drive
Milton, XY 12345-0001
Telephone: 555-656-7890

Tricia   03/18/1972
Adam   11/04/1999
Karen   04/28/2002

TRICIA LAMBERT
14276 VALLEY VIEW LANE
HOPKINS, XY 98765

20XX

DATE	PROFESSIONAL SERVICE DESCRIPTION	CHARGE		CREDITS			CURRENT BALANCE	
				PAYMENTS	ADJUSTMENTS			

Due and payable within 10 days.   **Pay last amount in balance column**

Fig. 6-12 Ledger card (for Tricia Ann Lambert).

Performance Objective 6-2—Patient Case Study 6-1

Conditions: Complete a CMS-1500 form using the information provided in Case Study 6-1.

Supplies/Equipment: CMS-1500 form (paper or electronic) (Fig. 6-13)/pen; patient information form, ID card, encounter form (see Fig. 6-11), ledger card (see Fig. 6-12)

Guided Completion: For this claim form exercise, you also can use the Guided Completion software found on the Student CD to help you complete this CMS-1500 claim form.

Time Allowed: 50 minutes

Accuracy Needed to Pass: 80%

Broadmoor Medical Clinic 4353 Pine Ridge Drive Milton, XY 12345-0001 Clinic NPI X100XX1000 Telephone: 555-656-7890	Clinic EIN # 42-1898989 Dr. R.G. Jones NPI 1234567890 Dr. Marilou Lucero NPI 2907511822 Group # GRW0000 Date claim 1 day after examination

Procedural Steps	Points Earned	Comments
Evaluator: Note time began: _____		
1. Carefully read and study the applicable documents.		
2. Using the Blue Cross and Blue Shield template from Fig. 6-13, generate a clean claim for Karen Ebers' office visit. (100)		
Optional: May deduct points for taking more time than allowed.		

Total Points = 100

Student's Score: _____

Evaluator: _____

Comments: _____

_____

_____

_____

_____

1500

HEALTH INSURANCE CLAIM FORM

APPROVED BY NATIONAL UNIFORM CLAIM COMMITTEE 08/05

PICA | PICA

CARRIER

1. MEDICARE (Medicare #) | MEDICAID (Medicaid #) | TRICARE CHAMPUS (Sponsor's SSN) | CHAMPVA (Member ID#) | GROUP HEALTH PLAN (SSN or ID) | FECA BLK LUNG (SSN) | OTHER (ID)

1a. INSURED'S I.D. NUMBER (For Program in Item 1)

2. PATIENT'S NAME (Last Name, First Name, Middle Initial)

3. PATIENT'S BIRTH DATE MM | DD | YY SEX M F

4. INSURED'S NAME (Last Name, First Name, Middle Initial)

5. PATIENT'S ADDRESS (No., Street)

6. PATIENT RELATIONSHIP TO INSURED Self Spouse Child Other

7. INSURED'S ADDRESS (No., Street)

CITY STATE

8. PATIENT STATUS Single Married Other

CITY STATE

ZIP CODE TELEPHONE (Include Area Code) ( )

Employed Full-Time Student Part-Time Student

ZIP CODE TELEPHONE (Include Area Code) ( )

9. OTHER INSURED'S NAME (Last Name, First Name, Middle Initial)

10. IS PATIENT'S CONDITION RELATED TO:

11. INSURED'S POLICY GROUP OR FECA NUMBER

a. OTHER INSURED'S POLICY OR GROUP NUMBER

a. EMPLOYMENT? (Current or Previous) YES NO

a. INSURED'S DATE OF BIRTH MM | DD | YY SEX M F

b. OTHER INSURED'S DATE OF BIRTH MM | DD | YY SEX M F

b. AUTO ACCIDENT? YES NO PLACE (State)

b. EMPLOYER'S NAME OR SCHOOL NAME

c. EMPLOYER'S NAME OR SCHOOL NAME

c. OTHER ACCIDENT? YES NO

c. INSURANCE PLAN NAME OR PROGRAM NAME

d. INSURANCE PLAN NAME OR PROGRAM NAME

10d. RESERVED FOR LOCAL USE

d. IS THERE ANOTHER HEALTH BENEFIT PLAN? YES NO *If yes*, return to and complete item 9 a-d.

READ BACK OF FORM BEFORE COMPLETING & SIGNING THIS FORM.

12. PATIENT'S OR AUTHORIZED PERSON'S SIGNATURE I authorize the release of any medical or other information necessary to process this claim. I also request payment of government benefits either to myself or to the party who accepts assignment below.

SIGNED DATE

13. INSURED'S OR AUTHORIZED PERSON'S SIGNATURE I authorize payment of medical benefits to the undersigned physician or supplier for services described below.

SIGNED

PATIENT AND INSURED INFORMATION

14. DATE OF CURRENT: MM | DD | YY ILLNESS (First symptom) OR INJURY (Accident) OR PREGNANCY(LMP)

15. IF PATIENT HAS HAD SAME OR SIMILAR ILLNESS. GIVE FIRST DATE MM | DD | YY

16. DATES PATIENT UNABLE TO WORK IN CURRENT OCCUPATION FROM MM | DD | YY TO MM | DD | YY

17. NAME OF REFERRING PROVIDER OR OTHER SOURCE

17a.

17b. NPI

18. HOSPITALIZATION DATES RELATED TO CURRENT SERVICES FROM MM | DD | YY TO MM | DD | YY

19. RESERVED FOR LOCAL USE

20. OUTSIDE LAB? YES NO $ CHARGES

21. DIAGNOSIS OR NATURE OF ILLNESS OR INJURY (Relate Items 1, 2, 3 or 4 to Item 24E by Line)

1. ___ . ___

2. ___ . ___

3. ___ . ___

4. ___ . ___

22. MEDICAID RESUBMISSION CODE ORIGINAL REF. NO.

23. PRIOR AUTHORIZATION NUMBER

24. A. DATE(S) OF SERVICE From MM DD YY To MM DD YY	B. PLACE OF SERVICE	C. EMG	D. PROCEDURES, SERVICES, OR SUPPLIES (Explain Unusual Circumstances) CPT/HCPCS MODIFIER	E. DIAGNOSIS POINTER	F. $ CHARGES	G. DAYS OR UNITS	H. EPSDT Family Plan	I. ID. QUAL.	J. RENDERING PROVIDER ID. #
1								NPI	
2								NPI	
3								NPI	
4								NPI	
5								NPI	
6								NPI	

25. FEDERAL TAX I.D. NUMBER SSN EIN

26. PATIENT'S ACCOUNT NO.

27. ACCEPT ASSIGNMENT? (For govt. claims, see back) YES NO

28. TOTAL CHARGE $

29. AMOUNT PAID $

30. BALANCE DUE $

31. SIGNATURE OF PHYSICIAN OR SUPPLIER INCLUDING DEGREES OR CREDENTIALS (I certify that the statements on the reverse apply to this bill and are made a part thereof.)

SIGNED DATE

32. SERVICE FACILITY LOCATION INFORMATION

a. NPI b.

33. BILLING PROVIDER INFO & PH # ( )

a. NPI b.

PHYSICIAN OR SUPPLIER INFORMATION

NUCC Instruction Manual available at: www.nucc.org

APPROVED OMB-0938-0999 FORM CMS-1500 (08/05)

Fig. 6-13 Blank CMS-1500 form (for Karen Ebers).

Scoring Rubric for CMS-1500 Performance Objective

BLOCK NO.	POINTS ALLOWED	STUDENT'S SCORE	COMMENTS
1	1		
1a	2		
2	5		
3	1		
4	2		
5	5		
6	1		
7	3		
8	2		
9	5		
10	3		
11d	1		
14	1		
17	2		
17b	2		
21	5		
24a	2 × 4		
24b	1 × 4		
24d	2 × 4		
24e	1 × 4		
24f	1 × 4		
24g	1 × 4		
24j	1 × 4		
25	2		
26	1		
27	1		
28	4		
31	3		
32	4		
32a	1		
33	5		
33a	1		
33b	1		
TOTAL	100		

Performance Objective 6-3—Interpreting an Explanation of Benefits

Conditions: Student will interpret an EOB generated from Case Study 6-1.
Supplies/Equipment: Pen, EOB form from Blue Cross and Blue Shield claim (Fig. 6-14)
Time Allowed: 20 minutes
Accuracy Needed to Pass: 100%

Procedural Steps	Points Earned	Comments
Evaluator: Note time began: _____		
1. Carefully read and study the EOB document provided in Fig. 6-14.		
2. Using the ledger card generated in Performance Objective 6-1, post the insurance payment rec'd 10/30. (10)		
3. Calculate the amount that must be adjusted off. (10)		
4. Calculate the amount still owed by the patient (the last figure in the column "Current Balance" should reflect the amount the patient owes). (10)		
Optional: May deduct points for taking more time than allowed.		

Total Points = 30

Student's Score: _____

Evaluator: _____

Comments: _____

_____

_____

_____

_____

EXPLANATION OF BENEFITS

(THIS IS NOT A BILL)

This is your Explanation of Health Care Benefits. This statement shows how we applied your coverage to claim(s) submitted to us. If you have any questions, please call our Customer Service Department at 555-666-0000 or 800-222-1111 weekdays between the hours of 8 a.m. and 5 p.m.

Insured Name: Tricia Ann Lambert
14276 Valley View Lane
Hopkins, XY 98765

ID # XYZ511110022

Patient: Karen S. Ebers

Service Date(s): 10-07-20XX

Provider: Broadmoor Medical Clinic

Billed Charges	Provider Savings	Amount Insurance Paid	Amount Patient Owes
$220.00	$28.50	$136.45	$55.05

CLAIM DETAILS

Billed Charge	125.00	20.00	35.00	40.00
Allowed Charge	111.00	17.50	23.00	-- *
Copayment (−)	11.00	1.75	2.30	-- *
Deductible (−)	-- **	-- **	-- **	-- **
Sub-Total	100.00	15.75	20.70	40.00
Insurance Paid	100.00	15.75	20.70	--

Group Number	Claim Number	Account Number	Provider Number	Date Received	Date Processed
000GRW0000	000050505011	1818181XZ	00234543	10-10-20XX	10-11-20XX

NOTES:

*D – Patient has met yearly deductible

**L – Contract Limitation(s)

A check in the amount of ___$136.45___ **has been mailed to your provider.**

Fig. 6-14 Explanation of benefits for Tricia Lambert. (Courtesy the Blue Cross Blue Shield Association.)

Chapter Check List

Student name: _____

Chapter completion date: _____

1.	Record	Your start time and date: _____
2.	Read	The assigned chapter in the text
3.	View	PowerPoint slides (if available)
4.	Complete	Exercises in the Workbook as assigned
5.	Compare	Your answers with the answers posted on the bulletin board/website/handout
6.	Correct	Your answers
7.	Complete	All tests and required activities
8.	Read	Assigned readings (if any)
9.	Complete	Chapter performance objectives (competencies), if any
10.	Evaluate	Chapter performance and submit to your instructor
11.	Record	Your ending time and date: _____
12.	Move on	Begin next chapter as assigned

PERFORMANCE EVALUATION

Student name: _____

Chapter completion date:_____

Evaluate your classroom performance. Complete the self-evaluation, and submit it to your instructor. When your instructor returns this form to you, compare your self-evaluation with the evaluation completed by your instructor.

Skill	Student Self-Evaluation			Instructor Evaluation		
	Good	Average	Poor	Good	Average	Poor
Attendance/punctuality						
Personal appearance						
Applies effort						
Is self-motivated						
Is courteous						
Has positive attitude						
Completes assignments in timely manner						
Works well with others						

Student's initials:_____

Date: _____

Points Possible: _____

Points Awarded: _____

Chapter Grade: _____

Instructor's initials: _____

Date: _____

Composing a Patient Letter

You have received a letter from Tricia Lambert inquiring why there is a balance owing on Karen Ebers' account. Compose a letter of explanation. (*Instructor's hint:* The insurance policy does not cover routine eye examinations.)

Health Insurance Professional's Notebook

Figs. 6-3 and 6-4 in your textbook illustrate a template for required fields on the CMS-1500 form along with block-by-block guidelines for completion of claims for Wellmark Blue Cross and Blue Shield (Iowa and South Dakota). Research the guidelines in your state/area, and compare them with these documents. Note any differences your Blue Cross and Blue Shield carrier requires, then create a new template reflecting a correctly completed Blue Cross and Blue Shield claim form for your area. Incorporate these pages under the "commercial claims" section in your notebook.

7 Unraveling the Mysteries of Managed Care

Chapter 7 deals with the "mysteries" of managed care. Because managed care can present a greater challenge than some of the other topics in the textbook, the activities in this chapter of the student workbook focus on helping the student "unravel" the mysteries and, in doing so, gain a better understanding of how managed care functions.

Managed care includes medical plans in which access to healthcare services is structured in such a way as to provide quality medical care, while attempting to limit healthcare costs. Premiums are typically lower with managed care policies than for traditional fee-for-service healthcare plans, and the charge for each provider visit is comparatively small. As we learned from Chapter 7 in the textbook, a common form of managed care is the health maintenance organization (HMO), which restricts patients to the HMO's own group of medical professionals. Other forms of managed care include point of service (POS) and preferred provider organization (PPO) plans. Although these plans typically charge the low per-visit fee of an HMO for treatment by healthcare professionals within the plan's network, they also allow out-of-network treatment at a lower reimbursement rate.

WORKBOOK CHAPTER OBJECTIVES

After completing the workbook activities for Chapter 7, the student should be able to:
- Define the terms used in the chapter.
- Answer the review questions to within the evaluation criteria set by the instructor.
- Demonstrate higher order thinking (e.g., the ability to synthesize and evaluate critically new information).
- Integrate knowledge, and transfer it from one document to another.
- Access the information needed from the Internet to complete workbook activities.
- Perform basic math calculations for billing purposes.
- Abstract applicable information from healthcare documents necessary for completion of various forms used in healthcare billing and the claims process.
- Complete specific forms common to managed care organizations (MCOs).
- Generate information and documents for inclusion in the student's personal Health Insurance Professional's Notebook.
- Undertake self-criticism and evaluation, including seeking and responding to feedback and comments and setting realistic targets.

DEFINING CHAPTER TERMS

Using the computer (or typewriter), students should key an accurate definition for each of the chapter terms listed. These definitions should be in the students' own words. When finished, students should compare their definitions with those listed in the glossary at the back of the textbook, correcting any inaccuracies.

capitation
closed panel HMO
consultation
copayment
direct contract model
enrollees
grievance
group model
health maintenance organization (HMO)
iatrogenic effects
individual practice association (IPA)
managed care
network

network model
open panel plan
point of service (POS)
preauthorization
precertification
predetermination
preferred provider organization (PPO)
primary care physician (PCP)
referral
specialist
staff model
utilization review

Multiple Choice

Directions: In the questions/statements presented, choose the response that **best** answers/completes the stem, and circle the letter that precedes it.

1. An organized, interrelated system of people and facilities that communicate with one another and work together as a unit is commonly referred to as a(n):
   a. Network
   b. Community
   c. Demograph
   d. Organizational unit

2. Individuals belonging to a managed healthcare plan are referred to as:
   a. Beneficiaries
   b. Enrollees
   c. Receivers
   d. Entities

3. The two most common types of MCOs are:
   a. PPOs and individual practice associations (IPAs)
   b. IPAs and HMOs
   c. HMOs and PPOs
   d. PPOs and POSs

4. A specific provider who oversees an HMO member's total healthcare treatment is called a(n):
   a. Specific provider
   b. Attending physician
   c. Complete care provider
   d. Primary care physician (PCP)

5. The amount of money a patient has to pay out-of-pocket per visit is referred to as a(n):
   a. Copayment
   b. Deductible
   c. Premium
   d. Allowable fee

6. When an individual first enrolls in an HMO, he or she chooses a(n):
   a. Specialist
   b. Insurance carrier
   c. Fiscal intermediary
   d. PCP

7. Most managed healthcare plans emphasize:
   a. Small copayments
   b. Frequent physician visits
   c. Preventive healthcare
   d. Paying premiums on time

8. A multispecialty group practice where all healthcare services are provided within the building(s) owned by the HMO is called a:

   a. Staff model

   b. Group model

   c. Network model

   d. Direct contact model

9. An HMO that contracts with independent, multispecialty physician groups that provide all healthcare services to its members and usually share the same facility, support staff, medical records, and equipment is called a:

   a. Staff model

   b. Group model

   c. Network model

   d. Direct contact model

10. A reimbursement system in which healthcare providers receive a fixed fee for every patient enrolled in the plan, regardless of how many or few services the patient uses, is called a(n):

    a. Usual, customary, and reasonable

    b. Capitation

    c. Misallocation

    d. Allowed fee system

11. A managed care system composed of individual healthcare providers who offer healthcare services for HMO and non-HMO patients, but maintain their own offices and identities, is called a(n):

    a. Network model

    b. Open-panel IPA

    c. Direct-contact model

    d. POS plan

12. A plan that allows patients to use the HMO provider or go outside the plan and pay a higher copayment and deductible is a(n):

    a. Network model

    b. Open-end HMO

    c. Direct-contact model

    d. POS plan

13. A system designed to determine the medical necessity and appropriateness of a requested medical service, procedure, or hospital admission prior, concurrent, or retrospective to the event is called:

    a. Accreditation

    b. Certification

    c. Utilization

    d. Endorsement determination

14. If a particular medical service or procedure is determined not to be "medically necessary," a patient may file a(n):

    a. Grievance

    b. Objection

    c. Lawsuit

    d. Appeal

15. A procedure required by third-party payers that requires permission before a provider can carry out specific procedures and treatments is:

   a. Referral

   b. Certification

   c. Adjudication

   d. Preauthorization

True/False

Directions: Place a "T" in the blank preceding the sentence if it is true; place an "F" if it is false.

_____ 1.   An HMO provides its members with basic healthcare services for a fixed price and for a given period of time.

_____ 2.   PPOs typically do not require authorization from a PCP for a referral to a specialist.

_____ 3.   PPOs are more tightly controlled by government regulations than HMOs.

_____ 4.   HMOs typically have no deductibles or plan limits.

_____ 5.   The federal government requires that HMOs operate their own facilities, staffed with salaried physicians.

_____ 6.   HMOs are neither accredited nor certified.

_____ 7.   Preauthorization pertains to medical necessity and appropriateness and guarantees payment.

_____ 8.   Precertification involves collecting information before inpatient admissions or performance of selected ambulatory procedures and services.

_____ 9.   A referral is a request by a healthcare provider for a patient under his or her care to be evaluated or treated or both by another provider.

_____ 10. In all managed care situations, for the healthcare plan to recognize the referral, it must come from the patient's designated PCP.

Fill-in-the-Blank

Directions: Select the word or word groups from the box on the next page to complete the following statements correctly. (**Note:** Some word or word groups can be used more than once.)

1. _____ describes types of health insurance that control the use of health services by their members so that they can contain healthcare costs, the quality of care, or both.

2. An interrelated system where people and facilities communicate with one another and work together as a unit is

   referred to as a(n) _____.

3. Individuals who are eligible for healthcare services and benefits under a specific managed care plan are called

   _____.

4. The two most common types of MCOs are _____ and _____.

5. _____ are groups of healthcare providers who work under one umbrella to provide medical services at a discount to individuals who participate in the managed care plan.

6. A(n) _____ is a specific provider who oversees an HMO member's total healthcare treatment.

7. When a patient's problem exceeds the expertise of his or her PCP, the PCP can arrange a(n) _____ to a specialist to take over the patient's care.

8. _____ typically have no deductibles or plan limits.

9. Managed care plans emphasize _____ healthcare.

10. A(n) _____ HMO is a multispecialty group practice where all healthcare services are provided within the building(s) owned by the HMO.

11. In a(n) _____, the HMO contracts with independent, multispecialty physician groups who provide all healthcare services to its members.

12. _____ is a fixed fee per member per specified time period (usually monthly).

13. The staff model is a(n) _____ HMO.

14. The _____ HMO is similar to an IPA except the HMO contracts directly with the individual physicians.

15. An IPA is a(n) _____.

16. The _____ HMO is one that has multiple provider arrangements, including staff, group, or IPA structures.

17. The _____ is a "hybrid" type of managed care (also referred to as an open-ended HMO) that allows patients to use the HMO provider or go outside the plan and use any provider they choose.

18. _____ is a system designed to determine the medical necessity and appropriateness of a medical service, procedure, or hospital admission.

19. _____ is a procedure required by most managed healthcare and indemnity plans before a provider is able to carry out specific procedures or treatments for a patient.

20. A(n) _____ is when the PCP requests another physician to provide his or her expert opinion regarding the patient's condition.

capitation	closed panel
consultation	direct contract model
enrollees	group model
health maintenance organizations (HMOs)	open-panel plan
managed care	preauthorization
network model	preventive
point of service (POS) model	referral
preferred provider organizations (PPOs)	utilization review
primary care physician (PCP)	network
staff model	

Short Answer

1. An MCO typically performs three main functions, which are:

   _____

   _____

   _____

2. Explain briefly in your own words each of the following types of managed care systems:

   PPO: _____

   HMO: _____

   IPA: _____

   POS: _____

3. Under the Federal HMO Act, an entity must have three characteristics to call itself an HMO. List them.

   _____

   _____

   _____

4. List three advantages and three disadvantages of HMOs.

   _____

   _____

   _____

   _____

   _____

5. For a particular managed healthcare plan to become accredited by the National Committee for Quality Assurance (NCQA), it first must undergo a survey and meet certain standards designed to evaluate the facility's clinical and administrative systems. These standards fall into five broad categories. List them.

   _____

   _____

   _____

   _____

6. The Joint Commission's standards outline performance expectations for activities that affect the safety and quality of patient care. List the six categories these standards include.

_____

_____

_____

_____

_____

_____

7. List four types of actions that a patient can file a grievance against.

_____

_____

_____

_____

8. Explain the difference between a referral and a consultation.

_____

9. How do the Health Insurance Portability and Accountability Act's (HIPAA's) regulations affect managed care?

_____

10. In your own opinion, what is the future of managed care?

_____

CRITICAL THINKING ACTIVITIES

A. New patient Dorothy Scoval comes to the medical facility with a knee injury. She informs you that she is a current enrollee of Envision, a local HMO. Would the procedure for gathering demographic and insurance information differ with this patient compared with one who is insured under a traditional commercial plan? Explain why or why not.

B. Examine the ID card shown in Fig. 7-1, then answer the following questions from the information printed on the card.

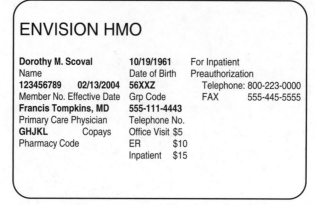

ENVISION HMO

Dorothy M. Scoval	**10/19/1961**	For Inpatient
Name	Date of Birth	Preauthorization
123456789 02/13/2004	**56XXZ**	Telephone: 800-223-0000
Member No. Effective Date	Grp Code	FAX 555-445-5555
Francis Tompkins, MD	**555-111-4443**	
Primary Care Physician	Telephone No.	
GHJKL Copays	Office Visit $5	
Pharmacy Code	ER $10	
	Inpatient $15	

Fig. 7-1 Health maintenance organization ID card for Scoval.

1. What is the name of the insured individual?
2. What is the name of the patient's PCP?
3. What dollar amount should you collect from the patient for an office visit?
4. What type of HMO is this?
5. If the patient was seen on February 2, 2004, would the HMO pay for the visit?

C. Established patient Dorothy Scoval telephones 1 week after her initial encounter complaining of chest pain and shortness of breath. She asks if she can schedule an appointment with an Envision cardiologist. The scheduling receptionist refers the call to you, the health insurance professional. How should this request be handled?

D. The medical facility in which you work as a health insurance professional is part of Envision, a staff model HMO. The healthcare providers are employees of the HMO and see patients on a "capitated" (per patient) basis. How does this payment structure affect claims submission for the plan's enrollees?

E. Healthcare reform has been a popular topic in the United States for many years; however, not everyone has a clear picture of exactly what managed care is and how it functions. Following are several statements regarding managed care, particularly HMOs. Place a "T" in the blank preceding all true statements; place an "F" in the blank if the statement is false.

_____ 1.   Most HMOs typically offer substandard healthcare to keep costs under control.

_____ 2.   MCOs encourage members to take a proactive or "preventive" role in their own healthcare.

_____ 3.   All HMOs are the same.

_____ 4.   The primary differences among managed care plans are found in the type of plan, what benefits it covers, and the out-of-pocket costs members will pay for services.

_____ 5.   The NCQA has developed standards to evaluate the medical and quality systems in HMOs.

_____ 6.   The main role of the PCP in HMOs is to serve as a "gatekeeper," rationing treatment options simply to contain costs.

_____ 7.   The best physicians do not participate in HMO networks; members cannot be sure they are getting quality medical care.

_____ 8.   Most healthcare providers participate in some type of managed care plan.

_____ 9.   Most HMO members are dissatisfied with their plans.

_____ 10.   Managed care plans are able to keep costs low because of an emphasis on disease prevention and wellness.

PROBLEM-SOLVING/COLLABORATIVE (GROUP) ACTIVITIES

A. Create a page for an Office Procedures Manual outlining the course of action to follow for obtaining preauthorization for a managed care patient who is to be admitted to the hospital for a surgical procedure. Include an example of a typical preauthorization form.

B. There are four main HIPAA regulations that affect healthcare:

1. Maintaining patient confidentiality

2. Implementing standards for electronic transmission of transactions and code sets

3. Establishing national provider and employer identifiers

4. Resolving security and privacy issues arising from the storage and transmission of healthcare data

Select one of the above-listed regulations, and prepare a 5-minute group presentation expanding it as follows:
- Its impact on patients
- Its impact on healthcare providers
- Its impact on business and community in general
- Pros and cons

C. Group study topics:
1. Compare benefit structures offered in managed care with benefits in traditional indemnity insurance.
2. Explain how capitation might lead to underuse of healthcare services.

PROJECTS/DISCUSSION TOPICS

A. There are four main federal laws that govern health insurance; you already have learned about three of them:

ERISA—places critical limitations on health plan liability
COBRA—provides substantial protection for preserving an individual's insurance coverage after job or life changes
HIPAA—protects an individual's privacy and his or her ability to maintain healthcare coverage
The fourth one is the **Federal HMO Act.** Conduct in-depth research to learn about this important act. Then write a brief synopsis explaining what this act involves and how it affects today's healthcare market.

B. **Discussion forum:** Study and prepare for a discussion regarding one or more of the following:

What is managed care?
What do "capitation" and other managed care systems involve?
What ethical concerns does managed care raise?
What specific impact does managed care have on physician-patient relationships?
What should providers consider when evaluating managed care contracts?

C. Generate a chart comparing managed care with traditional (indemnity) insurance.

CASE STUDIES

A. Eric Thomas has healthcare coverage with a PPO. His deductible is $500, which he has met for the current year. According to his policy, if he is treated by a PPO member physician, his coinsurance ratio is 90/10. If he is treated by a non-PPO physician, the coinsurance ratio is 80/20. Calculate the amount Eric would have to pay either of the two following physicians.

PPO Member Physician	Non-PPO Physician
Benjamin P. Moore, M.D.	Lydia R. Davis, M.D.
Est. Pt. Level II OV = $90	Est. Pt. Level II OV = $65
Eric's payment: _____	Eric's payment: _____

Chapter **7** Unraveling the Mysteries of Managed Care

B. The following case study is for patient Judith Kelley. Read it thoroughly and complete the referral authorization form in Fig. 7-2.

Patient Name: Judith A. Kelley
DOB: 03/14/1955
Med. Record No.: 10445
Health Insurance: Zenith HMO
Member No.: 444661112

Judith Kelley visited Kayla Parsons, her PCP, on 08/22/20XX, complaining of nausea, loss of appetite, and unexplained weight loss, which began about 2 months before this visit after a bout of the flu. After taking a detailed history and performing a complete examination, including a urinalysis and complete blood count, Dr. Parsons suspects Mrs. Kelley's symptoms point to a serious underlying condition and warrants a referral to a specialist for evaluation and treatment. Dr. Marvel Sutton is an endocrinologist and practices within the patient's HMO system. Initially, Dr. Parsons has authorized two visits with Dr. Sutton, and the first appointment date is 08/30/20XX.

Diagnoses: (1) Loss of weight—783.21; (2) Nausea—787.02
Referral No.: 032425
Provider ID No.: 6544355
Dr. Parson's phone number: 555-876-2123; fax: 555-876-2110

Note: Students should use their own name as a contact person.

HEALTH Referral Authorization Form

This facsimile transmission is private, confidential and intended only of the recipient named hereon. If you receive this transmission in error, please contact Iowa Health's Medical Management Dept. at (555) 333-XXXX or (800) 222-XXXX.

FAX THIS COMPLETED FORM TO: (555) 333-XXXX or (800) 222-XXXX

Referral #: _____   **ALL REFERRALS EXPIRE IN 60 DAYS**

Patient Information

Member Name	Member #	DOB	Refer to Provider	Specialty

Please check the requested services:	☐ Evaluation and recommendation	☐ Evaluate and treat
☐ OPS ☐ One follow-up visit	☐ Send report to PCP	
Number of Visits:	Appointment Date:	

Medical Information

Diagnosis:	ICD-9 Code:

Symptoms: _____
_____
_____

Previous Treatment (if pertinent for referral): _____
_____

Lab/X-Ray Finding (if pertinent for referral): _____
_____

Medical Record #:

Authorization

PCP Name	Phone # (Include Area Code)
Contact Name	Fax #

For Office use only

PCP Provider #		Refer to Provider	
Member Effective Date	Auth Type		Extent of Care
Auth Start Date	Auth End Date		# of Visits Approved
Approved by:		Date:	
Entered by:		Date:	

This referral does not constitute a payment agreement. Coverage is based on the eligibility of the member at the time of service is rendered.

Fig. 7-2 Referral authorization form (Kelley).

C. The following case study is for patient Fredric Basquez. From this information, complete the prior authorization request form in Fig. 7-3.

Patient Name: Fredric M. Basquez
DOB: 09/26/1972
Health Insurance Plan: OutReach Plus
Subscriber ID No.: QST99442
Med. Record No.: BA092662
Social Security No.: 222-00-9999

Fredric Basquez comes to see Dr. Eric Woods, an orthopedic surgeon, for complaints of head and neck pain accompanied by numbness and tingling in his right arm after an all-terrain vehicle (ATV) accident. The patient reports he was riding on the back of his brother's ATV, when the vehicle came into contact with a concealed tree stump. He was subsequently thrown from the vehicle, landing on the right side of his head. A 2-cm laceration of the right cheek was sutured in the emergency department yesterday, and débridement of minor abrasions and contusions of the face and shoulder was performed. X-rays of the head and neck, done at the time of the emergency department visit, were inconclusive. He was given prescriptions for naproxen. An emergency department staff member scheduled an appointment with this office for follow-up. A detailed history was taken, and a complete physical examination was done. Suspected herniated disk with progressive objective neurologic deficits.

Diagnosis: Neck injury—959.09
Provider ID No.: 6577890113
Dr. Woods' phone number: 555-232-0987; fax: 555-232-0980

Dr. Woods asks you to arrange an MRI for Mr. Basquez. You note from the patient's insurance ID card that prior authorization must be obtained for any outside diagnostic testing. From the information above, complete the Prior Authorization Request form for Mr. Basquez's MRI. (*Note:* You will be attaching a copy of the initial history and physical examination [H & P] with this form.)

Note: Do not complete the area below the heavy black line.

Prior Authorization Request for MRI/CT Scan of the Neck and Spine

To Be Completed By Ordering Provider / *Date:*

Patient Name:	Patient Subscriber ID:	Patient Date of Birth:
Provider Name:	Provider ID Number:	Provider Phone: Provider Fax:

Please Indicate the Study Ordered:	☐ MRI	☐ Neck ☐ Spine	☐ CT	☐ Neck ☐ Spine
Diagnosis (ICD-9 Code):			Scheduled Date:	

MRI Indications		CT Indications
☐ Myelopathy ☐ Infection of spine/cord/disk ☐ Spinal trauma ☐ Grossly abnormal plain films ☐ Co-existing systemic illness	☐ Congenital anomalies of spine ☐ Spinal stenosis ☐ Post-op spinal surgery w/residua ☐ Where contrast is required ☐ Known malignancy/suspected mets	☐ Spinal fracture

Conditional Indications		
Suspected herniated disk with one or more of the following:	☐ Progressive objective neurological deficits (sensory/motor loss, reflex change, fasciculations, wasting) ☐ Cauda equina syndrome	☐ Serious systemic illness (malignancy, TB, etc.) ☐ Spinal cord compression
Uncomplicated back pain or sciatica only after 4–6 weeks of the conservative treatment with:	☐ Home self-care ☐ Analgesics ☐ PT or chiropractic care ☐ Spinal exercises	
If none of the above, rationale for exception (all exceptions must have supporting documentation):		

Supporting Documentation: ☐ Initial Evaluation (H & P) ☐ Treatment Plan ☐ Office Notes

To Be Completed By	☐ Approved	☐ Denied

Comments: _____

This notice is not a guarantee payment will be provided and only approves the medical necessity and appropriateness of the medical services requested and authorized. The determination on payment of claims will be made when the claim is received. The claim will be subject to the terms and limitations of the member's benefit plan, including applicable deductibles and copayments. Additionally, prior authorization will be honored only if the member is a covered member and dues are paid at the time the services are provided. Payment will not be allowed if the member is not covered at the time of service.

Reviewed by: _____ Date: _____

Fig. 7-3 Prior authorization request (Basquez).

A. Log on to the Internet, and using the search words "managed healthcare," locate a website that provides current information regarding new managed healthcare issues. Prepare a 1-page essay or a 3-minute oral presentation entitled "What's New in Managed Healthcare." Your instructor will provide specific guidelines for this activity.

B. Research The Joint Commission website **(http://www.jointcommission.org)** and identify current updates regarding HIPAA compliance standards. At The Joint Commission home page, enter HIPAA in the search box located in the top right corner.

C. Explore the Kaiser Permanente website **(http://www.kaiserpermanente.org).** Note the various informational areas. Click on "a prospective member," choose a region of interest to you, and check out the various plan options.

Performance Objective 7-1—Completing a Preauthorization Form

Conditions: Student will complete a preauthorization/admission form from the information provided on the forms illustrated in Figs. 7-4 and 7-5.

Supplies/Equipment: Pen/typewriter, Envision HMO preauthorization request form (see Fig. 7-4), patient registration data form (see Fig. 7-5), blank preauthorization/admission form (Fig. 7-6).

Time Allowed: 20 minutes

Accuracy Needed to Pass: 90%

Procedural Steps	Points Earned	Comments
Evaluator: Note time began: _____		
1. Carefully read and study the above-named forms, then correctly complete the preauthorization form; 1 point is awarded for each correctly completed blank on the form.		
2. Patient information (3)		
3. Provider information (8)		
4. Physician information (6)		
5. Procedure information (10)		
6. Student used a pen/wrote legibly (3)		
Optional: May deduct points for taking more time than allowed.		

Total Points = 30

Student's Score: _____

Evaluator: _____

Comments: _____

_____

_____

_____

_____

ENVISION HMO

PREAUTHORIZATION REQUEST FORM

PATIENT INFORMATION

Last Name: Scoval First Name: Dorothy M

DOB: 10/16/1961 Member #: 123456789 Group #: 56XXZ

PREAUTHORIZATION REQUEST INFORMATION

Please list *both* procedure/product code and narrative description:

CPT/HCPCS Code(s): 27407 Durable Medical Equipment: ☐ Rental ☐ Purchase

Description: Repair, primary, torn anterior cruciate ligament (Ⓛ Knee) CPT 27407

Date of Service: 12-23-20XX Length of Stay (if applicable): 24-48 hrs

Place of Service or Vendor Name: Broadmoor Medical Center

Assistant Surgeon Requested? ☐ Yes ☒ No Please list *both* diagnosis(es) code and narrative description:

1. ICD-9 Code: 717.83

   Description: Sprain/tear anterior cruciate ligament Ⓛ knee

2. ICD-9 Code: _____

   Description: _____

Ordering Physician/Provider: John Langley, MD Office Location: Suite 416 So. Vine
FIRST *AND* LAST NAMES PLEASE
SSS-988-6604

Referring Physician/Provider: Francis Tompkins, MD Milton, XY 12345.
FIRST *AND* LAST NAMES PLEASE; REQUIRED FOR PRIME PLANS FAX SSS-987-6540

Date: 11-14-20XX Contact Person: Celia Reeves Phone: SSS-987-6543

> ### *Please note: Incomplete forms will delay the preauthorization process.*
> **Requests received after 3:00 PM are processed the next working day.**
>
> PacificSource responds to preauthorization requests within 2 working days.
> A determination notice will be mailed to the requesting provider, facility, and patient.
>
> Please attach pertinent chart notes as appropriate.

FOR INTERNAL OFFICE USE ONLY:

STATUS: APPROVED / DENIED / PENDING / EXPLANATION ENVISION Phone No.

DATE: 11-15-20XX ACUITY: UKN INITIALS: JIB 800-223-0000

Reason/Status R Code S6 S Code 114 Px Auth #004X39SRM

Hosp Auth #HSP003111

Field 11 Notes See pt record LOS Approved F.W. Samules

☑ Chart notes filed with preauthorization

Notes Authorization numbers expire after 60 days

Field 10 Facility Copy 416 Suite 9 Bldg 4

Fig. 7-4 Preauthorization request form (Scoval).

Registration Data

1. Your Name __Scoval Dorothy M__   Sex ☐ Male   Date of Birth __10/16/1961__
   (Last)   (First)   (Middle)   ☒ Female
2. Social Security #: __123-45-6789__   Marital Status: (S) M D Se W
3. Address: __320 Pine Grove__   4. __SSS-342-1110__
   (Street)   (Phone)
   __Milton   XY   12345__
   (City)   (State)   (Zip)
5. Employer: __Kemper Engineering Inc__   Occupation: __Eng. Asst.__
   Employer Address: __63 Highway 6West__   __SSS-342-6780__
   (Work Phone)
   Spouse: _____   Employer: _____   Occupation: _____
   Employer Address: _____   (Work Phone)

6.
Other Household Members	Date of Birth	Relationship
	/ /	
	/ /	
	/ /	
	/ /	
	/ /	

7. Medical Insurance Information

	Ins. Company Name	Policy No.	Policy Holder	Sgl.	Fmly.	Primary	Sec.
( )	Envision HMO	123456789	Self	☒	☐	☐	☐
( )				☐	☐	☐	☐
( )				☐	☐	☐	☐

(Type of Coverage)

8. Person to Contact in an Emergency __Henry Barton__ Relationship to you __brother__
   Their Work Phone _____ Their Home Phone __SSS-342-1177__

9. Party with primary responsibility for payment: ☒ Self ☐ Other
   Name _____   Relationship to you _____
   Address _____   Home Phone _____

For Office Use Only

Date Completed _____   Account No. _____   Patient No. _____

Household Status ☐ Head of Household

☐ Spouse   ☐ Child   ☐ Other: _____

Head of Household Name _____

Fig. 7-5 Registration data sheet (Scoval).

Chapter **7** Unraveling the Mysteries of Managed Care

PREAUTHORIZATION/ADMISSION FORM

Orders must be faxed to appropriate department. History and Physicals are required on all invasive procedures with conscious sedation. **If you have any questions, please call 555-992-XXXX.**

PATIENT INFORMATION

Patient Name: _____ SSN: _____ DOB: _____

PROVIDER INFORMATION

Policy Holder's Name: _____ SSN: _____

Policy Holder's Employer: _____ Employer's Phone Number: _____

Name of Health Plan: _____ Health Plan Phone Number: _____

Policy/ID#: _____ Group #: _____

PHYSICIAN INFORMATION

Physician Contact Person: _____ Coordinator's Phone Number: _____

Fax Number: _____ Primary Care Physician: _____

Requesting Physician: _____ Requesting Physician's Phone Number: _____

PROCEDURE INFORMATION

Procedure: _____ CPT Code: _____

Diagnosis: _____

Department(s) Involved *(Please check all appropriate areas.)*

OR_____ GI _____ RAD _____ Cath _____ CP _____ Women's Center_____ Day Surgery _____

Date of Procedure: _____ Authorized by: _____

Physician's Authorization Number: _____ Expiration Date: _____

Hospital Authorization Number: _____ Expiration Date: _____

Inpatient: _____ Outpatient: _____ Approximate Length of Stay: _____

Comments: _____

_____

_____

Fig. 7-6 Preauthorization/admission form (Scoval).

Performance Objective 7-2—Completing a Precertification Form

Conditions: Student will complete a precertification form (Fig. 7-7) for the upper gastrointestinal series from the information provided in the case study in Fig. 7-8. This is an outpatient procedure (length of stay is less than 24 hours). H & P and laboratory reports are to be attachments submitted with the precertification form. (*Note:* Student will be the "office contact person.")

Supplies/Equipment: Pen, Envision HMO precertification request form (see Fig. 7-7), case study (see Fig. 7-8)

Time Allowed: 20 minutes

Accuracy Needed to Pass: 90%

Procedural Steps	Points Earned	Comments
Evaluator: Note time began: _____		
1. Carefully read and study the information provided, then complete the precertification form; 1 point is awarded for each correctly completed blank on the form.		
2. Patient information (7)		
3. Hospital information (3)		
4. Physician information (4)		
5. Procedure information (8)		
6. Diagnostic information (3)		
7. Student used a pen/wrote legibly (3)		
Optional: May deduct points for taking more time than allowed.		

Total Points = 28

Student's Score: _____

Evaluator: _____

Comments: _____

_____

_____

_____

_____

ENVISION HMO

REQUEST FOR INITIAL PRECERTIFICATION REVIEW
PHONE: 555-992-XXXX/FAX: 555-992-XXXX

Date: _____   Outpatient _____   Inpatient _____

Patient's Name _____ Member # _____ Group # _____

Patient's Address _____ DOB _____

Hospital Name _____ Phone # _____

Hospital Address _____

Physician Name _____ Phone # _____

Physician Address _____

Office Contact Person _____

Admission Date _____ Anticipated Length of Stay _____

Admitting DX/ICD-9 Code _____

Surgery/CPT Code _____ Date of Surgery _____

Related HX/Current Signs/Symptoms _____

_____

_____

_____

_____

Lab Findings _____

X-Ray/Diagnostic Findings _____

Current Medications/Freq. _____

Plan of Treatment: _____

_____

_____

FOR ENVISION USE ONLY: Date Received _____ by (initials) Date Referred for Review _____

Rev. Initials _____ Reference ID # _____ Date of PX Notification _____ Office Contact _____

Fig. 7-7 Request for initial precertification review (Oliver).

Case Study: Before performing certain diagnostic tests, it is customary to contact the patient's insurance carrier to make sure the procedure/service will be covered under his or her policy. This is referred to as *precertification*, which differs from preauthorization. This case study involves notifying the patient's insurance carrier of a planned diagnostic procedure.

Date: 4/19/20XX

Patient Name: Justin C. Oliver   DOB: 7/22/67   Record # OL72267
                916 No. Court   SS # 666-77-8888
                Milton, XY 12345

Patient is in the office today with continuing complaints of severe heartburn. He has been seen in the office by me on several occasions prior to this for treatment of GERD. He is currently on Naprosyn 500 mg BID with food PRN and Prevacid 15 mg one daily. He was advised on his last visit that if his stomach keeps bothering him with this heartburn, we may need to do a UGI or other testing. He is back in the office today requesting this procedure. He will be going to Envision Laboratory tomorrow for a CBC, CMP, lipid panel, and possibly a TSH. We will request a UGI to be performed at Broadmoor Medical Center on 4/22 and will see him back in 1 week.

Diagnosis: GERD 530.81   CPT Code for Upper Gastrointestinal (UGI) Series 91032

(s) Dennis R. Mulligan, MD   Broadmoor Medical Center
4353 Pine Ridge Drive, Suite 233   4500 Pine Ridge Drive
Milton, XY 12345   Milton, XY 12345
                                           Phone: 555-876-5433
                                           Fax: 555-876-5400

ENVISION HMO

Justin C. Oliver   **07/22/1967**   For Inpatient Preauthorization
Name   Date of Birth   Telephone: 800-223-0000
123654998   01/17/2000   92LMQ   FAX   555-445-5555
Member No.   Effective Date   Grp Code
Dennis R. Mulligan, MD   555-544-6601
Primary Care Physician   Telephone No.
GHJKL   Copays   Office Visit $5
Pharmacy Code   ER/Outpatient $10
                                  Inpatient $15

Fig. 7-8 Case study (Oliver).

Chapter **7   Unraveling the Mysteries of Managed Care**

Generate a Document for a Nonroutine HMO Patient

Morris Bennett comes to Broadmoor Medical Clinic, where you are employed as a health insurance professional, complaining of severe pain in the right lower quadrant accompanied by cramping, mild fever, and constipation of 4 days' duration. Morris is employed by John Deere Health, an HMO in Illinois, and became ill while visiting relatives over the Thanksgiving holiday in the city where your office is located. You contact his insurance carrier, and they fax Mr. Bennett the following instruction sheet for claims purposes:

If you need to pay for care because of an emergency or urgent (nonroutine) situation when traveling outside of our network, or on vacation, send an itemized bill including the following information:

1. Member's name and member ID
2. Date of service or supplies provided
3. State or country in which services were rendered or supplies obtained
4. Description of services/supplies
5. The provider's name, address, and tax identification number
6. An interpretation of the claim, if in a foreign language (any information provided will assist in making the proper payment determination and prevent delays)
7. Accident details (if applicable)

The chart notes indicate that Mr. Bennett has been under the care of Dr. Edgar Billingham for treatment of diverticulosis for quite some time. Today, he was prescribed ampicillin, 500 mg TID #30 and was instructed to drink only clear fluids for 2 to 3 days for bowel rest. He was given instructions regarding prevention and control of this disorder and told to see his family physician on returning home.

The claim address is: John Deere Health, 4000 16th Avenue, Moline, XY, 61265

Include patient name, patient ID, and a daytime phone number where the patient can be reached. Payment is subject to the terms and conditions of the Plan Administrator's benefit plan.

From the information on Mr. Bennett's registration and encounter forms (Figs. 7-9 and 7-10), (1) generate an itemized bill (using the blank ledger card in Fig. 7-11), and (2) compose a brief explanatory cover letter to accompany the bill.

Registration Data

1. Your Name **Bennett Morris T.**   Sex ☒ Male   Date of Birth **10-21-46**
   (Last)   (First)   (Middle)   ☐ Female
2. Social Security #: **333-44-SSSS**   Marital Status: S ⓜ D Se W
3. Address: **2900 Sunnylawn**   4. **SSS-343-2222**
   (Street)   (Phone)
   Moline   **IL**   **SSS66**
   (City)   (State)   (Zip)
5. Employer: **John Deere Enterprises**   Occupation: **Inspector**

   Employer Address: **4910 John Deere Blvd. Moline, IL SSS66**   **SSS-343-8762**
   (Work Phone)
   Spouse: **Frieda**   Employer: **N/A**   Occupation: **Housewife**

   Employer Address: _____   _____
   (Work Phone)

6.

Other Household Members	Date of Birth	Relationship
	/ /	
	/ /	
	/ /	
	/ /	

7. Medical Insurance Information

Ins. Company Name	Policy No.	Policy Holder	Sgl.	Fmly.	Primary	Sec.
John Deere Health	333XLM	Morris Bennett	☐	☒	☐	☐
			☐	☐	☐	☐
			☐	☐	☐	☐

Type of Coverage

8. Person to Contact in an Emergency **Frieda Bennett** Relationship to you **spouse**
   Their Work Phone _____   Their Home Phone **SSS-343-2229**

9. Party with primary responsibility for payment: ☒ Self ☐ Other

   Name _____   Relationship to you _____
   Address _____   Home Phone _____

For Office Use Only

Date Completed _____   Account No. _____   Patient No. _____

Household Status ☐ Head of Household

☐ Spouse ☐ Child ☐ Other: _____

Head of Household Name _____

Fig. 7-9 Registration data sheet (Bennett).

Chapter **7 Unraveling the Mysteries of Managed Care**

BROADMOOR MEDICAL CLINIC

ACCT. #: 32100	DATE OF SERVICE: 11-26-20XX	CATEGORY: GA	DIAGNOSIS: diverticulitis
PATIENT'S NAME: Morris T. Bennett			Rec #11336

CPT	✔	DESCRIPTION	FEE	CPT	✔	DESCRIPTION	FEE	CPT	✔	DESCRIPTION	FEE
OFFICEVISIT - NEW PATIENT				**IMMUNIZATIONS**				**INJECTIONS (CONT'D.)**			
99201		Focused		90701		DtaP		J3410		Vistaril	
99202		Expanded		90632		Hep A (Adult)		J3420		Vitamin B12	
99203	✔	Detailed	185 00	90633		Hep A (Ped)		J2000		Xylocaine	
99204		Comprehensive		90744		Hep B (Ped)		**PROCEDURES**			
99205		Complex		90746		Hep B (Adult)		46600		Anoscopy	
OFFICEVISIT - ESTABLISHED PATIENT				90737		Hib		92551		Audio Screening	
99211		Minimal		90657		Influenza		11730		Avulsion Nail, Partial or	
99212		Focused		90707		MMR				Complete, Single	
99213		Expanded		90732		Pneumococcal		11200		Rem. of Skin Tags up to 15	
99214		Detailed		90718		Td		11201		Each Additional 10	
99215		Comprehensive		90703		Tetanus Toxoid		10060		I & D Simple Abscess	
				90716		Varicella		10120		Removal FB Skin	
PHYSICAL EXAM - NEW PATIENT								11740		I & D Subung. Hematoma	
99381		Age Under 1 Year		**INJECTIONS**				58310		IUD Removal	
99382		Age 1 - 4 Years		J1200		Benadryl up to 50 mg		94010		Spirometry	
99383		Age 5 - 11 Years		J0540		Bicillin up to 1,200,000 mg		A4570		Splint	
99384		Age 12 - 17 Years		J0690		Cefazolin Sodium 250 mg		99173		Vision Screening	
99385		Age 18 - 39 Years		J0704		Celestone		**LABORATORY**			
99386		Age 40 - 64 Years		J0780		Compazine		82270	✔	Blood Occult	30 00
99387		Age 65+ Years		J1100		Decadron		85680		TB Intradermal	
				J0970		Delestrogen		81000	✔	Urine Dip Stick	15 00
PHYSICAL EXAM - ESTABLISHED PATIENT				J1050		Depo Provera		84703		Serum Pregnancy Test	
99391		Age Under 1 Year		J1510		Gamma Globulin		87082		Strep Screen	
99392		Age 1 - 4 Years		J3301		Kenalog					
99393		Age 5 - 11 Years		J1940		Kasix		36415	✔	Venipuncture	25 00
99394		Age 12 - 17 Years		J2550		Phenergan		99000	✔	Handling	10 00
99395		Age 18 - 39 Years		J3490		Rocephin					
99396		Age 40 - 64 Years		J1070		Testosterone		**MISCELLANEOUS**			
99397		Age 65+ Years		J3250		Tigan					
				J1885		Torodol					

ICD-9 ☐ **DIAGNOSIS**
CARDIOLOGY
794.31 ☐ Abn Ekg
786.50 ☐ Chest Pain, Nos
780.4 ☐ Dizziness And Giddiness
787.1 ☐ Heartburn
272.0 ☐ Hypercholesterolem
272.4 ☐ Hyperlipidemia Nec/Nos
401.1 ☐ Hypertension Benign
401.9 ☐ Hypertension Nos
401.0 ☐ Hypertension, Malig.
785.1 ☐ Palpitations
ENDOCRINE
250.01 ☐ IDDM Controlled
250.03 ☐ IDDM Uncontrolled
250.02 ☐ NIDDM Uncontrolled
250.00 ☐ NIDDM Controlled
251.2 ☐ Hypoglycemia
244.9 ☐ Hypothyroidism
242.90 ☐ Hyperthyroidism
EAR, NOSE, THROAT
386.30 ☐ Labyrinthitis Nos
382.9 ☐ Otitis Media, Ac./Chr.
462. ☐ Pharyngitis Acute
477.9 ☐ Rhinitis, Allergic
461.9 ☐ Sinusitis, Ac Nos
473.9 ☐ Sinusitis, Chronic
528.0 ☐ Stomatitis
034.0 ☐ Strep Throat

388.30 ☐ Tinnitus Nos
463. ☐ Tonsillitis, Acute
474.0 ☐ Tonsillitis, Chronic
FEMALE / GYNECOLOGY
795.0 ☐ Abn Pap Smear-Cervix
793.8 ☐ Abn Findings-Breast
626.0 ☐ Amenorrhea
611.72 ☐ Breast Mass/Lump
616.0 ☐ Cervicitis
V25.09 ☐ Contracept. Mgmt.
625.3 ☐ Dysmenorrhea
626.4 ☐ Menstruation, Irreg.
625.2 ☐ Menstruation, Excessive
614.9 ☐ Pelvic Inflam Dis
V22.2 ☐ Preg State, Incidental
616.10 ☐ Vaginitis
PHYSICAL EXAM
V20.1 ☐ Well Child
V72.84 ☐ Pre-Op Exam
GASTRO-INTESTINAL
789.06 ☐ Abnormal Pain, Epigastric
794.3 ☐ Abn. Liver Function Study
578.1 ☐ Blood in Stool
564.0 ☐ Constipation
787.91 ☐ Diarrhea
562.11 ☒ Diverticulitis
530.81 ☐ Esophageal Reflux
535.5 ☐ Gastritis/Duodenitis Nos
455.6 ☐ Hemorrhoids

787.0 ☐ Nausea And Vomiting
533.90 ☐ Peptic Ulcer Nos
569.3 ☐ Rectal Bleeding
GENITO-URINARY
585. ☐ Chronic Renal Failure
595.0 ☐ Cystitis Acute
788.1 ☐ Dysuria
599.7 ☐ Hematuria
601.0 ☐ Prostatitis Acute
599.0 ☐ UTI
HEMATOLOGY
790.6 ☐ Abn Blood Chemistry Nec
285.9 ☐ Anemia Nos
280.1 ☐ Anemia, Iron Def
INFECTIOUS
616.3 ☐ Abcess: Bartholin Gland
682.9 ☐ Abcess: Skin
780.6 ☐ Fever: Unkn. Origin
IMMUNOLOGY - ALLERGIES
995.3 ☐ Allergic Reaction Nos
477.0 ☐ Allergy, Hay Fever
042. ☐ Human ImmunoVirus Dis.
ORTHOPEDICS
716.90 ☐ Arthritis Unspec.
724.5 ☐ Backache Nos
727.3 ☐ Bursitis Nec
354.0 ☐ Carpal Tunnel Syndrome
719.40 ☐ Joint Pain-Unspec.
729.1 ☐ Myalgia And Myositis Nos.

733.00 ☐ Osteoporosis
845.00 ☐ Sprain: Ankle
847.2 ☐ Sprain: Back
847.0 ☐ Sprain: Cervical
840.9 ☐ Sprain: Shoulder
729.81 ☐ Swelling of Limb
726.00 ☐ Tendonitis
NEUROLOGY
784.0 ☐ Headache
346.9 ☐ Migraine Nos
724.3 ☐ Sciatica
307.81 ☐ Tension Headache
780.4 ☐ Vertigo
OPHTHALMOLOGY
373.00 ☐ Blepharitis Nos
372.30 ☐ Conjunctivitis
918.1 ☐ Corneal Abrasion
PULMONARY / RESPIRATORY
493.9 ☐ Asthma Nos
466.0 ☐ Bronchitis Acute
490. ☐ Bronchitis Nos
486. ☐ Pneumonia
786.2 ☐ Cough
786.0 ☐ Dyspnea/Resp Abn
487. ☐ Influenza
786.52 ☐ Painful Respiration
786.09 ☐ S O B
465.9 ☐ URI
079.9 ☐ Viral Syndrome

PSYCH / MENTAL HEALTH
303.9 ☐ Alcoholism
300.00 ☐ Anxiety State Nos
300.00 ☐ Depression
SKIN / DERMATOLOGIC
706.1 ☐ Acne Nec
691. ☐ Dermatitis, Atopic
692. ☐ Dermatitis, Contact
110.1 ☐ Dermatophytosis, Nail
691.0 ☐ Diaper Rash
054.9 ☐ Herpes Simplex Nos
053.9 ☐ Herpes Zoster Nos
054.19 ☐ Herpes Genital Nec
684. ☐ Impetigo
703.0 ☐ Ingrowing Nail
215.9 ☐ Nevus
110.1 ☐ Onychomycosis
696.1 ☐ Psoriasis
706.2 ☐ Sebaceous Cyst
708.8 ☐ Urticaria Nec
078.1 ☐ Warts, Viral
OTHER - MISC.
780.7 ☐ Malaise and Fatigue
780.2 ☐ Syncope
WRITE - IN

INSTRUCTIONS: Make appt w/PCP upon returning home	RETURN APPOINTMENT: ___ Days ___ Weeks ___ Months ___ PRN ___ 15 ___ 30 ___ 45	PAID ☒ CASH ☐ CHECK ☐ CR. CD.	PREV. BAL. — 0 —
			TODAY'S FEE 265 00
			AMT. REC'D. 5.00

Fig. 7-10 Encounter form (Bennett).

		STATEMENT		Spouse: Frieda

Insurance:
John Deere Health HMO
ID# 333XLM
DOB: 10/21/1946
A/C#32100

STATEMENT

BROADMOOR MEDICAL CLINIC
4353 Pine Ridge Drive
Milton, XY 12345-0001
Telephone: 555-656-7890

Spouse: Frieda

MORRIS T. BENNETT
2900 SUNNYLAWN
MOLINE, IL 55566

DATE 20XX	PROFESSIONAL SERVICE DESCRIPTION	CHARGE	CREDITS		CURRENT BALANCE
			PAYMENTS	ADJUSTMENTS	

Due and payable within 10 days.   Pay last amount in balance column ⇧

Fig. 7-11 Ledger card (Bennett).

Health Insurance Professional's Notebook

Continue construction of your notebook. In Chapter 7, you might want to include the following:

- A brief description of each of the HMO models
- An explanation of how HMOs in your area handle claims
- A description of how PPOs differ from HMOs
- A list of the PPOs in your area along with guidelines for completing CMS-1500 forms
- Examples of HMO and PPO cards with explanations of what each entry means (see Fig. 7-11)
- Examples of common forms used with managed care plans:
  - Preauthorization
  - Precertification
  - Referral
  - Request for consultation
  - Preadmission

ENRICHMENT ACTIVITIES

A. Contact an HMO or other managed care plan health insurance professional in your area. Interview the health insurance professional to determine (1) what benefits are offered and (2) how claims are handled. Request information brochures or fact sheets.

B. Visit a local medical facility that is a member of an HMO or other managed care plan. Interview the health insurance professional there to determine the differences in handling managed care cases compared with cases with traditional insurance. Request copies of any applicable office brochures and preauthorization/referral forms.

C. Generate a bulletin board collage of the various brochures, fact sheets, and forms you acquired from A and B.

Chapter Check List

Student name: _____

Chapter completion date: _____

1.	Record	Your start time and date: _____
2.	Read	The assigned chapter in the text
3.	View	PowerPoint slides (if available)
4.	Complete	Exercises in the Workbook as assigned
5.	Compare	Your answers to the answers posted on the bulletin board/website/handout
6.	Correct	Your answers
7.	Complete	All tests and required activities
8.	Read	Assigned readings (if any)
9.	Complete	Chapter performance objectives (competencies), if any
10.	Evaluate	Chapter performance, and submit to your instructor
11.	Record	Your ending time and date: _____
12.	Move on	Begin next chapter as assigned

Student name: _____

Chapter completion date: _____

Evaluate your classroom performance. Complete the self-evaluation, and submit it to your instructor. When your instructor returns this form to you, compare your self-evaluation with the evaluation completed by your instructor.

Skill	Student Self-Evaluation			Instructor Evaluation		
	Good	Average	Poor	Good	Average	Poor
Attendance/punctuality						
Personal appearance						
Applies effort						
Is self-motivated						
Is courteous						
Has positive attitude						
Completes assignments in timely manner						
Works well with others						

Student's Initials: _____

Date: _____

Points Possible: _____

Points Awarded: _____

Chapter Grade: _____

Instructor's Initials: _____

Date: _____

8 Understanding Medicaid

We learned in the textbook that Medicaid is a medical assistance program jointly financed by state and federal governments for low-income, blind, or disabled individuals. It was first enacted in 1965 as an amendment to the Social Security Act of 1935. Today, Medicaid is a major social welfare program and is administered by the Centers for Medicare and Medicaid Services (CMS) under the direction of the Department of Health and Human Services.

The student workbook presents activities and work assignments to familiarize students with the structure of Medicaid and important issues and functions involved with the healthcare of Medicaid recipients. Because Medicaid health benefits differ from state to state, it is difficult to generate exercises that represent all states. The author uses a fictitious state—Xtra (XT)—and applies some of the more general rules to this state. It is important, however, for health insurance professionals to keep in mind that benefits, forms, and claims completion guidelines used herein are generic. On-the-job health insurance professionals should become familiar with the actual Medicaid guidelines in their area.

WORKBOOK CHAPTER OBJECTIVES

After completing the workbook activities for Chapter 8, the student should be able to:
- Define the terms used in the chapter.
- Answer the review questions to within the evaluation criteria set by the instructor.
- Demonstrate the ability to think logically and draw conclusions from facts and evidence.
- Explore websites to acquire information needed to complete workbook activities.
- Abstract applicable information from healthcare documents necessary for completion of various forms used in Medicaid claims.
- Complete specific forms common to the health insurance professional's role in Medicaid claims.
- Generate information and collect documents for inclusion in the student's personal Health Insurance Professional's Notebook relative to Medicaid.
- Undertake self-analysis/evaluation in completed workbook activities.

DEFINING CHAPTER TERMS

Using the computer (or typewriter), students should key an accurate definition for each of the chapter terms listed. These definitions should be in the students' own words. When finished, students should compare their definitions with those listed in the glossary at the back of the textbook, correcting any inaccuracies.

balance billing
budget period
categorically needy
comprehensive
cost avoid(ance)
cost sharing
countable income
disproportionate share hospitals
dual coverage (Medi-Medi)
dual eligibles
Early and Periodic Screening, Diagnosis, and Treatment (EPSDT) program
federal poverty level (FPL)
fiscal intermediary (FI) (fiscal agent)
mandated services
Medicaid
Medicaid "simple" claim
medically necessary
medically needy
Medicare hospital insurance (Medicare HI)

Medicare-Medicaid crossover claims
optional services
pay-or-chase claims
payer of last resort
Program of All-Inclusive Care for the Elderly (PACE)
Qualified Disabled and Working Individuals
Qualified Medicare Beneficiaries
reciprocity
remittance advice (RA)
Specified Low-Income Medicare Beneficiaries
spend down
State Children's Health Insurance Program (SCHIP)
Supplemental Security Income (SSI)
supplementary medical insurance (SMI)
Temporary Assistance for Needy Families (TANF)
third-party liability

125

Multiple Choice

Directions: In the questions/statements presented, choose the response that **best** answers/completes the stem and circle the letter that precedes it.

1. Title XIX of the Social Security Act of 1965 established:
   a. Social Security benefits to people older than 65
   b. Workers' compensation
   c. Medicare
   d. Medicaid

2. Medicaid is administered by:
   a. Congress
   b. CMS
   c. The Social Security Administration
   d. The Federal Insurance Advisory Board

3. Supplemental Security Income (SSI) is a cash benefit program controlled by:
   a. The Social Security Administration
   b. CMS
   c. Individual state governments
   d. The Federal Insurance Advisory Board

4. Categorically needy individuals typically include:
   a. Low-income families with children
   b. Individuals receiving SSI
   c. Pregnant women, infants, and children with incomes less than a specified percent of the federal poverty level (FPL)
   d. Qualified Medicare Beneficiaries (QMBs)
   e. All of the above

5. The term used for the process of depleting private or family finances to the point where the individual/family becomes eligible for Medicaid assistance is:
   a. Cataloging
   b. Spend down
   c. Asset reduction
   d. Diminution

6. The program that provides comprehensive alternative care for noninstitutionalized elderly who otherwise would be in a nursing home is known as:
   a. SSI
   b. Social Security Disability Insurance
   c. Program of All-Inclusive Care for the Elderly
   d. Long-term care

7. Medicaid coverage should be verified:
   a. Every time a patient comes to the office
   b. No less than once a month
   c. At least annually
   d. Biannually

8. Aged or disabled individuals who are very poor are covered under the Medicaid and Medicare programs, which are commonly referred to as:

   a. Dual eligibles

   b. Medi-Medi

   c. Supplemental coverage

   d. a and b

9. Medicare beneficiaries who qualify for certain Medicaid benefits if they have incomes below the FPL and resources at or below twice the standard allowed under the SSI program are known as:

   a. QDWIs

   b. QMBs

   c. SLMBs

   d. SMIs

10. When one state allows Medicaid beneficiaries from other states to be treated in its medical facilities, this exchange of privileges is referred to as:

   a. Reciprocity

   b. Medi-Medi

   c. Coinsurance

   d. Dual coverage

True/False

Directions: Place a "T" on the blank preceding the statement if it is true; place an "F" if the statement is false.

_____ 1.   Medicaid benefits are the same from state to state.

_____ 2.   All states have a Medicaid program.

_____ 3.   In 1972, federal law established the SSI program, which provides federally funded cash assistance to unmarried pregnant women with dependent children.

_____ 4.   To be eligible for SSI, an individual must be at least 65 years old, blind, or disabled, and have limited resources.

_____ 5.   Eligibility for SSI benefits is based on an individual's employment record.

_____ 6.   All states must cover the cost of prescription drugs for all categories of Medicaid recipients.

_____ 7.   All providers must accept and treat all categories of Medicaid patients.

_____ 8.   Providers must agree to accept what Medicaid pays as payment in full for covered services and are prohibited by law to "balance bill."

_____ 9.   Medicaid, by law, is intended to be the "payer of last resort."

_____ 10. The time limit for filing Medicaid claims in all states is 1 year.

_____ 11. Providers are never allowed to ask a Medicaid-eligible patient to make a copayment.

_____ 12. Assignment should be accepted on all Medicaid claims.

Short Answer/Fill-in-the-Blank

Directions: Read the statements, and then using the textbook for review, insert the correct word or words that complete the sentence or answer the question.

1. Medicaid originally was created to give _____ access to healthcare.

2. The Medicaid program, formerly referred to as Aid to Families with Dependent Children, is now called _____

   _____ in many states.

3. Under Medicaid guidelines, families, pregnant women, and children fall under the _____ classification.

4. Persons receiving institutional or other long-term care in nursing and intermediate care facilities fall under the

   _____ classification.

5. _____ classification includes low-income individuals who lose employer healthcare coverage.

6. List the services that categorically needy individuals must be provided with according to federal standards.

   _____

   _____

   _____

7. List some of the optional coverage that individual states can provide.

   _____

   _____

   _____

8. Define and explain the function of a fiscal intermediary (FI).

   _____

9. List common responsibilities of an FI.

   _____

   _____

   _____

10. List the federally mandated services specified in law that Medicaid must cover.

_____

_____

_____

_____

_____

11. List four optional services commonly covered by states to their categorically needy population not provided to other groups.

_____

_____

_____

_____

_____

_____

12. Explain the basic differences between Medicare and Medicaid.

_____

_____

_____

_____

_____

13. List four examples of third-party liability.

_____

_____

_____

_____

A. Explain the difference between "categorically needy" and "medically needy," and give examples of individuals who fall into each group.

B. You are a health insurance professional employed by Generic Family Practice. On September 7, 20XX, Emily Carson brought her 4-year-old son, Cory, to the office. Cory, complaining of ear pain and a sore throat, is new to the practice. Ms. Carson, a single mother, states that she and Cory are on Medicaid. After greeting Ms. Carson, what is the first thing you should do?

C. Brice Samuels, a 9-year-old girl, comes to Generic Family Practice on a monthly basis for follow-up treatment for a severe case of asthma. Gina Peters, a temp who is filling in for you during an absence, notes that Brice was eligible for Medicaid every month for the last 2 years. Assuming that Brice also is eligible for Medicaid benefits on this visit, Gina neglects to verify current eligibility.

   1. What, if any, possible problems could result from Gina's failure to follow proper procedures?
   2. If Brice's visits have been covered by Medicaid for the past 2 years, what possible reasons might there be for Medicaid to discontinue benefits?

D. Lamont Frasier, the senior physician at Generic Family Practice and a Medicaid participating provider, tells you that because he is getting close to retirement, he does not want you to accept any more Medicaid patients. "I have a total of 50 Medicaid patients, and that's enough," he tells you. What might be an appropriate response to Dr. Frazier's statement?

E. Dr. Frasier has several patients (age 65 or older) that he sees periodically at the Sunshine Nursing Home. You do not see these patients, but you are responsible for the billing. Two of them are on Medicaid. How do you process Dr. Frasier's fees for these two Medicaid patients?

F. Dr. Alexandra Parsons, a psychiatrist, charges $250 for 1 hour of psychotherapy and $175 for a 30-minute session. She knows that Medicaid's allowable charge is $200 and $150, so she cuts the time she spends with her patients accordingly. When she counsels Wayne Gerber, she spends 40 minutes with him and charges Medicaid the full hour. She sees Tabitha Enrich for 20 minutes and charges Medicaid for the full 30 minutes. Dr. Parsons rationalizes that, by doing this, she does not lose so much money and really does not cheat the patient. You are Dr. Parsons' health insurance professional. Is this fraud? If so, what should you do?

A. Beverly Franklin was driving her 8-year-old daughter Suzie to school on a foggy morning in April when her car was rear-ended by Tim Wright, father of another third-grade student. Suzie, suffering from cuts and bruises and complaining of neck pain, was brought to the SunnyDay Medical Clinic where you are employed as a health insurance professional. You verify that Suzie is eligible for Medicaid for the month of April, and after the encounter, you submit a claim to Medicaid.

1. Create a template for a Medicaid "simple" claim form by shading out all blocks that do not require completion. Use one of the blank universal CMS-1500 forms, provided in the back of the workbook, for this activity.

2. Using the top half of a blank CMS-1500 form, enter the correct information in all required blocks to generate a claim for Suzie Franklin. Use the information on the Medicaid ID card in Fig. 8-1.

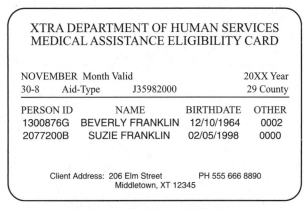

Fig. 8-1 Medicaid ID card (Franklin).

B. A week after you submit the claim for Suzie Franklin, Medicaid denies the claim. Answer the following questions for clarification and understanding of why Medicaid denied the claim.

1. In a situation such as this, why did Medicaid deny the claim, and what is the technical term for Medicaid's denial?
2. Who carries primary liability in this case?
3. What are your options for getting the claim paid?
4. If your state's policy allows Medicaid to "pay-and-chase," how would this affect payment of this claim?

C. Study the sample Medical Assistance ID card in Fig. 8-2 and its accompanying key in Fig. 8-3. Then answer the following questions (answers can be keyed on a computer or typewriter and printed out):

1. What are the name and address of the client, head of household, or guardian?
2. What are the dates of eligibility?
3. How can you determine if this client is on Medicare?
4. What is the client's birth date?
5. Is this individual a client of the Division of Developmental Disabilities?
6. Is this individual covered under a private insurance plan?
7. Is this client restricted to one provider?
8. How would you know if this client has elected hospice care?
9. What do the alpha characters "CNP" indicate?

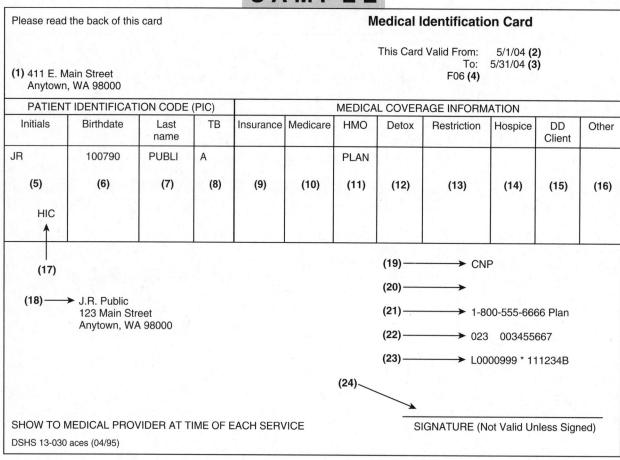

Fig. 8-2 Sample medical assistance ID card.

Key to Medical Assistance ID Card

Top Portion of the MAID Card:

1. Address of CSO
2. Date eligibility begins
3. Date eligibility ends
4. Medical coverage group

Patient Identification Code (PIC) Includes:

5. First and middle initials (or a dash [-] if the middle initial is not known)
6. Six-digit birth date, consisting of numerals only (MMDDYY)
7. First five letters of the last name (and spaces if the name is fewer than five letters)
8. Tie breaker (an alpha or numeric character)

Medical Coverage Information:

9. **Insurance carrier code:** A four-character alphanumeric code (insurance carrier code) in this area indicates the private insurance plan information
10. **Medicare:** An X indicates the Client has Medicare coverage
11. **HMO** (health maintenance organization): Alpha code indicates enrollment in an MAA Healthy Options managed healthcare plan. **Managed healthcare plan is the same as HMO.** This area may also contain the alpha code PCCM (Primary Care Case Manager)
12. **Detox:** An X indicates eligibility for a 3-day alcohol or a 5-day drug detoxification program
13. **Restriction:** An X indicates the Client is assigned to one Provider and one pharmacist. The words "Client on review" in Field 20 will also indicate restricted Clients
14. **Hospice:** An X indicates the Client has elected hospice care
15. **DD Client:** An X indicates this person is a Client of the Division of Developmental Disabilities
16. **Other:** This area is not currently in use

Lower Portion of the MAID Card:

17. Alpha Code HIC indicates the Client is on Medicare
18. Indicates name and address of Client, head of household, or guardian
19. Indicates medical program and scope of care indicators
20. Space reserved for other messages (e.g., Client on review, delayed certification, emergency hospital only)
21. Indicates phone number and name of PCCM or Healthy Options plan
22. Indicates local field office (3 digits) and ACES assistance unit number (9 digits)
23. Internal control numbers for MAA use only
24. Client's signature may be used to verify identity of Client

Fig. 8-3 Key to medical assistance ID card.

PROJECTS/DISCUSSION TOPICS

A. The textbook discussed the terms "cost avoid" and "pay-and-chase." These terms may be foreign to most health insurance students and may need further explanation for a better understanding. Research the meaning of these terms, and prepare for an in-class discussion. Have examples to illustrate their meaning ready for presentation. *Note:* See the article, "States struggle to recover Medicaid pharmacy payments from third parties," *Healthcare Financial Management*, October 2001 (**http://www.findarticles.com**).

B. Another term that may cause confusion is "adjudicated." Prepare a clear and concise explanation of this term as it pertains to health insurance claims. Compare your definition with others in the class. With the help of your classmates, choose the five definitions you think are best. From this list, generate one final, all-inclusive definition.

C. Determine the **statute of limitations** regarding the retention of copies of Medicaid claims in your state by logging onto your state Medicaid website, contacting your local Medicaid FI, or telephoning a medical facility in your area that provides services to Medicaid-eligible patients.

D. Fig. 8-4 shows a sample Medicaid ID card for the state of Utah. Study it and be prepared for an in-class discussion regarding what information can be gathered from this document.

1. Dates of Medicaid eligibility
2. Types of services covered
3. *Health Maintenance Organization indicator
4. Third Party Liability (insurance) indicator
5. Client name
6. Medicaid Identification Number
7. Sex is M or F: male/female
8. Date of birth
9. Age
10. *Medical Provider: HMO or Primary Care Provider
11. **Pharmacy provider
12. **Dental care provider
13. *Mental health services provider
14. Copayment/co-insurance indicators for certain types of services
15. TPL information
16. Additional Medicaid clients
17. (F) indicates a client entitled to the FULL scope of Medicaid services
18. Information for Medicaid client
19. Information for Medicaid Provider

*When a healthcare provider is identified for a service type, the client must use that provider.
**Managed care plans do not cover pharmacy, dental, or chiropractic services. Card states "A participating physician/pharmacist/dentist." The client may choose a provider who accepts Medicaid for the service needed.

DEPARTMENT OF WORKFORCE SERVICES
158 SOUTH 200 WEST
P.O. BOX 45490
SALT LAKE CITY UT 84145

NON-NEGOTIABLE

JANE DOE
1TEERTSTSRIF432
ANYTOWN UT 84000

NELBAITOGEN-NO

MEDICAID IDENTIFICATION CARD
UTAH DEPARTMENT OF HEALTH

1 ELIGIBLE FROM - JUNE1, 2002 THRU JUNE30, 2002

2 THIS ID CARD ENTITLES THE FOLLOWING NAMED PERSONS TO MEDICAL/DENTAL/PHARMACY SERVICES.

3 HMO   4 TPL   HMO   TPL   HMO

5 NAME	6 ID	7 SEX	8 DOB	9 AGE	10 11 MEDICAL/PHARMACY
DOE, JANE	9999999999	F	01APR60	42	HMO or Primary CarePhysician

12 DENTAL
Dental care provider
13 MENTAL HEALTH SERVICES
Mental health services provider

14 COPAY/CO-INS FOR: NON EMERGENCY USE OF ER, OUTPAT HOSP & PHYSICIAN SVCS, PHARMACY INPAT HOSP
15 THIRD PARTY: MAILHANDLERS
POLICY HOLDER: DOE, JOHN

---

16 DOE, JOHN 9999999999 M   01APR82   20   MEDICAL/PHARMACY
TSRELDNAHLIAM:YTRAPDRIH   HnaicisyhPeraCyramirProOM
PNHOJ,EOD:REDLOHYCILO   DLATNE
14 NO CO-PAYMENT REQUIRED   Dental care provider
                                                    MENTAL HEALTH SERVICES
                                                    Mental health services provider

---

16 DOE, BLANE 9999999999 (F)   M   01APR87   15   MEDICAL/PHARMACY
TSRELDNAHLIAM:YTRAPDRIH   HnaicisyhPeraCyramirProOM
PNHOJ,EOD:REDLOHYCILO   DLATNE
14 NDERIUQERTNEMYAP-OCO   Dredivorperaclatne
                                                         MENTAL HEALTH SERVICES
                                                         Mental health services provider

* *

18 CLIENT: THIS CARD MUST BE PRESENTED BEFORE RECEIVING MEDICAID SERVICES. PLEASE KEEP THIS CARD FOR YOUR RECORDS. IF YOU HAVE QUESTIONS ON MEDICAL COVERAGE CALL MEDICAID AT 1-800-662-XXXX. IF YOU HAVE QUESTIONS ON MENTAL HEALTH COVERAGE CALL [Prepaid Mental Health Plan] AT [PMHP phone number]. FOR NON-EMERGENCY TRANSPORTATION SERVICES CALL 1-888-822-1XXXX. IF YOU HAVE QUESTIONS REGARDING THE USE OF THIS CARD OR QUESTIONS ON DENTAL OR PHARMACY, PLEASE CONTACT MEDICAID INFORMATION AT 538-6155 OR TOLL FREE AT 1-800-662-XXXX. ANY ATTEMPT TO MODIFY THIS CARD IN ANY WAY OR ALLOW USE BY UNAUTHORIZED PERSONS CONSTITUTES FRAUD.
19 PROVIDER: IF THERE ARE ANY CHANGES ON INSURANCE COVERAGE, CALL THE TPL UNIT AT 1-800-821-XXXX. PLEASE KEEP A COPY OF THIS CARD FOR YOUR RECORDS. THIS IS THE END OF THE MEDICAID IDENTIFICATION CARD. **000191919 FM

Fig. 8-4 Utah Medicaid ID card.

Complete a CMS-1500 for each of the following case studies using the patient record, the Medicaid ID card, and the ledger card. Use a blank CMS-1500 form, located in the back of the workbook or the electronic CMS-1500 forms located on the CD. Post the charge(s) on the ledger card. (Date claim form submissions *1 day after encounter*.) Use the information in the Broadmoor Medical Clinic provider box for claims completion.

Provider Box	
Broadmoor Medical Clinic	Clinic EIN No. 42-1898989
4353 Pine Ridge Drive	Dr. R. L. Jones NPI 1234567890
Milton, XY 12345-0001	Dr. Marilou Lucero NPI 2907511822
Clinic NPI X100XX1000	Group # GRW0000
Telephone: 555-656-7890	Date claims 1 day after examination

A. Medicaid patient Pricilla Atkins—Record No. 052541 (Figs. 8-5, 8-6, and 8-7).
   Electronic Forms: For this claim form exercise, you also can use the Electronic Forms found on the Student CD.

B. Medicaid patient Hattie Lawrence—Record No. 052544 (Figs. 8-8, 8-9, and 8-10).
   Electronic Forms: For this claim form exercise, you also can use the Electronic Forms found on the Student CD.
   Note: This patient has Medicare and Medicaid.

C. Using the Medicare/medical insurance record tracking form (Fig. 8-11), post the two Medicaid claims generated in Case Studies A and B.
   Note: Remember to post the Medicaid claim filing notation on the ledger card.

Patient Record No. _052541_

Name: _Pricilla Atkins_   Birth Date: _06/15/99_   Sex: _F_

Address: _456 Summer Street_   City/State/Zip: _Middletown, XT 12345_

Employer/Occupation: _____

Employer Address/Phone No.: _____

Responsible Party (Spouse/Parent/Guardian): _Sherril Atkins_

Relationship to Patient: _mother_

Occupation/Employer: _custodian Silver Creek Shopping Center_

Employer Address/Phone No.: _4500 Highway 406 W., Middletown, XT 12345_

Primary Insurance: _____   Subscriber: _____

Policy No.: _____   Group No.: _____   Effective Date: _____

Other Insurance: _____   Subscriber: _____

Policy No.: _____   Group No.: _____   Effective Date: _____

Medicare No.: _____   Medicaid No.: _169426G_   SSN: _____

Name/NPI of Referring Provider: _____

Referring Provider's Address/Phone No.: _____

PROGRESS NOTES

02/13/20XX   Pricilla returns to the office today for destruction of two flat warts on her left hand. The lesion that was removed from her right hand two weeks ago is healing nicely. RTN 2 wks.

DIAGNOSIS   Juvenile warts (078.19)   *R. L. Jones, M.D.*

CHARGES: 17110 Ex Les. x 2 (L) $ 80.00

Fig. 8-5 Patient record (Atkins).

Chapter **8** **Understanding Medicaid**

Fig. 8-6 Medicaid ID card (Atkins).

XTRA DEPARTMENT OF HUMAN SERVICES
MEDICAL ASSISTANCE ELIGIBILITY CARD

FEBRUARY Month Valid			20XX Year
30-8 Aid-Type	J35982000		29 County

PERSON ID	NAME	BIRTHDATE	OTHER
169426G	PRICILLA ATKINS	06/15/1999	0000
2899123B	JACOB ATKINS	11/22/2002	0000

Client Address: 456 Summer Street   PH 555 666 7377
Middletown, XT 12345

Ins: Medicaid
Ph # 555-666-7377

STATEMENT

169426G Pricilla 6/15/99
2899123B Jacob 11/22/02

BROADMOOR MEDICAL CLINIC
4353 Pine Ridge Drive
Milton, XY 12345-0001
Telephone: 555-656-7890

Mrs. Sherrill Atkins
456 Summer Street
Middletown, XT 12345

DATE 20XX	PROFESSIONAL SERVICE DESCRIPTION	CHARGE	CREDITS		CURRENT BALANCE
			PAYMENTS	ADJUSTMENTS	
1/31	99212 OV EST (Pricilla)	65 00			65 00
1/31	17000 EX LES (RT)	45 00			110 00
2/3	Medicaid Claim	—			
2/10	Medicaid Ck#0317004		110 00		— 0 —

Due and payable within 10 days.   Pay last amount in balance column ⬆

Fig. 8-7 Ledger card (Atkins).

Patient Record No. 052544

Name: Hattie Lawrence   Birth Date: 06/02/1939   Sex: F

Address: 2925 Aspen Road   City/State/Zip: Milton, XT 12345

Employer/Occupation: unemployed

Employer Address/Phone No.: _____

Responsible Party (Spouse/Parent/Guardian): self

Relationship to Patient: _____

Occupation/Employer: _____

Employer Address/Phone No.: _____

Primary Insurance: _____   Subscriber: _____

Policy No.: _____   Group No.: _____   Effective Date: _____

Other Insurance: _____   Subscriber: _____

Policy No.: _____   Group No.: _____   Effective Date: _____

Medicare No.: 111223333A Medicaid No.: 788244F   SSN: 111-22-3333

Name/NPI of Referring Provider: Everette Barclay, MD 0045557111

Referring Provider's Address/Phone No.: 19 Royal Circle, Ste 440, Milton, XY 23456

PROGRESS NOTES

10/03/20XX	This elderly woman is in the office today complaining of mild pain in the R ear. This has been bothering her for about a week now. She has tried home remedies, which help some, but do not relieve the pain for more than a few hours. Today, she is having some associated dizziness. See H&P in health record.
	Patient was given a prescription for E-Mycin and Benadryl OTC.
PLAN:	Patient is to return in one week for recheck. If not improved, we will do a head CT scan and arrange for hearing test.
DX	Labyrinthitis (386.30) M. Lucero
CHARGES:	99212 OV EST PT $60.00

Fig. 8-8 Patient record (Lawrence).

XTRA DEPARTMENT OF HUMAN SERVICES
MEDICAL ASSISTANCE ELIGIBILITY CARD

| OCTOBER Month Valid | | | 20XX Year |
| 31-6 | MM-Type | J35982000 | 29 County |

| PERSON ID | NAME | BIRTHDATE | OTHER |
| 788244F | HATTIE LAWRENCE | 06/02/1939 | 0003 |

Client Address: 2925 Aspen Road   PH 555 666 2244
Middletown, XT 12345

Fig. 8-9 Medicaid ID card (Lawrence).

Medicaid 788244F
Medicare 111223333A
Ph # 555-666-2244

STATEMENT

BROADMOOR MEDICAL CLINIC
4353 Pine Ridge Drive
Milton, XY 12345-0001
Telephone: 555-656-7890

Ms. Hattie Lawrence
2925 Aspen Road
Middletown, XT 12345

DATE 20XX	PROFESSIONAL SERVICE DESCRIPTION	CHARGE	CREDITS PAYMENTS	ADJUSTMENTS	CURRENT BALANCE

Due and payable within 10 days.   Pay last amount in balance column ⇧

Fig. 8-10 Ledger card (Lawrence).

**Medical Insurance
Record Tracking Form**

Service Provided			Medicare/Medicaid						Private Insurance			Patient Responsibility	
Date of Service	Patient Name & ID Number	CPT Service Codes	Assign-ed Y or N	Amount Billed	Amount Approved	Applied To Deductible	Amount Paid Provider	Amount Paid Patient	Date Sent	Amount Paid Provider	Amount Paid Patient	Amount Patient Paid	Date Paid Check #

Fig. 8-11 Insurance tracking form.

INTERNET EXPLORATION

A. Using the website **http://cms.hhs.gov/medicaid/consumer.asp,** locate the Medicaid office in your state. Determine the following:

- Current FI
- Optional covered benefits for your state
- Required claim form

B. Some states provide a choice of Medicaid plans—fee-for-service and managed care. Log on to **http://www.cms.hhs. gov/home/medicaid.asp** to see if your state offers a managed care choice. If so, generate a chart comparing the two plans. If your state does not have a managed care plan, choose one that does.

C. Log on to the CMS fraud website at **http://www.cms.hhs.gov/FraudAbuseforProfs** (in addition, students should also research the "Related Links" at the bottom of the page). Create a page for the Office Procedures Manual giving step-by-step instructions for reporting suspected fraud and abuse in your state. Include a list of pertinent names, addresses, and telephone numbers.

D. Log on to the CMS website at **http://www.cms.hhs.gov,** and click on SCHIP. Under the SCHIP Summary, choose the SCHIP Resource Index. Next, under State Information, click on Fact Sheets. Locate the fact sheet for your state. Study and compare how children qualify for coverage and the cost sharing of your SCHIP with that of other states.

PERFORMANCE OBJECTIVES

Use the blank CMS-1500 forms and ledger cards (back of workbook), paper or electronic (found on your Student Software CD), for the exercises in these performance objectives.

Performance Objective 8-1—Medicaid Simple Claim

Conditions: Student will complete a Medicaid "simple" claim and ledger card using the information in Patient Record No. 052547.

Supplies/Equipment: Patient Record No. 052547 (Fig. 8-12), CMS-1500 claim form (paper or electronic), blank ledger card (paper or electronic)

Guided Completion: For this claim form exercise, you also can use the Guided Completion software found on the Student CD to help you complete this CMS-1500 form.

Time Allowed: 50 minutes

Accuracy Needed to Pass: 90%

Procedural Steps	Points Earned	Comments
Evaluator: Note time began: _____		
1. Carefully read and study Patient Record No. 052547.		
2. Complete *all* blocks required for a Medicaid simple claim. (30)		
3. Generate a ledger card; post date of office visit, CPT code/description, fee, and balance. (14)		
4. Note Medicaid claim submission. (1)		
5. Proofread claim for accuracy.		
Optional: May deduct points for taking more time than allowed.		

Total Points = 45

Student's Score: _____

Evaluator: _____

Comments: _____

_____

_____

_____

_____

Patient Record No. 052547

Name: Charles T. Brown   Birth Date: 07/30/2000   Sex: M

Address: 55 N. Winston Dr.   City/State/Zip: Middletown, XT 12345

Employer/Occupation: student

Employer Address/Phone No.: _____

Responsible Party (Spouse/Parent/Guardian): Marvel Brown   Phone: 555-334-3344

Relationship to Patient: father   (Same address)

Occupation/Employer: janitor – Washington Heights Apartments

Employer Address/Phone No.: 3939 Belview Ct., Middletown, XT 12345

Primary Insurance: BCBS**   Subscriber: Marvel Brown

Policy No.: _____ Group No.: _____ Effective Date: _____

Other Insurance: _____ Subscriber: _____

Policy No.: QKZ111006666 Group No.: _____ Effective Date: _____

Medicare No.: _____ Medicaid No.: 5748392 SSN: _____

Name/NPI of Referring Provider: _____

Referring Provider's Address/Phone No.: _____

PROGRESS NOTES

11/09/20XX

CC   Charles is a new patient in the office today with complaints of pain and swelling in the R ankle. Applying weight on the ankle causes the pain to increase. He reports that he "crashed into another player" during soccer practice at the YMCA today.

PX   See patient's health record. X-ray revealed no fracture.

ASSESSMENT Sprain, R ankle (845.00)

PLAN   Charles was referred to Dr. Jamie Richards in the Orthopedic Clinic for treatment. *M. Lucero*

Charges: 99202   OV New PT $65.00
          73600   X-ray R ankle   40.00

**Pt not covered under father's BCBS plan.

Fig. 8-12 Medical record (Brown).

Performance Objective 8-2—Medicaid Secondary Claim

Conditions: Student will complete a Medicaid secondary claim and ledger card using the information in Patient Record No. 052545.

Supplies/Equipment: Patient Record No. 052545 (Fig. 8-13), CMS-1500 claim form (paper or electronic), blank ledger card (paper or electronic)

Guided Completion: For this claim form exercise, you also can use the Guided Completion software found on the Student CD to help you complete this CMS-1500 form.

Time Allowed: 50 minutes

Accuracy Needed to Pass: 90%

Procedural Steps	Points Earned	Comments
Evaluator: Note time began: _____		
1. Carefully read and study Patient Record No. 052545.		
2. Complete *all* blocks required for a Medicaid secondary (Blue Cross and Blue Shield) claim. (32)		
3. Generate a ledger card; post date of office visit, CPT code/description, fee, and balance. (4)		
4. Note Blue Cross and Blue Shield claim submission. (1)		
5. Proofread claim for accuracy.		
Optional: May deduct points for taking more time than allowed.		

Total Points = 37

Student's Score: _____

Evaluator: _____

Comments: _____

_____

_____

_____

_____

Patient Record No. 052545

Name: Tyler Swanson   Birth Date: 01/04/2001   Sex: M

Address: 529 Parkway   City/State/Zip: Middletown, XT 12345

                                       Phone: 555-766-1100
Employer/Occupation: student

Employer Address/Phone No.: _____

Responsible Party (Spouse/Parent/Guardian): Connie Templeton (same address)

Relationship to Patient: legal guardian   DOB: 04/22/1968

Occupation/Employer: Administrative Assistant

Employer Address/Phone No.: Superior Insurance Adjustment Bureau

Primary Insurance: Blue Cross/Blue Shield** Subscriber: Connie Templeton

Policy No.: QXY654321100 Group No.: XYZ12   Effective Date: 12/31/1998

Other Insurance: _____ Subscriber: _____

Policy No.: _____ Group No.: _____ Effective Date: _____

Medicare No.: _____ Medicaid No.: 13647780 SSN: 654-00-1111

Name/NPI of Referring Provider: _____

Referring Provider's Address/Phone No.: _____

PROGRESS NOTES

2/04/20XX	Tyler is a new patient to the practice. He complains of ear pain and sore throat of two days' duration.
PX	See health record
ASSESSMENT	Acute tonsillitis
PLAN	Bedrest and fluids. Amoxicillin, 250 mg. x 12. Rtn 1 wk PRN.
DX	Otitis media, acute (382.9) *M. Lucero*
Charges:	99202 OV New PT $65.00

**Patient is covered under his guardian's BCBS plan.

Fig. 8-13 Medical record (Swanson).

Chapter **8** **Understanding Medicaid**

Conditions: Student will complete a Medicare/Medicaid claim and ledger card using the information in Patient Record No. 052548.

Supplies/Equipment: Patient Record No. 052548 (Fig. 8-14), CMS-1500 claim form (paper or electronic), blank ledger card (paper or electronic)

Time Allowed: 50 minutes

Accuracy Needed to Pass: 90%

Procedural Steps	Points Earned	Comments
Evaluator: Note time began: _____		
1. Carefully read and study Patient Record No. 052545.		
2. Complete *all* blocks required for a Medicare/Medicaid claim. (30)		
3. Generate a ledger card; post date of office visit, CPT code/description, fee, and balance. (14)		
4. Note insurance claim submission. (1)		
5. Proofread claim for accuracy.		
Optional: May deduct points for taking more time than allowed.		

Total Points = 45

Student's Score: _____

Evaluator: _____

Comments: _____

_____

_____

_____

_____

Patient Record No. 052548

Name: Margaret R. Phillips   Birth Date: 03/21/1940   Sex: F

Address: 1893 Edgewood Place   City/State/Zip: Middletown, XT 12345

                                               Phone: 555-985-2318

Employer/Occupation: retired

Employer Address/Phone No.: _____

Responsible Party (Spouse/Parent/Guardian): Frederick Phillips (son)

Relationship to Patient: son

Occupation/Employer: farmer – self-employed

Employer Address/Phone No.: _____

Primary Insurance: _____ Subscriber: _____

Policy No.: _____ Group No.: _____ Effective Date: _____

Other Insurance: _____ Subscriber: _____

Policy No.: _____ Group No.: _____ Effective Date: _____

Medicare No.: 666554444B   Medicaid No.: 123321456   SSN: 666-55-4444

Name/NPI of Referring Provider: Olin Swenson, MD   0814551100

Referring Provider's Address/Phone No.: _____

PROGRESS NOTES

4/22/20XX

CC	Margaret is here again today complaining of redness and "crusting" of the L eyelid, which began yesterday morning. She is accompanied by her son who reports that several of the residents at WondraCare Assisted Living are suffering from similar complaints.
PX	See patient's health record for PX
ASSESSMENT	Conjunctivitis (372.30)
PLAN	Patient was advised not to rub her eyes. Apply cool compresses to the affected eye several times a day. Trifluridine 1%. Rtn 1 wk PRN. *R. L. Jones*
Charges:	99212 OV Est Pt. $60.00

Fig. 8-14 Medical record (Phillips).

Performance Objective 8-4—Medicaid/Commercial Claim

Conditions: Student will complete a Medicaid/commercial claim and ledger card using the information in Patient Record No. 052543.

Supplies/Equipment: Patient Record No. 052543 (Fig. 8-15), CMS-1500 claim form (paper or electronic), blank ledger card (paper or electronic)

Time Allowed: 50 minutes

Accuracy Needed to Pass: 90%

Procedural Steps	Points Earned	Comments
Evaluator: Note time began: _____		
1. Carefully read and study Patient Record No. 052543.		
2. Complete *all* blocks required for a Medicare/Medicaid claim. (30)		
3. Generate a ledger card; post date of office visit, CPT code/description, fee, and balance. (14)		
4. Note insurance claim submission. (1)		
5. Proofread claim for accuracy.		
Optional: May deduct points for taking more time than allowed.		

Total Points = 45

Student's Score: _____

Evaluator: _____

Comments: _____

_____

_____

_____

Patient Record No. 052543

Name: Inga M. Jones   Birth Date: 8/10/1962   Sex: F

Address: 600 Lincoln Way   City/State/Zip: Middletown, XT 12345

Employer/Occupation: Daycare aide at Babes R Us DayCare

Employer Address/Phone No.: 2551 Ridgemont, Middletown, XT 12345

Responsible Party (Spouse/Parent/Guardian): self   (NO PHONE)

Relationship to Patient: _____

Occupation/Employer: _____

Employer Address/Phone No.: _____

Primary Insurance: Allgood Life & Health   Subscriber: Inga Jones

Policy No.: 44355QWP   Group No.: 55X9L   Effective Date: 01/01/1999

Other Insurance: _____ Subscriber: _____

Policy No.: _____ Group No.: _____ Effective Date: _____

Medicare No.: _____ Medicaid No.: 44637620011   SSN: 444-44-4444

Name/NPI of Referring Provider: _____

Referring Provider's Address/Phone No.: _____

PROGRESS NOTES

11/06/20XX

CC	New pt Inga Jones is in the office today with complaints of headache, fever, and cough of 2 days' duration. Pt works at a daycare center and reports that many of the children have colds and flu.
PX	See H&P in patient health record.
ASSESSMENT	Influenza w/cold (487.1)
PLAN	Bedrest, fluids and OTC cold remedies. No prescriptions at this time. Rtn 1 wk PRN if symptoms don't improve.

11/07/20XX   Pt returns today with worsening symptoms of a "tight feeling" in her chest, nausea, and sore throat. Reported fever of 102.3 last night. Chest x-ray was clear.

ASSESSMENT   Acute bronchitis (466.0)   *R. L. Jones*

PLAN   Penicillin 5cc IM. Rtn 1 wk PRN.

CHARGES: 99202   OV New Pt. $55.00
              99214   OV Est. PT $170.00

Fig. 8-15 Medical record (Jones).

Performance Objective 8-5—Posting Payments from Medicaid Remittance Advice

Conditions: Student will post payments from a Medicaid RA on ledger cards for five patients.

Supplies/Equipment: Pen, RA No. 433900 (Fig. 8-16) from XT Department of Human Services; five patient ledger cards (Figs. 8-17 through 8-21)

Time Allowed: 50 minutes

Accuracy Needed to Pass: 90%

Procedural Steps	Points Earned	Comments
Evaluator: Note time began: _____		
1. Carefully read and study remittance advice #433900; note the Medicaid patients in this clinic must pay 10% copay for office visits on the day they are seen.		
2. Remittance advice and Medicaid check was received on 11/28/20XX.		
3. Correctly post payments on the ledger cards for the following patients:		
I. M. Jones (8)		
C. T. Brown (8)		
J. L. Doe (8)		
E. Martin (8)		
Juan Ruiz (3)		
4. Proofread each ledger card for accuracy.		
Optional: May deduct points for taking more time than allowed.		

Total Points = 35

Student's Score: _____

Evaluator: _____

Comments: _____

_____

_____

_____

_____

XT DEPARTMENT OF HUMAN SERVICES
MEDICAID MANAGEMENT INFORMATION SYSTEM

REMITTANCE ADVICE

RA No. 433900
MMIS Ck No. 0098887

TO: HARPER, DANIEL, MD
606 BRIDGE STREET
MIDDLETOWN, XT 12345

PROVIDER NO. 12345678
POLICY/BILLING 800-555-0987

REPORT SEQ NUMBER: 3
R/S NUMBER 987654343

DATE: 11/24/20XX
PAGE 1

PATIENT NAME/ID NO. SERVICE DATES FROM TO	PERF PROV NO.	DAYS QTY	PROC CODE	PROCEDURE DESCRIPTION	AMOUNT BILLED	AMOUNT ALLOWED	COPAY	PAID AMOUNT	EOB CODES
PAID OR DENIED CLAIMS									
JONES, I.M./44637620011 110620XX 110720XX	81234123 81234123	1 1	99202 99214	OFFICE/OP VISIT–NEW PT OFFICE/OP VISIT–ESTABL PT	55.00 170.00	49.50 152.00	5.50 17.00	44.00 134.50	12 12
BROWN, C.T./44637112001 110920XX	12345678	1	99202	OFFICE/OP VISIT–NEW PT XRAY ® ANKLE	65.00 40.00	49.50 38.00	6.50 4.00	44.00 36.00	12 12
			73600						
DOE, J.L./44637220887 11/11/20XX	12345678	1	99218	INITIAL OBSERVATION CARE	110.00	110.00	N/A	110.00	14
MARTIN, E./4463771124 11/15/20XX 11/15/20XX 11/15/20XX	12345678 81234123 81234123	1 1 1	99215 99175 99401	OFFICE/OP VISIT–NEW PT IPECAC/SIM ADMIN FOR IND EMESIS COUNSELLING/RISK FX (15 MIN)	225.00 35.00 50.00	212.00 35.00 25.00	22.50 N/A 5.00	189.50 35.00 20.00	12 14 13
RUIZ, JUAN/446375566 11/19/20XX	81234123	1	96900	ACTINOTHERAPY (UV)	25.00	0.00	2.50	0.00	15
TOTALS					775.00	671.00	63.00	613.00	

EOB CODES:
12 Service paid at the maximum amount allowed by Medical Assistance Reimbursement policies
13 Service paid at 50% of amount allowed by Medical Assistance Reimbursement policies
14 Service paid at 100% by Medical Assistance Reimbursement policies
15 Service not allowed by Medical Assistance Reimbursement policies

Fig. 8-16 Medicaid remittance advice.

STATEMENT

BROADMOOR MEDICAL CLINIC
4353 Pine Ridge Drive
Milton, XY 12345-0001
Telephone: 555-656-7890

INGA M. JONES
600 LINCOLN WAY
MIDDLETOWN, XT 12345

DATE 20XX	PROFESSIONAL SERVICE DESCRIPTION	CHARGE	CREDITS		CURRENT BALANCE
			PAYMENTS	ADJUSTMENTS	
11/06	99202 OV NP	55 00	5 50		49 50
11/07	99214 OV EST PT	170 00	17 00		202 50
11/08	Medicaid claim				

Due and payable within 10 days.   **Pay last amount in balance column** ⇧

Fig. 8-17 Ledger card (Jones).

STATEMENT

BROADMOOR MEDICAL CLINIC
4353 Pine Ridge Drive
Milton, XY 12345-0001
Telephone: 555-656-7890

MARVEL BROWN
55 NORTH WINSTON DR.
MIDDLETOWN, XT 12345

DATE 20XX	PROFESSIONAL SERVICE DESCRIPTION	CHARGE	CREDITS		CURRENT BALANCE
			PAYMENTS	ADJUSTMENTS	
11/09	99202 Charles OV NP	65 00	6 50		58 50
11/09	73600 X-ray ® ankle	40 00	4 00		94 50
11/10	Medicaid claim				

Due and payable within 10 days.   Pay last amount in balance column ⇧

Fig. 8-18 Ledger card (Brown).

STATEMENT

BROADMOOR MEDICAL CLINIC
4353 Pine Ridge Drive
Milton, XY 12345-0001
Telephone: 555-656-7890

JERAMIAH L. DOE
14 HILLCREST CIRCLE
MIDDLETOWN XT 12345

DATE 20XX	PROFESSIONAL SERVICE DESCRIPTION	CHARGE	CREDITS		CURRENT BALANCE
			PAYMENTS	ADJUSTMENTS	
11/11	99218 Init Obs. Care	110 00			110 00
11/12	Medicaid claim				

Due and payable within 10 days.   **Pay last amount in balance column** ⇧

Fig. 8-19 Ledger card (Doe).

STATEMENT

BROADMOOR MEDICAL CLINIC
4353 Pine Ridge Drive
Milton, XY 12345-0001
Telephone: 555-656-7890

MRS. ELOISE C. MARTIN
543 MAPLE STREET
MIDDLETOWN, XT 12345

DATE 20XX	PROFESSIONAL SERVICE DESCRIPTION	CHARGE	PAYMENTS	ADJUSTMENTS	CURRENT BALANCE
11/15	99215 OV NP	225 00	22 50		202 50
11/15	99175 Ipecac Adm.	35 00	—		237 50
11/15	99401 couns./Risk FX	50 00	5 00		282 50
11/16	Medicaid claim				

Due and payable within 10 days. **Pay last amount in balance column** ⇧

Fig. 8-20 Ledger card (Martin).

STATEMENT

BROADMOOR MEDICAL CLINIC
4353 Pine Ridge Drive
Milton, XY 12345-0001
Telephone: 555-656-7890

JUAN RUIZ
1500 SOUTH 9TH ST.
MIDDLETOWN, XT 12345

DATE 20XX	PROFESSIONAL SERVICE DESCRIPTION	CHARGE	CREDITS PAYMENTS	ADJUSTMENTS	CURRENT BALANCE
11/19	96900 Actinotherapy	25 00	2 50		22 50
11/20	Medicaid claim				

Due and payable within 10 days.   Pay last amount in balance column ⇧

Fig. 8-21 Ledger card (Ruiz).

Performance Objective 8-6—Posting Claims to Medical Insurance Record Tracking Form

Conditions: Student will post the claims generated in Performance Objectives 8-1 through 8-4 and patient payments and payments received from the third-party insurers, using the insurance tracking form begun in Case Study C (see Fig. 8-11).

Supplies/Equipment: Pen/typewriter, medical insurance record tracking form

Time Allowed: 50 minutes

Accuracy Needed to Pass: 90%

Procedural Steps	Points Earned	Comments
Evaluator: Note time began: _____		
1. Assemble the four claims generated in Performance Objectives 8-1 through 8-4.		
2. Post the applicable information to the insurance tracking form begun in Case Study C.		
3. Correctly post the applicable information from the claims for:		
Brown (5)		
Swanson (5)		
Phillips (5)		
Jones (5)		
4. Proofread your entries for accuracy.		
Optional: May deduct points for taking more time than allowed.		

Total Points = 20

Student's Score: _____

Evaluator: _____

Comments: _____

_____

_____

_____

_____

Health Insurance Professional's Notebook

Generate a section in your notebook for Medicaid information. You should include the following information and documents as well as other information or forms that you find pertinent:

- Medicaid's FI in your state
- Names/telephone numbers of Medicaid FI
- Sample Medicaid ID cards with explanations
- List of procedures/services covered by Medicaid in your state
- Sample claim form required by Medicaid's FI
- Guidelines for completing the required claim form
- Template showing blocks on the claim that require completion
- Sample completed claims for:
  - Medicaid simple
  - Medicaid secondary
  - Medicare/Medicaid
- Helpful websites for additional provider information

Chapter Check List

Student name: _____

Chapter completion date: _____

1.	Record	Your start time and date: _____
2.	Read	The assigned chapter in the text
3.	View	PowerPoint slides (if available)
4.	Complete	Exercises in the Workbook as assigned
5.	Compare	Your answers to the answers posted on the bulletin board/website/handout
6.	Correct	Your answers
7.	Complete	All tests and required activities
8.	Read	Assigned readings (if any)
9.	Complete	Chapter performance objectives (competencies), if any
10.	Evaluate	Chapter performance, and submit to your instructor
11.	Record	Your ending time and date: _____
12.	Move on	Begin next chapter as assigned

Student name: _____

Chapter completion date: _____

Evaluate your classroom performance. Complete the self-evaluation, and submit it to your instructor. When your instructor returns this form to you, compare your self-evaluation with the evaluation completed by your instructor.

Skill	Student Self-Evaluation			Instructor Evaluation		
	Good	Average	Poor	Good	Average	Poor
Attendance/punctuality						
Personal appearance						
Applies effort						
Is self-motivated						
Is courteous						
Has positive attitude						
Completes assignments in timely manner						
Works well with others						

Student's Initials: _____   **Instructor's Initials:** _____

Date: _____   **Date:** _____

Points Possible: _____

Points Awarded: _____

Chapter Grade: _____

9 Conquering Medicare's Challenges

Medicare is the U.S. health insurance program for people age 65 or older, certain people with disabilities who are younger than age 65, and people of any age who have permanent kidney failure. Medicare provides basic protection against the cost of healthcare, but it does not cover all medical expenses or the cost of most long-term care. The Medicare program is financed by a portion of the Federal Insurance Contributions Act (FICA) taxes paid by workers and their employers. It also is financed partly by monthly premiums paid by beneficiaries. The Centers for Medicare and Medicaid Services (CMS) (formerly the Health Care Financing Administration) is the federal agency in charge of the Medicare program. The Social Security Administration determines who is eligible for Medicare, enrolls individuals in the program, and distributes general Medicare information.

Medicare may be the most challenging of all healthcare reimbursement programs. It is composed of several different components (Parts A, B, C, and D), and these parts and what is covered under each tend to change frequently. It is important that health insurance professionals understand the ins and outs of Medicare not only for their own benefit and the benefit of the providers with whom they are employed, but also for the sake of the patients who are beneficiaries of this program. The exercises and activities in this workbook chapter reinforce your understanding of and ability to deal with Medicare's challenges.

WORKBOOK CHAPTER OBJECTIVES

After completing the workbook activities for Chapter 9, the student should be able to:
- Define the terms used in the chapter.
- Answer the review questions to within the evaluation criteria set by the instructor.
- Demonstrate the ability to think critically and draw conclusions from facts and information provided in scenarios and performance objectives.
- Explore websites to acquire information needed to complete workbook activities successfully.
- Abstract applicable information from healthcare documents necessary for completion of Medicare claims.
- Complete specific forms common to the health insurance professional's role in Medicare claims and billing.
- Compute arithmetic calculations to arrive at correct patient statement balances.
- Generate information and collect documents for inclusion in the student's personal Health Insurance Professional's Notebook.
- Undertake self-analysis/evaluation in completed workbook activities.

DEFINING CHAPTER TERMS

Using the computer (or typewriter), students should key an accurate definition for each of the chapter terms listed. These definitions should be in the students' own words. When finished, students should compare their definitions with those listed in the glossary at the back of the textbook, correcting any inaccuracies.

adjudicated
advance beneficiary notice (ABN)
allowable charges
beneficiary
benefit period
biologicals
claims adjustment reason codes
Clinical Laboratory Improvement Act (CLIA)
coordination of benefits contractor
coverage requirements
credible coverage
crosswalks
demand bills
denial notice
downcoding
dual eligibles
electronic funds transfer (EFT)

electronic Medicare Summary Notice
electronic remittance advice (ERA)
end-stage renal disease (ESRD)
Federal Insurance Contributions Act
Health Care Quality Improvement Program
health insurance claim number (HICN)
HMO with point-of-service (POS) option
initial claims
lifetime (one-time) release of information form
local coverage determinations (LCDs)
local medical review policies (LMRPs)
mandated Medigap transfer
medically necessary
Medicare
Medicare Beneficiary Protection Program
Medicare gaps
Medicare HMOs

161

Medicare limiting charge
Medicare managed care plan
Medicare nonparticipating provider (nonPAR)
Medicare Part A
Medicare Part A fiscal intermediary (FI)
Medicare Part B
Medicare Part B carrier
Medicare Part B Crossover Program
Medicare Part C (Medicare Advantage Plans)
Medicare Part D (Prescription Drug Plan)
Medicare participating provider (PAR)
Medicare Secondary Payer (MSP)
Medicare Summary Notice (MSN)
Medicare supplement policy
Medigap insurance
Medi-Medi

network
noncovered services
open enrollment period
peer review organization (PRO)
Program of All-Inclusive Care for the Elderly
  (PACE)
prospective payment system (PPS)
provider sponsored organization (PSO)
quality improvement organization
quality review study
remittance remark codes
resource based relative value system
self-referring
standard paper remittance advice (SPRA)
trading partner agreement

ASSESSMENT

Multiple Choice

Directions: In the statements presented, choose the **best** response, and circle the letter that precedes it.

1. Medicare was established by Congress in 1966 to provide financial assistance with medical expenses to:
   a. People older than 65
   b. People with end-stage renal disease
   c. People younger than 65 with disabilities
   d. All of the above

2. Medicare requires its beneficiaries to pay premiums, deductibles, and coinsurance, which is referred to as:
   a. Medigap
   b. Taxation
   c. Cost sharing
   d. Allowable charges

3. Medicare Part A, the hospital insurance part of Medicare, is funded through:
   a. Taxes withheld from employees' wages
   b. Taxes paid by employers
   c. State funds
   d. a and b are correct

4. Coverage requirements under Medicare state that for a service to be covered, it must be considered:
   a. Proper and timely
   b. Reasonable and customary
   c. Medically necessary
   d. Medicare has no coverage requirements

5. Part A coverage is available free of charge to eligible Medicare beneficiaries who:
   a. Have no other insurance
   b. Are "dual eligibles"
   c. Are eligible to receive Social Security benefits
   d. Medicare Part A is not free of charge to anyone

6. A private organization that contracts with Medicare to pay Part A and some Part B bills and determines payment to Part A facilities is called a:

   a. Fiscal intermediary (FI)

   b. Part A negotiator

   c. Beneficiary

   d. Participating provider (PAR)

7. Medicare Part B helps pay for:

   a. Medically necessary physician's services

   b. Acute care hospitalization

   c. Custodial and long-term care

   d. All of the above

8. Medicare pays _____% of allowable charges after the annual deductible is met.

   a. 20

   b. 50

   c. 80

   d. 100

9. The _____ is the duration of time during which a Medicare beneficiary is eligible for Part A benefits for services incurred in a hospital or skilled nursing facility (SNF) or both.

   a. Donut hole

   b. Medicare gap

   c. Benefit period

   d. Open enrollment period

10. Managed Healthcare plans that offer regular Part A and Part B Medicare coverage and additional coverage for certain other services are called:

    a. Medicare Part A

    b. Medicare Part B

    c. Medicare Part C

    d. Medicare Part D

11. The prescription drug coverage plan, which began in January 2006, is called:

    a. Medicare Part A

    b. Medicare Part B

    c. Medicare Part C

    d. Medicare Part D

12. The period during which a Medicare beneficiary is responsible for all prescription drug expenses until a total of $3850 (2007 figure) is spent out-of-pocket is referred to as the:

    a. Medigap

    b. Donut hole

    c. Crosswalk

    d. Nonbenefit period

13. An individual qualifying for Medicare and Medicaid benefits is referred to as a:
    a. Dual eligible
    b. MediMax
    c. Medical qualifier
    d. Categorically eligible

14. The program that provides community-based acute and long-term care services to Medicare beneficiaries is called:
    a. FICA
    b. PACE
    c. CLIA
    d. LMRP

15. A health insurance plan sold by private insurance companies to help pay for healthcare expenses not covered by Medicare is called a:
    a. Commercial policy
    b. Trading partner plan
    c. Prospective payment plan
    d. Supplemental policy

16. The term used when another insurance policy is primary to Medicare is:
    a. Medigap
    b. Medicare Supplement Insurance
    c. Medicare Secondary Payer (MSP)
    d. Other health insurance

17. Some Medicare health maintenance organization (HMO) enrollees are allowed to see specialists outside the "network" without going through a primary care physician. This is called:
    a. Self-referring
    b. Open enrollment
    c. Noncovered services
    d. Not medically necessary

18. A group of medical providers that skips the insurance company middleman and contracts directly with patients is referred to as a:
    a. Coordination of benefits (COB)
    b. Nonparticipating provider (nonPAR)
    c. Trading partner agreement
    d. Provider sponsored organization

19. Local medical review policies (LMRPs) were replaced in 2003 by:
    a. CLIAs
    b. LCDs
    c. COBs
    d. QIOs

20. A form that Medicare requires all healthcare providers to use when Medicare does not pay for a service is the:
    a. SPRA
    b. COB
    c. ABN
    d. EOB

True/False

Directions: Place a "T" in the blank preceding the sentence if it is true; place an "F" if it is false.

_____ 1. Medicare Parts A and B are provided free of charge for qualifying individuals.

_____ 2. Part A covers custodial and long-term care.

_____ 3. Neither Medicare Part A nor Part B covers any preventive care services.

_____ 4. For durable medical equipment to qualify for Medicare payment, it must be ordered by a physician for use in the home, and items must be reusable.

_____ 5. Most Medicare Part B beneficiaries pay for Part B coverage in the form of a premium deducted from their monthly Social Security check.

_____ 6. Medicare beneficiaries are allowed only one "benefit period" per year.

_____ 7. An individual must be eligible for Part A or B to enroll in a Medicare Advantage Plan.

_____ 8. If a beneficiary has a Medicare Advantage Plan, he or she still needs a supplemental policy.

_____ 9. An individual who has Medicare Parts A and B must have a supplement policy.

_____ 10. The private organization that determines payment of Part B covered items and services is called a peer review organization.

_____ 11. If individuals do not sign up for Medicare Part B when first becoming eligible and later decide to enroll, the monthly premiums may be higher because of penalties.

_____ 12. When an individual turns 65 and enrolls in Medicare, federal law forbids insurance companies from denying eligibility for Medigap policies for 6 months.

_____ 13. Workers' compensation would likely be a primary payer to Medicare.

_____ 14. Medicare HMOs typically screen potential enrollees for preexisting conditions.

_____ 15. Under certain circumstances, a signed release of information form for Medicare beneficiaries can be valid for more than 1 year.

_____ 16. Medicare's definition of medical necessity must meet specific criteria.

_____ 17. Medicare health insurance claim numbers are typically in the format of nine numeric characters followed by one alpha character.

_____ 18. The Medicare fee schedule is now based on a resource-based relative value system.

_____ 19. Medicare nonPARs do not have to submit claims for their Medicare patients.

_____ 20. The process of matching one set of data elements or category of codes to their equivalents within a new set of elements or codes is called a crossover.

Short Answer/Fill-in-the-Blank

1. The second cost sharing requirement in Medicare Part B is an annual deductible of $_____, after which

   Medicare pays _____% of _____.

2. The duration of time Medicare uses for hospital and SNF services is called a(n) _____.

3. This duration of time begins the day an individual is _____ to a hospital or SNF and ends when the

   beneficiary has not received care in a hospital or SNF for _____ days in a row.

4. Medicare Part C, previously called _____, was renamed _____ _____ by the Medicare Prescription Drug, Improvement, and Modernization Act of 2003.

5. The Balanced Budget Act of 1997, which went into effect in January 1999, expanded the role of private plans to

   include _____ _____ plans.

6. List the various managed care choices included under Medicare Part C.

   _____

   _____

   _____

7. Medicare managed care plans (Medicare Part C) coverage not only includes Part A and Part B coverage, but also
   pays for services not covered under the original Medicare plan, such as

   _____

   _____

   _____

8. What main change did Medicare Part D introduce in January 2006?

   _____

9. Explain Medicare's basic payment structure for Medicare Part D.

   _____

10. How does Medicare's Part D payment structure differ for dual eligibles compared with that for Medicare beneficia-
    ries who do not qualify for dual eligibility?

    _____

Matching
Directions: Place the letter that precedes the word or words that correctly answer the question/statement. (**Note:** Not all
answers will be used.)

_____ 1.   The program that provides community-
              based acute and long-term care services.

_____ 2.   A health insurance plan sold by private
              insurance companies to help pay for
              expenses not covered by Medicare.

_____ 3.   The time period Medicare allows for
              enrolling in a Medicare supplement
              plan without penalty.

_____ 4.   The term used when Medicare is not the
              primary payer, and the beneficiary is
              covered under another insurance policy.

_____ 5.   The individual responsible for initial
              MSP development activities formerly
              performed by Medicare FIs and carriers.

a. COB contractor

b. MSP

c. Program of All-Inclusive Care for the
   Elderly

d. Medigap

e. Open enrollment

f. Medi/Medi

g. Preferred provider organization

CRITICAL THINKING ACTIVITIES

A. You are employed as a health insurance professional at Broadmoor Medical Clinic where there is a standing policy that patients cannot be seen until they produce "proof of insurance." When you ask Averil Potter, a 76-year-old new patient, for his Medicare ID card, he informs you that he does not carry it with him because he is afraid of "identity theft." He informs you that he has memorized his Medicare number, which is his Social Security number with an ending alpha character. In light of the growing incidence of identity theft and the fact that many insurance companies use Social Security numbers as policy identifiers, would you recommend that the clinic's policy be changed? If so, how; if not, why not?

B. Members of the healthcare team of the Broadmoor Medical Center's emergency department are not allowed to ask for proof of insurance before treating a patient who has arrived for emergency treatment. What is the rationale for this difference in policy as opposed to that of the Clinic?

C. Because a Medicare nonPAR can charge 15% over and above the Medicare allowable charge and bill the patient for this excess amount, why do many providers become Medicare PARs?

D. Frieda Dawson is a 66-year-old Medicare established patient. She was seen on March 16, 20XX, and had a mammogram the next day. Frieda returns on November 30 of that same year for treatment of a severe urinary tract infection, at which time she requests another mammogram. She is worried because her 73-year-old sister was recently diagnosed with breast cancer. You schedule the second mammogram as Frieda requests; however, Medicare disallows it as not being "medically necessary." You failed to get an advance beneficiary notice because you thought Medicare paid for mammograms. How should you handle this situation?

PROBLEM-SOLVING/COLLABORATIVE (GROUP) ACTIVITIES

Study Table 9-1. Then solve the following problems.

Table 9-1 2006 Medicare Benefits Table—Part A	
	Beneficiary Pays
Inpatient Hospital Days 1-60	Deductible of $952 per benefit period*
Days 61-90	$238 per day
Days 91-150	$476 per day
After 150 days	All charges
Skilled Nursing Facility Days 1-20	Nothing
Days 21-100	$119 per day
Beyond 100 days	All charges
Home Health Part-time care	Nothing (if approved)
Hospice	Nothing if physician certifies care except limited costs for drug and respite care
Blood	First 3 pints

*A benefit period begins when an individual is admitted to a hospital and ends 60 days after discharge from a hospital or a skilled nursing facility.

Note: For more detailed information on preventive and other benefits, see http://www.Medicare.gov.

A. Alfred Winters was admitted to Broadmoor Medical Center on November 11, 20XX, which began a new inpatient benefit period for him. Alfred's hospital stay was 98 days.

1. How much of the cost for Alfred's hospital stay is his responsibility?

   Days 1-60: _____

   Days 61-90: _____

   Days 91-98: _____

   Total due from Alfred: _____

2. How many days would be left if Alfred were to be admitted again as an inpatient?

   1 month later: _____

   6 months later: _____

B. Sylvia Thompson is a Medicare beneficiary with Medicare Parts A and B. Follow her through a series of hospitalizations and subsequent care, and write the Medicare inpatient hospital deductible amount at each point Sylvia was responsible for, using Table 9-1 for calculating Part A Benefits and Table 9-2 for Part B benefits. Write the Medicare inpatient hospital deductible amount at each point Sylvia was responsible for in the blanks in Table 9-3. Assume this is her first hospitalization.

Table 9-2 2006 Medicare Benefits Table—Part B	
Benefits	**Individual Pays**
Premium	$88.50 per month
Deductible	$124 per year

Physician and other medical services
    Physician accepts assignment
    Physician does not accept assignment
	
	20% coinsurance
	20% coinsurance plus up to 15% over Medicare-approved fee*

Outpatient hospital care	20% coinsurance
Ambulatory surgical services	20% coinsurance
X-rays	20% coinsurance
Durable medical equipment	20% coinsurance
Physical, occupational, and speech therapy	20% coinsurance†
Clinical diagnostic laboratory services	No coinsurance
Home health care	No coinsurance
Outpatient mental health services	50% coinsurance

Preventive services
    Flu shots, pneumococcal vaccines,
        colorectal and prostate cancer screenings,
        Pap smears, mammograms
    Bone mass measurement, diabetes
        monitoring, glaucoma screening
	Part B deductible and 20% coinsurance are waived for certain preventive services
	
	20% coinsurance

*Referred to as the Medicare Limiting Charge Law, the limit on the percentage above the Medicare-approved amount that a physician can charge is less than 15% in some states.

†Coverage limit on Medicare outpatient therapy services ($1590 limit per year for occupational therapy services, $1590 limit per year for physical and speech-language therapy services combined).

Note: For more detailed information on preventive and other benefits, see http://www.Medicare.gov.

Table 9-3 Inpatient Hospital Benefits Exercise	
	Day of Admission
February 27, Sylvia is admitted to the hospital as an inpatient for removal of her gallbladder. She remains in the hospital for 5 days before being discharged.	February 27 (5 days) _____
March 11, Sylvia returns to the hospital with a severe infection. This time, her hospital stay is 10 days.	March 11 (10 days) _____
April 20, Sylvia returns to the hospital for chest pains. Her stay for this problem is 3 days.	April 20 (3 days) _____
August 22, Sylvia is admitted to the hospital for bladder cancer surgery. She remains for 7 days.	August 22 (7 days) _____
November 17, Sylvia is hospitalized with complications from the cancer surgery. She remains in the hospital for 60 days before being transferred to a skilled nursing facility.	November 17 (60 days) _____

C. Louise Mayfair visits Broadmoor Medical Clinic on January 2, 20XX, and sees two different PAR providers. Dr. Aldrich charges $85; Dr. Bennett charges $78. Medicare approves $55 for Dr. Aldrich and $45 for Dr. Bennett.

1. If these were Mrs. Mayfair's first medical expenses of the year, and she has no other insurance, calculate how much Mrs. Mayfair owes each provider. *Note:* Use the information in Table 9-2 for this exercise.

   Dr. Aldrich: $_____

   Dr. Bennett: $_____

2. If Mrs. Mayfair's visits were to PAR providers, and Medicare pays 80% of the "approved" charges, why must she pay these fees?

3. If Drs. Aldrich and Bennett had been nonPARs, how much more could they have charged Mrs. Mayfair?

4. Mrs. Mayfair's next visit to Broadmoor Medical Clinic on March 23, 20XX, was to Dr. Carbolla, also a PAR provider. Dr. Carbolla's charge for services was $130, and the Medicare approved amount was $100. Calculate the amount Mrs. Mayfair owes for this encounter. (Assume she has now met her deductible.)

Amount charged by Dr. Carbolla	$_____
Medicare-approved amount	$_____
Medicare will pay	$_____
Mrs. Mayfair owes	$_____

5. Is Mrs. Mayfair responsible for the difference between the amount Dr. Carbolla charged ($130) and the Medicare-approved amount ($100)? Why or why not?

6. Do you as the health insurance professional need to address this $30 difference on Mrs. Mayfair's account? If so, how do you handle it?

Chapter **9 Conquering Medicare's Challenges**

7. Mrs. Mayfair was referred to Dr. Dykstrom on April 14, 20XX, a nonPAR provider (does not accept assignment). Dr. Dykstrom's charge was $115, of which Medicare approves $100. How much does Mrs. Mayfair owe in this scenario?

Dr. Dykstrom's charge (limiting)	$115
Medicare-approved amount	$100
Medicare pays	$_____
Mrs. Mayfair's coinsurance amount	$_____
Allowed excess charge	$_____
Total owed by Mrs. Mayfair	$_____

D. Alicia Freemont, a 66-year-old patient with Medicare Part B, comes to see Dr. Beverly Carson, a dermatologist at Broadmoor Medical Clinic, and asks for dermabrasion treatments to reduce an unsightly scar on her face. You advise Ms. Freemont that this procedure may not covered by Medicare; however, she insists that she wants it anyway.

1. What do you do?
2. Ms. Freemont remarks, "Well, if Medicare won't pay for it, my Medigap supplement policy will." Is she correct? Why or why not?

E. What is the deadline for submitting Medicare claims for services rendered October 1, 2006, through September 30, 2007?

PROJECTS/DISCUSSION TOPICS

A. The Medicare fee schedule is published yearly by CMS. According to the fee schedule, a medical practice is reimbursed a prespecified rate for each service identified on the fee schedule. Discuss the pros and cons of such a method of determining Medicare's payment for healthcare services.

B. Debate the advantages and disadvantages of a PAR versus a nonPAR Medicare provider.

C. Prepare a 1-page paper suitable for display in a medical facility's information library explaining the Qualified Medicare Beneficiary (QMB) and the Specified Low-Income Medicare Beneficiary (SLMB) programs.

D. Generate a chart comparing traditional fee-for-service Medicare with Medicare managed care options (Medicare Advantage).

E. Search the Internet and find a good website for information on how to appeal a denied Medicare claim. Create a page for the Office Procedures Manual detailing a step-by-step procedure for appealing a denied Medicare claim.

A. **Medicare Part B benefits:** When Phyllis Trent, age 72, was in the hospital, she received services from several providers in addition to the hospital. Some providers were PAR; some were nonPAR.

1. The first provider to visit Phyllis was Dr. Frank McDonald, her internist and her regular physician. Dr. McDonald examined Phyllis and referred her to a surgeon, Dr. Maxwell Leonard. (**Note:** Phyllis has not met her deductible for the year.) Dr. McDonald's charges to Medicare were processed as follows:

   Charged for professional services: $500
   Medicare-approved charges: $400

   Phyllis owes deductible of _____

   Medicare paid _____% × $_____ = _____

   Phyllis owes coinsurance of _____% × $_____ = $_____

2. Dr. Leonard, the surgeon, is a Medicare PAR provider. He bills Medicare as follows:

   Charges for professional services: $1800
   Medicare-approved charges: $1200

   Medicare paid _____% × $_____ = _____

   Phyllis owes deductible of _____

   Phyllis owes coinsurance of _____% × $_____ = $_____

3. Phyllis received a statement from the anesthesiologist, who is nonPAR with Medicare and does not accept assignment. The anesthesiologist billed Medicare as follows:

   Charges for professional services: $920
   Medicare-approved charges: $800

   Medicare paid _____% × $_____ = _____

   Phyllis owes deductible of _____

   Phyllis owes coinsurance of _____% × $_____ = $_____

   Plus **excess** charges of _____% × $_____ = $_____

4. Phyllis was transported to the hospital by ambulance. Medicare determined it was medically necessary because it was an emergency. The ambulance claim was processed as follows:

   Charges for ambulance transport: $720
   Medicare-approved charge: $300

   Medicare paid _____% × $_____ = _____

   Phyllis owes deductible of _____

   Phyllis owes coinsurance of _____% × $_____ = $_____

   Plus **excess** charges of _____% × $_____ = $_____

5. Before her surgery, Phyllis had several procedures performed on an outpatient basis at the hospital. The hospital billing was processed as follows:

Hospital charges	$3000
Medicare paid	$1215
Beneficiary copay	$571

What is the total amount Phyllis owes?

6. Phyllis had a series of clinical diagnostic laboratory tests while in the hospital. This claim was processed as follows:

Blood series charge: $280
Medicare-approved charge: $220

Phyllis owes coinsurance of _____% × $_____ = $_____

Plus **excess** charges of _____% × $_____ = $_____

7. How would Phyllis' responsibility for the laboratory tests change if she had not yet satisfied her Part B deductible?

8. Medicare denied one laboratory test as "not medically necessary." What was Phyllis' responsibility for this charge?

B. **Interpreting a Medicare Summary Notice (MSN):** Study the MSN in Fig. 9-1, then answer the following questions.

1. What does the "A" indicate following this patient's Medicare ID number?
2. If the alpha character had been a "D," what would that indicate?
3. This claim was for a _____ day _____.
4. Has the patient met the deductible for this benefit period?
5. What is the total amount the patient may have to pay out-of-pocket?

Medicare Summary Notice

Customer Service Information

Your Medicare Number: 123-45-6789A

If you have questions, write or call:
Medicare
555 Medicare Blvd.
Suite 200
Medicare Building
Medicare, US XXXXX-XXXX

Local: (XXX)XXX-XXXX
Toll-free: 1-800-XXX-XXXX
TTY for Hearing Impaired: 1-800-XXX-XXXX

Jane Beneficiary
123 Any Street
Anytown, Iowa 50000

HELP STOP FRAUD: Beware of door-to-door solicitors offering free or discounted Medicare items or services.

This is a summary of claims processed from 09/15/2000 through 10/15/2000.

PART A HOSPITAL INSURANCE – INPATIENT CLAIMS

Dates of Service	Benefit Days Used	Amount Charged	Non-Covered Charges	Deductible and Coinsurance	You May Be Billed	See Notes Section
Claim number 0000-0000-0000 Broadmoor Medical Clinic Milton, XY 12345 R. L. Jones, MD						a
09/06/00-09/08/00	2 days	$2,399.55	$34.00	$776.00	$810.00	b,c,d

Notes Section:

a. This information is being sent to your private insurer(s). Send any questions regarding benefits to them.

b. $776.00 was applied to your inpatient deductible.

c. Days used are being subtracted from your total inpatient benefits for this benefit period.

d. $34.00 for noncovered charges for which you are liable.

Deductible Information:

You have now met the Part A deductible for this benefit period.

General Information:

If you were offered free items or services but Medicare was billed, please call your local Customer Service at (XXX)XXX-XXXX or toll-free 1-800-XXX-XXXX.

Appeals Information – Part A

If you disagree with any claims decision on this notice, you can request an appeal by **December 15, 2000.** Follow the instructions below:

1) Circle the item(s) you disagree with and explain why you disagree.

2) Send this notice, or a copy, to the address in the "Customer Service Information" box on Page 1.

3) Sign here _____ Phone number (____)_____

THIS IS NOT A BILL – Keep this notice for your records.

Fig. 9-1 Medicare Summary Notice.

C. Elizabeth Franklin has a Medicare supplement policy with Blue Cross and Blue Shield of Iowa. Study the explanation of benefits (EOB) in Fig. 9-2 and answer the following questions.

1. What was the date of service? _____

2. Milton Gastroenterology charged _____.

3. Medicare-approved charge is _____.

4. How much did Medicare pay? _____

5. How much did Blue Cross and Blue Shield pay? _____

6. How much does Ms. Franklin owe on this claim? _____

D. Study the EOB from the Medicare Supplemental Policy in Fig. 9-3.

1. Dr. Jones charged Harold Shalladay $32 for an office visit on 01/03/20XX, and Medicare approved $17.17. Did Medicare pay anything on this claim? If so, why? If not, why not?

2. Medicare sent Mr. Shalladay's claim to his Medicare supplemental carrier, Mutual of Omaha Companies. How much, if anything, did Mutual of Omaha pay toward this claim?

3. What amount can you bill Mr. Shalladay after Medicare and Mutual of Omaha have paid their share of the claim?

4. Can you determine from the EOB if Dr. Jones is Medicare PAR or nonPAR?

5. If Mr. Shalladay were eligible for the QMB program, how much would he have to pay out-of-pocket for this claim?

INTERNET EXPLORATION

A. Log on to **http://www.medicare.gov** and choose "Learn More About Plans in Your Area." Enter your state and county and click "Continue." Study the relevant information about Medigap plans in your state. Compare this information to plans in neighboring states.

B. Local coverage determinations have replaced LMRPs. Log on to **http://www.cms.hhs.gov/coverage/lmrp_contractors_index.asp.** Find the contractor who administers Medicare in your state. Research the site to learn what resources are available to learn more about this topic.

BlueCross BlueShield of Iowa

Explanation of Health Benefits
Medicare Supplement

Page   1

Identification Number:

Claim Number: 43900190CLJX

Provider Number: 4486942

Provider Name: MILTON GASTROENTEROLOGY CLINIC

This is not a bill. It is a statement showing how we applied your Blue Cross and Blue Shield of Iowa coverage to claims submitted to us. If you have a question, please detach the top of this form and send it to us with a letter or call: Customer Service is available to answer calls Mon.–Fri. 8:00 a.m.–4:00 p.m.

Date of Service		SER-VICE CODE	Charge		Medicare Approved		Medicare Benefit Amount		BC/BS Benefit Amount		Notes	Claim Summary
From	Through											
11-01	11-01-20XX	3G	50	00	26	99	21	59	5	40		Total Charges Submitted
												50.00
												Medicare Approved
												26.90
												Medicare Benefit Amount
												21.50
												Noncovered Services
												.00
												Amount You Owe*
												.00
												Blue Cross Blue Shield Benefit Amount For This Claim
This is not a bill and you should not send us money. However, if you have not paid for the service shown here, you may owe the provider. You may want to keep this statement for your records.												5.40

Notes

*This is the amount you owe the provider indicated above. If you have already paid this provider, please disregard this amount.

Identification Number	Group Number	Claim Number	Account Number
Claim Received 12-22-20XX	**Claim Processed** 01-13-20XX	**Provider Name** MILTON GASTROENTEROLOGY CLINIC	**Patient Name**

Fig. 9-2 Blue Cross and Blue Shield explanation of benefits.

175

Medicare Summary Notice

Customer Service Information

Your Medicare Number: 123-45-6789A

If you have questions, write or call:
Medicare
555 Medicare Blvd.
Suite 200
Medicare Building
Medicare, US XXXXX-XXXX

Local: (XXX)XXX-XXXX
Toll-free: 1-800-XXX-XXXX
TTY for Hearing Impaired: 1-800-XXX-XXXX

Harold Shalladay
1552 Airline Drive
Milton, XY 12345

HELP STOP FRAUD: Beware of door-to-door solicitors offering free or discounted Medicare items or services.

This is a summary of claims processed from 02/15/2000 through 03/15/2000.

PART B MEDICAL INSURANCE – ASSIGNED CLAIMS

Dates of Service	Services Provided	Amount Charged	Medicare Approved	Medicare Paid Provider	You May Be Billed	See Notes Section
Claim number 0000-0000-0000 Broadmoor Medical Clinic Milton, XY 12345 R. L. Jones, MD						a
01/31/00	1 Office/Outpatient visit, Est. (99212)	$32.00	$17.17	$0.00	$17.17	b

Notes Section:

a. This information is being sent to your private insurer(s). Send any questions regarding benefits to them.

b. $17.17 of this approved amount has been applied toward your deductible

Deductible Information:

You have now met $38.73 of your Part B deductible.

General Information:

If you were offered free items or services but Medicare was billed, please call your local Customer Service at (XXX)XXX-XXXX or toll-free 1-800-XXX-XXXX.

Appeals Information – Part B

If you disagree with any claims decision on this notice, you can request an appeal by **September 15, 2000.** Follow the instructions below:

1) Circle the item(s) you disagree with and explain why you disagree.

2) Send this notice, or a copy, to the address in the "Customer Service Information" box on Page 1.

3) Sign here _____ Phone number (__) _____

THIS IS NOT A BILL – Keep this notice for your records.

Fig. 9-3 Medicare Summary Notice (Shalladay).

Use a blank claim form at the back of the workbook or the electronic forms found on your Student CD for these exercises. After you have completed each Performance Objective, remove the scoring sheet from the workbook, and attach your completed exercise to it for submission.

Special Notes:

1. The providers at Broadmoor Medical Clinic are PARs.
2. All patients have a current release of information on file.
3. All claims are assigned.
4. Names and addresses of FIs or carriers are listed in Fig. 9-4.

Names and Addresses of FIs and/or Insurance Carriers	
Medicare FI/Carrier	TRISTATE MEDICARE CARRIER PO BOX 8885A ZENOBIA, ZT 5555-8885
Blue Cross/Blue Shield XY	BLUE CROSS AND BLUE SHIELD OF XTRA PO BOX 1212 DUBUQUE, XT 44444-1212
Medicaid FI	MEDICAID FISCAL INTERMEDIARY PO BOX 4692J PORT HURON, XY 51111-0002

Fig. 9-4 Names/addresses of fiscal intermediaries/carriers.

Provider Block	
Broadmoor Medical Clinic 4353 Pine Ridge Drive Milton, XY 12345-0001 Telephone: 555-656-7890 Clinic NPI X100XX1000	Clinic EIN No. 42-1898989 Dr. R. L. Jones NPI 1234567890 Dr. Marilou Lucero NPI 2907511822 Date claims 1 day after encounter

Performance Objective 9-1—Medicare-Only Claim

Conditions: Student will complete a Medicare-only claim using the information in Patient Record No. 052547.
Supplies/Equipment: Patient Record No. 052547, CMS-1500 claim form (paper or electronic)
Guided Completion: For this claim form exercise, you also can use the Guided Completion software found on the Student CD to help you complete this CMS-1500 claim form.
Time Allowed: 50 minutes
Accuracy Needed to Pass: 90%

Procedural Steps	Points Earned	Comments
Evaluator: Note time began:_____		
1. Carefully read and study Patient Record No. 052547.		
2. Complete *all* blocks required for a Medicaid claim. (35)		
3. Proofread claim for accuracy.		
Optional: May deduct points for taking more time than allowed.		

Total Points = 35

Student's Score: _____

Evaluator: _____

Comments:_____

_____

_____

_____

_____

Patient/Insurance Information	Billing Information
Vivian R. Ross	Record No. 052547
DOB: 04/15/1952; widow	02/03/20XX; 99203—$81.00
688 Plum Street	02/03/20XX; 73560—$98.00
Middletown, XT 12345	Diagnosis: Knee Pain (719.46)
555-455-6009	Attending Physician: Marilou Lucero, M.D.
Med. No. 200-00-2222D	
No secondary insurance	

178

Performance Objective 9-2—Medicare Secondary Claim

Conditions: Student will complete a Medicare secondary claim using the information in Patient Record No. 052548.
Supplies/Equipment: Patient Record No. 052548, CMS-1500 claim form (paper or electronic)
Guided Completion: For this claim form exercise, you also can use Guided Completion software found on the Student CD, to help you complete this CMS-1500 form.
Time Allowed: 50 minutes
Accuracy Needed to Pass: 90%

Procedural Steps	Points Earned	Comments
Evaluator: Note time began:_____		
1. Carefully read and study Patient Record No. 052548.		
2. Complete *all* blocks required for a Medicaid secondary claim. (45)		
3. Proofread for accuracy.		
Optional: May deduct points for taking more time than allowed.		

Total Points = 45

Student's Score: _____

Evaluator: _____

Comments:_____

_____

_____

_____

_____

Patient/Insurance Information	Billing Information
Paul C. Robertson	Record No. 052548
DOB: 06/22/1948	02/03/20XX; 99213—$75.00
1555 Westlawn	02/03/20XX; 11730—$40.00
Middletown, XT 12345	02/03/20XX; 85025—$25.00
555-455-2333	Diagnosis: Ingrowing Nail (703.0)
Med. No. 122-00-4444A	Anemia NOS (285.9)
Group insurance through spouse's employer	Attending Physician: R. L. Jones, M.D.
Employer: R & T Bottling Company	
Nelda S. Robertson (wife); DOB: 10/04/1950	
Blue Cross Blue Shield XQZ122004444	
Group No. 544XXL	

Performance Objective 9-3—Medicare/Medicaid Claim

Conditions: Student will complete a Medicare/Medicaid claim using the information in Patient Record No. 052549.
Supplies/Equipment: Patient Record No. 052549, CMS-1500 claim form (paper or electronic)
Time Allowed: 50 minutes
Accuracy Needed to Pass: 90%

Procedural Steps	Points Earned	Comments
Evaluator: Note time began: _____		
1. Carefully read and study Patient Record No. 052549.		
2. Complete *all* blocks required for a Medicare/Medicaid claim. (50)		
3. Proofread claim for accuracy.		
Optional: May deduct points for taking more time than allowed.		

Total Points = 50

Student's Score: _____

Evaluator: _____

Comments:_____

_____

_____

_____

_____

Patient/Insurance Information	Billing Information
Dorothy R. Stevens (single)	Record No. 052549
DOB: 02/26/1939	02/03/20XX; 99213—$75.00.
2934 Valley View	02/03/20XX; 82270—$25.00
Middletown, XT 12345	02/03/20XX; 81000—$15.00
555-478-9011	02/04/20XX; 90732—$10.00
Medicare No. 134-55-6666D	Diagnosis: Hypertension, benign (401.1)
Medicaid No. 22334567HIJ	Palpitations (785.1)
	Heartburn (727.1)
	Attending Physician: R. L. Jones, M.D.

180

Performance Objective 9-4—Medicare/Medigap Claim

Conditions: Student will complete a Medicare/Medigap claim using the information in Patient Record No. 052550.
Supplies/Equipment: Patient Record No. 052550, CMS-1500 claim form (paper or electronic).
Time Allowed: 50 minutes
Accuracy Needed to Pass: 90%

Procedural Steps	Points Earned	Comments
Evaluator: Note time began: _____		
1. Carefully read and study Patient Record No. 052550.		
2. Complete *all* blocks required for a Medicare/Medigap claim. (35)		
3. Proofread claim for accuracy.		
Optional: May deduct points for taking more time than allowed.		

Total Points = 35

Student's Score: _____

Evaluator: _____

Comments:_____

_____

_____

_____

_____

Patient/Insurance Information	Billing Information
Lewis A. Barnes (married)	Record No. 052550
DOB: 10/22/1950	02/03/20XX; 99251—$150.00
92 Hwy 34 West	Diagnosis: Chest pain (786.50)
Middletown, XT 12345	Dyspnea/Resp Abn (786.00)
555-452-8888	Attending Physician: Marilou Lucero, M.D.
Med. No. 211-11-2222A	
Medigap Policy Carrier: Bankers' Life	
Medigap Policy No. 8299466J	

181

Performance Objective 9-5—Interpreting a Medicare Remittance Advice

Conditions: Student will correctly answer questions using the information found on the Medicare remittance advice (RA) #09876 shown in Fig. 9-5.

Supplies/Equipment: Pen/typewriter/computer/printer, Medicare RA #09876

Time Allowed: 30 minutes

Accuracy Needed to Pass: 90%

Procedural Steps	Points Earned	Comments
Evaluator: Note time began: _____		
1. Carefully read and study Medicare RA No. 09876.		
2. Correctly answer the following:		
Question No. 1 (2)		
Question No. 2 (2)		
Question No. 3 (2)		
Question No. 4 (2)		
Question No. 5 (2)		
Question No. 6 (2)		
Question No. 7 (2)		
Question No. 8 (5)		
3. Proofread/recheck your answers. (2)		
Optional: May deduct points for taking more time than allowed.		

Total Points = 21

Student's Score: _____

Evaluator: _____

Comments:_____

_____

_____

_____

_____

GREAT PLAINS HEALTH CARE ALLIANCE
REMITTANCE ADVICE

Broadmoor Medical Clinic
4353 Pine Ridge Drive
Milton, XY 12345-0001

PO Box 89774
Omaha, NE 66677

RA # 09876
Check No./Date: 23445 09/01/20XX
Page 1 of 1
EIN # 42-1898989

Recipient Name/ID	Service Dates	Days/ Units	Paid Claims – Medical	Total Billed	Total Allowed	Paid Amount	Reason Codes
Ross, Vivian R. 200002222D		1	Claim Number: 10202020999CLIXX MEDREC 052547				100
	02/03/20XX	1	99203	81.00	77.00	00.00	100
	02/03/20XX	1	73560	98.00	80.00	26.40	101
Robertson, Paul C. 122004444A			Claim Number: 102020201000CLIXX MEDREC 052548				
	02/03/20XX	1	99213	75.00	72.50	58.00	
	02/03/20XX	1	11730	40.00	30.00	24.00	
	02/03/20XX	1	85025	25.00	25.00	20.00	101
Stevens, Dorothy R. 134556666D CrOv Medicaid22334567HIJ			Claim Number: 102020201001CLIXX MEDREC 052549				
	02/03/20XX	1	99213	75.00	72.50	58.00	
	02/03/20XX	1	82270	25.00	22.50	18.00	
	02/03/20XX	1	81000	15.00	15.00	12.00	
	02/04/20XX	1	90732	10.00	10.00	10.00	102
			Suspended Claims - Medical				
Barnes, Lewis A. 211112222A CrOv Medigap 8299466J	02/03/20XX	1	Claim Number: 102020201002LIXX MEDREC 052550 99251	150.00	00.00	00.00	103
			Denied Claims - Medical				
Goodman, Julia B. 143880909B	01/15/20XX		Claim Number: 10202020925XX MEDREC 052533				
		1	99253	200.00	00.00	00.00	104
		1	99261	150.00	00.00	00.00	104
TOTALS				**944.00**	**404.50**	**226.40**	

RA Reason/Remark Codes:
100 = applied to patient deductible
101 = Medicare allows 100% of charge
102 = Beneficiary copay doesn't apply
103 = Claim under review
104 = Claim denied (second provider filed claim on same service date)

Fig. 9-5 Remittance advice No. 09876.

1. Medicare allowed $77 for Mrs. Ross' office visit on 02/03/20XX; however, they paid nothing toward this charge. Explain why Medicare did not pay 80% of this service.

   _____

2. Show your calculations to prove that the $26.40 Medicare paid on Mrs. Ross' second charge (73560) was correct.

   _____

3. Has Mr. Robertson met his deductible for 20XX? If so, how do you know?

   _____

4. Explain why Medicare paid 100% of Mr. Robertson's procedure No. 85025.

   _____

5. What rationale can you give for the RA to include Ms. Stevens' Medicaid number and her Medicare number?

   _____

6. The RA shows that Mr. Barnes' claim was "suspended." What does that tell you?

   _____

7. Ms. Goodman's claim (from the previous month) was denied. Explain why.

   _____

8. If you determine that Ms. Goodman's claim should be appealed, what is the first step you should take to begin the appeal process?

   _____

Performance Objective 9-6—Appealing a Denied Medicare Claim

Instructions: According to the RA 09876 in Fig. 9-5, the claim for Julia Goodman was denied. On your telephone/written inquiry, the Medicare carrier has advised you that the reason the claim was denied was because "more than one physician filed a claim for similar services for this beneficiary on the same date." The Medicare carrier states further that they will review the claim "if the provider employed at Broadmoor Medical Clinic has documented proof that these services were medically necessary and different from the second claim."

Generate a written response to the Medicare carrier explaining the following facts:

- Dr. Jones was called in for a consultation by the surgeon because the patient, who had had a cholecystectomy, developed a severe reaction to an antibiotic the surgeon had prescribed.
- Dr. Jones saw the patient in his office 1 week later for follow-up.
- You are enclosing documentation (Dr. Jones' consultation report and clinical notes of follow-up visit) to substantiate Dr. Jones' charges.
- You are requesting the Medicare carrier to review the claim for reconsideration.

Note: Ensure that your correspondence includes all of the necessary information for a proper review. List all letter enclosures correctly, and note that a copy is being sent to Ms. Goodman.

Conditions: Student will generate a letter to the Medicare carrier (Great Plains Healthcare Alliance) for the purpose of review and possible payment of Ms. Goodman's denied claim following the directions given in the Procedural Steps.

Supplies/Equipment: Pen/typewriter/paper/computer with word processor, blank document, instructions

Time Allowed: 50 minutes

Accuracy Needed to Pass: 90%

Procedural Steps	Points Earned	Comments
Evaluator: Note time began: _____		
1. Carefully read and study the instructions given for Performance Objective 9-6.		
2. Generate a "mailable" letter using full block style formatting. (10)		
3. Use correct sentence structure, grammar, punctuation, and verbiage. (10)		
4. Compose letter to explain clearly reason for review request. (10)		
5. Generate a letter that closes with courteous request to review claim. (5)		
6. Note enclosures listing required documents and copy notation. (5)		
7. Letter has "picture frame" symmetry. (5)		
Optional: May deduct points for taking more time than allowed.		

Total Points = 45

Student's Score: _____

Evaluator: _____

Comments:_____

_____

_____

Performance Objective 9-7—Posting Claims to Medical Insurance Record Tracking Form

Conditions: Student will post the claims generated in Performance Objectives 9-1 through 9-4 and patient payments and payments received from third-party insurers, using the insurance tracking form shown in Fig. 9-6.

Supplies/Equipment: Pen/typewriter, medical insurance record tracking form

Time Allowed: 50 minutes

Accuracy Needed to Pass: 90%

Procedural Steps	Points Earned	Comments
Evaluator: Note time began: _____		
1. Post the four claims created in Performance Objectives 9-1 through 9-4 to the insurance tracking form.		
Vivian R. Ross (8)		
Paul C. Robertson (13)		
Dorothy R. Stevens (16)		
Lewis A. Barnes (6)		
2. RA and Medicare check was received on 11/28/20XX. Correctly post payments on the insurance tracking form for the following patients:		
Vivian R. Ross (6)		
Paul C. Robertson (6)		
Dorothy R. Stevens (8)		
Lewis A. Barnes (2)		
3. Proofread each entry for accuracy.		
Optional: May deduct points for taking more time than allowed.		

Total Points = 65

Student's Score: _____

Evaluator: _____

Comments:_____

_____

_____

_____

_____

Name: <u>Broadmoor Med. Clinic</u> **Medical Insurance**
Year: <u>20XX</u> Page: <u>122</u> **Record Tracking Form**

Service Provided			Medicare/Medicaid						Private Insurance			Patient Responsibility	
Date of Service	Patient Name & ID Number	CPT Service Codes	Assign-ed Y or N	Amount Billed	Amount Approved	Applied To Deductible	Amount Paid Provider	Amount Paid Patient	Date Sent	Amount Paid Provider	Amount Paid Patient	Amount Patient Paid	Date Paid Check #

Fig. 9-6 Insurance tracking form.

Chapter **9** **Conquering Medicare's Challenges**

Health Insurance Professional's Notebook

A. Because this chapter covers Medicare, students should have accumulated information that would be helpful for filing Medicare claims when they become employed. The following are some suggestions for inclusion in the Health Insurance Professional's Notebook:

- Sample Medicare ID cards
- Charts/tables noting what Medicare Parts A and B cover
- Sample "lifetime" release of information forms
- Name, address, and telephone numbers along with specific personnel to contact for local/state:
  - Medicare Part A FI
  - Medicare Part B carrier
  - Medicare Advantage carrier(s)

- Templates and completed examples of:
  - Medicare-only claims
  - MSP (large group health plan)
  - Medicare/Medicaid claims
  - Medicare/Medigap claims
  - A sample of a current Medicare fee schedule along with an explanation of how PAR and nonPAR charges are calculated
  - An MSN (beneficiary) along with explanation for interpretation
  - A Medicare RA (with explanations)
  - Samples of miscellaneous forms
  - Samples of miscellaneous correspondence

Chapter Check List

Student name: _____

Chapter completion date: _____

1.	Record	Your start time and date: _____
2.	Read	The assigned chapter in the text
3.	View	PowerPoint slides (if available)
4.	Complete	Exercises in the Workbook as assigned
5.	Compare	Your answers with the answers posted on the bulletin board/website/handout
6.	Correct	Your answers
7.	Complete	All tests and required activities
8.	Read	Assigned readings (if any)
9.	Complete	Chapter performance objectives (competencies), if any
10.	Evaluate	Chapter performance and submit to your instructor
11.	Record	Your ending time and date: _____
12.	Move on	Begin next chapter as assigned

Student name: _____

Chapter completion date: _____

Evaluate your classroom performance. Complete the self-evaluation, and submit it to your instructor. When your instructor returns this form to you, compare your self-evaluation with the evaluation completed by your instructor.

Skill	Student Self-Evaluation			Instructor Evaluation		
	Good	**Average**	**Poor**	**Good**	**Average**	**Poor**
Attendance/punctuality						
Personal appearance						
Applies effort						
Is self-motivated						
Is courteous						
Has positive attitude						
Completes assignments in timely manner						
Works well with others						

Student's Initials: _____

Date: _____

Instructor's Initials: _____

Date: _____

Points Possible: _____

Points Awarded: _____

Chapter Grade: _____

10 Military Carriers: TRICARE and CHAMPVA

TRICARE (formerly CHAMPUS) provides coverage to the families of active duty service members, families of service members who died while on active duty, and retirees and their families, whether or not the veteran is disabled. TRICARE is administered by the Department of Defense.

CHAMPVA is a health benefits program in which the Department of Veterans Affairs (VA) shares the cost of certain healthcare services and supplies with eligible beneficiaries—qualifying disabled veterans and certain dependents of deceased veterans. CHAMPVA is managed by the VA's Health Administration Center (HAC) in Denver, Colorado. TRICARE and CHAMPVA are federal programs; however, an individual who is eligible for TRICARE is not eligible for CHAMPVA.

Some medical practices see few patients eligible for either the TRICARE or the CHAMPVA program; however, the health insurance professional still should be familiar with these two programs, what they cover, the rules and regulations for submitting claims, and how to interpret the explanation of benefits (EOB). The activities and exercises contained in this workbook chapter are designed to help prepare the health insurance professional for these tasks.

WORKBOOK CHAPTER OBJECTIVES

After completing the workbook activities for Chapter 10, the student should be able to:
- Define the terms used in the chapter.
- Answer the review questions to within the evaluation criteria set by the instructor.
- Demonstrate the ability to process information to find thoughtful solutions to problems, to make judgments or decisions, or to reason.
- Explore websites to acquire information needed to complete workbook activities.
- Complete specific forms common to the health insurance professional's role in military claims.
- Generate information and collect documents applicable to military claims for inclusion in the student's personal Health Insurance Professional's Notebook.
- Undertake self-analysis/evaluation in completed workbook activities.

DEFINING CHAPTER TERMS

Using the computer (or typewriter), students should key an accurate definition for each of the chapter terms listed. These definitions should be in the students' own words. When finished, students should compare their definitions with those listed in the glossary at the back of the textbook, correcting any inaccuracies.

accepting assignment
beneficiaries
catastrophic cap (cat cap)
CHAMPUS Maximum Allowable Charge
CHAMPVA for Life (CFL)
Civilian Health and Medical Program of the Department of Veterans Affairs (CHAMPVA)
Civilian Health and Medical Program of the Uniformed Services (CHAMPUS)
claims processor
covered charges
Defense Enrollment Eligibility Reporting System (DEERS)
lead agent (LA)
Military Health System (MHS)
military treatment facility (MTF)
nonavailability statement (NAS)

other health insurance (OHI)
primary care manager (PCM)
regional director
remote assignment
reserve components (RCs)
sponsor
TRICARE
TRICARE Extra
TRICARE for Life (TFL)
TRICARE Management Activity
TRICARE Prime
TRICARE Prime Remote
TRICARE Standard
TRICARE Standard Supplemental Insurance
TRICARE's allowable charge
XPressClaim

191

Multiple Choice

Directions: In the questions/statements presented, choose the response that **best** answers/completes the stem by circling the letter that precedes it.

1. TRICARE's two main objectives are:
   a. Health and welfare
   b. Accessibility and affordability
   c. Manageability and cost-effectiveness
   d. Supply healthcare during war and peace

2. TRICARE is administered regionally, serving ____ separate regions.
   a. 3
   b. 5
   c. 7
   d. 12

3. Each region is headed by an individual who is responsible for oversight of all healthcare delivery activities within his or her region and is called a:
   a. Claims review officer
   b. Fiscal intermediary
   c. Regional carrier
   d. Regional director

4. The name of the total healthcare system of the U.S. uniformed services is:
   a. Military Health System
   b. U.S. Military Insurance Program
   c. Federal Uniformed Services Program
   d. National Military Health Care System

5. TRICARE is administered by:
   a. The Department of Defense
   b. The Centers for Medicare and Medicaid Services (CMS) (formerly the Health Care Financing Administration)
   c. The VA
   d. Individual state governments

6. The main purpose of the TRICARE Management Activity (TMA) is to:
   a. Keep TRICARE premiums low
   b. Adjudicate TRICARE claims
   c. Coordinate TRICARE benefits with other health insurance (OHI)
   d. Enhance the performance of TRICARE worldwide

7. The computerized data bank that lists all active and retired military service members is called:
   a. TMA
   b. FEMA
   c. DEERS
   d. COBRA

8. Similar to Medicaid and Medicare, TRICARE-eligible individuals are referred to as:
   a. Enrollees
   b. Plan members
   c. Beneficiaries
   d. Covered employees

9. The fee-for-service option offer by TRICARE, which has basically the same benefits as the original CHAMPUS program, is:
   a. TRICARE Standard
   b. TRICARE Extra
   c. TRICARE Prime
   d. TRICARE for Life

10. The TRICARE option similar to preferred provider organization–type managed care is:
    a. TRICARE Standard
    b. TRICARE Extra
    c. TRICARE Prime
    d. TRICARE for Life

11. CHAMPVA is managed by:
    a. Social Security Administration
    b. CMS
    c. The VA's HAC
    d. Individual state governments

12. CHAMPVA eligibility can be lost if certain demographic changes occur, such as:
    a. A widow remarrying
    b. Divorcing the sponsor
    c. Becoming eligible for Medicare
    d. All of the above

13. CHAMPVA is the last payer after all other third-party payers have met their obligations except for:
    a. Medicaid
    b. CHAMPVA supplemental insurance
    c. OHI
    d. a and b are correct

14. The deadline for filing military claims is:
    a. 60 days
    b. 90 days
    c. 1 year
    d. 2 years

15. The annual catastrophic (cat) cap for CHAMPVA is:
    a. $1000
    b. $3000
    c. $5000
    d. $10,000

True/False

Directions: Place a "T" in the blank preceding the sentence if it is true; place an "F" if it is false.

_____ 1.   The sponsor's relationship to the beneficiary creates eligibility under TRICARE.

_____ 2.   Military retirees and their family members are not eligible for TRICARE.

_____ 3.   TRICARE pays for only their allowed services, supplies, and procedures.

_____ 4.   There is no "cost sharing" under TRICARE regulations.

_____ 5.   Active duty personnel are not CHAMPUS-eligible and are automatically enrolled in TRICARE Standard.

_____ 6.   TRICARE Prime is a health maintenance organization–type managed care option in which MTFs are the principal source of healthcare.

_____ 7.   Under TRICARE Prime's point of service (POS) option, enrollees are allowed to receive healthcare services only from providers within the POS network.

_____ 8.   Under TRICARE for Life, TRICARE pays Medicare deductibles and coinsurance or copayment amounts up to 115% of Medicare-allowable charges.

_____ 9.   Eligibility for patients claiming TRICARE and CHAMPVA coverage should be verified immediately.

_____ 10.   TRICARE participating providers (PARs) must accept the TRICARE allowable charge as payment in full for the healthcare services provided and cannot balance bill.

_____ 11.   Patients using TRICARE Standard are usually responsible for submitting their own claims.

_____ 12.   In the case of nonparticipating providers (nonPARs), TRICARE Standard patients must file their own claims; however, the reimbursement check is sent to the provider.

_____ 13.   Even though electronic claims submission is preferred by most major carriers, military carriers still prefer paper claims.

_____ 14.   The deadline for submitting military claims varies from region to region.

Short Answer/Fill-in-the-Blank

1. List the three basic plans available under the TRICARE program.

_____

_____

_____

2. The service member, whether in active duty, retired, or deceased, is called the _____.

3. List the various categories of TRICARE-eligible individuals.

_____

_____

_____

4. List three advantages of TRICARE Standard.

_____

_____

_____

5. List three responsibilities of a primary care manager.

_____

_____

_____

6. List the categories of individuals who are eligible for TRICARE Prime Remote.

_____

_____

_____

7. Explain the purpose of a nonavailability statement.

_____

_____

8. What are the eligibility criteria for TRICARE for Life?

_____

_____

_____

9. How might the health insurance professional verify eligibility for benefits under one of the military's healthcare programs?

_____

_____

_____

10. List the categories of individuals who are eligible for CHAMPVA.

_____

_____

_____

11. List four types of medical services where preauthorization may be required for CHAMPVA beneficiaries.

_____

_____

_____

_____

CRITICAL THINKING ACTIVITIES

A. Patient Betsy Froman has been referred to you, the health insurance professional at Broadmoor Clinic, with the following question: "I am currently participating in TRICARE Prime. Do I need to re-enroll in TRICARE Prime on a yearly basis?" What should you tell Ms. Froman?

B. Assume that the Broadmoor providers are nonPARs for military claims and require patients to file their own claims. Patient Arnold Chessworth, a CHAMPVA-eligible patient, asks you for help in getting claims filing information. Generate an instruction sheet for military patients on where to find this information; include online sources and toll-free telephone numbers.

CASE STUDIES

Refer to Tables 10-1 and 10-2 for help with the following case studies.

Table 10-1 TRICARE Cost Comparison Chart: Active Duty Family Members

	TRICARE Prime	TRICARE Extra	TRICARE Standard
Annual Deductible	None	$150/individual or $300/family for E-5 and above; $50/$100 for E-4 and below	$150/individual or $300/family for E-5 and above; $50/$100 for E-4 and below
Annual Enrollment Fee	None	None	None
Civilian Outpatient Visit	No cost	15% of negotiated fee	20% of negotiated fee
Civilian Inpatient Admission	No cost	Greater of $25 or $13.32/day	Greater of $25 or $13.32/day
Civilian Inpatient Mental Health	No cost	$20/day	$20/day
Civilian Inpatient Skilled Nursing Facility Care	$0 per diem charge per admission; no separate copayments/cost share for separately billed professional charges		

Chapter **10** **Military Carriers: TRICARE and CHAMPVA**

Table 10-2 TRICARE Cost Comparison Chart: Retirees, Their Families, and Others

	TRICARE Prime	TRICARE Extra	TRICARE Standard
Annual Deductible	None	$150/individual or $300/family	$150/individual or $300/family
Annual Enrollment Fee	$230/individual or $460/family	None	None
Civilian Copays	$12	20% of negotiated fee	25% of allowed charges for covered service
Emergency Care	$30		
Mental Health Visit	$25; $17 for group visit		
Civilian Inpatient Cost Share	Greater of $11/day or $25 per admission; no separate copayment for separately billed professional fees	Lesser of $250/day or 25% of negotiated charges plus 20% of negotiated fees	Lesser of $535/day or 25% of billed charges plus 25% of allowed professional fees
Civilian Inpatient Skilled Nursing Facility Care	Greater of $11/day or $25 per admission; no separate copayment for separately billed professional fees	$250 per diem cost share or 20% cost share of total charges, whichever is less; institutional services, plus 20% cost share of separately billed professional charges	25% cost share of allowed charges for institutional services, plus 25% cost share of allowable for separately billed professional charges
Civilian Inpatient Behavorial Health	$40/day; no charge for separately billed professional charges	20% of total charge. Plus, 20% of the allowable charge for separately billed professional services	**High volume hospitals:** 25% hospital specific per diem, plus 25% of the allowable charge for separately billed professional services **Low volume hospitals:** $175 per day or 25% of the billed charges, whichever is lower, plus 25% of the allowable charge for separately billed services

A. Christine Moss comes to Broadmoor Medical Clinic complaining of upper gastrointestinal pain. She subsequently is admitted to Broadmoor Medical Center on an outpatient basis for endoscopy. The following are the procedures performed on Mrs. Moss along with the charges:

Date of Service	CPT Code	Procedure/Service	TRICARE-Approved Charge
11/29/20XX	99244	Office consultation	$166.00
11/30/20XX	43239	Upper GI endoscopy with biopsy*	$625.00
11/30/20XX	43453-78	Dilate esophagus*	$670.00

*Outpatient procedure.

Aaron Moss, her husband, is currently on active duty in Afghanistan with an E-4 ranking. They have no children, so Mrs. Moss has "individual" coverage.

1. If Mrs. Moss is covered under TRICARE Prime, what is her annual deductible?

2. If she had TRICARE Extra, what would her annual (individual) deductible be?

3. Would Mrs. Moss' deductible be greater if she had enrolled in TRICARE Standard? If so, how much?

4. Assuming that Mrs. Moss has TRICARE Standard and she has met her deductible for the year, what would her copay be for (a) the office consultation, and (b) the outpatient procedures? Assume that the charges listed are the same as TRICARE's "allowable charges."

5. If Mrs. Moss was enrolled in TRICARE Extra, what would be the total amount she would have to pay out-of-pocket for the procedures and services rendered on 11/29/20XX and 11/30/20XX (a) if she had not yet met her annual deductible, and (b) if she had met her annual deductible?

B. Patrick Olson is a retired colonel of the U.S. Army. He is admitted as an inpatient to Broadmoor Medical Center for a knee replacement. The colonel only has to pay the individual deductible of $150. Other family members pay the balance. The orthopedic surgeon's bill for Col. Olson's hospitalization for $8825 is broken down as follows:

Date of Service	Procedure/Service	TRICARE-Approved Charge
11/29/20XX	Initial hospital visit	$150.00
11/30/20XX	Surgery (total knee replacement)	$8000.00
12/01/20XX through 12/05/20XX	Subsequent hospital visits × 5	$550.00
12/06/20XX	Discharge visit	$125.00

1. Assuming this patient has a family policy and has met any required annual deductibles, what would be the total out-of-pocket amount Col. Olson would have to pay for just the professional service listed (not including the enrollment fee) if he was enrolled in (a) TRICARE Prime, (b) TRICARE Extra, or (c) TRICARE Standard? Assume that the fees charged are the same as the "allowed fees."

2. Assuming this patient had not met his annual deductible, what would be the total out-of-pocket amount Col. Olson would have to pay if he was enrolled in (a) TRICARE Prime, (b) TRICARE Extra, or (c) TRICARE Standard?

3. In this scenario, after Col. Olson was discharged from Broadmoor Medical Center, he was transferred to a civilian inpatient skilled nursing facility (SNF) for a 10-day stay. If the SNF charges $180/day, how much did this stage of his rehabilitative care cost him if he was enrolled in (a) TRICARE Prime, (b) TRICARE Extra, or (c) TRICARE Standard?

INTERNET EXPLORATION

A. The health insurance professional should have ready access to the latest handbooks available for guidance in submitting claims. Log on to the following websites and peruse the electronic versions of the handbooks.

1. TRICARE website: **http://www.tricare.osd.mil/tricarehandbook**
2. CHAMPVA website: **http://www.va.gov/hac/forbeneficiaries/champva/handbook.asp**

B. Create a list of addresses where the various military claims (TRICARE and CHAMPVA) should be sent and a list of telephone numbers to call for questions and claims processing assistance.

C. The website **http://www.tricare.mil/faqs** provides extensive information and answers to frequently asked questions regarding TRICARE. Log on to this website and search for information that may be helpful to a health insurance professional.

Performance Objective 10-1—CMS-1500 Claim: TRICARE Standard Coverage Only

Conditions: Student will complete a CMS-1500 claim form for a patient with TRICARE Standard (only) using the information in Patient Record No. 052555.

Supplies/Equipment: Patient Record No. 052555, CMS-1500 claim form (paper or electronic)

Guided Completion: For this claim form exercise, you also can use the Guided Completion software found on the Student CD to help you complete this CMS-1500 claim form.

Time Allowed: 50 minutes

Accuracy Needed to Pass: 90%

Procedural Steps	Points Earned	Comments
Evaluator: Note time began: _____		
1. Carefully read and study Patient Record No. 052555.		
2. Complete *all* blocks required for a TRICARE claim.		
3. Proofread claim for accuracy.		
Optional: May deduct points for taking more time than allowed.		

Total Points = _____

Student's Score: _____

Evaluator: _____

Comments: _____

_____

_____

_____

_____

Note: Use the information in the provider block below for all CMS-1500 claims in this chapter.

Provider Block	
Broadmoor Medical Clinic	Clinic EIN # 421898989
4353 Pine Ridge Drive	Dr. R.L. Jones NPI 1234567890
Milton, XY 12345-0001	Dr. Marilou Lucero NPI # 2907511822
Clinic NPI X100XX1000	Date claims 1 day after examination
Telephone: 555-466-3422	

Patient/Insurance Information	Billing Information
Marie I. Carson	Record No. 052555
DOB: 08/29/1975	11/16/20XX; 99395—$150.00
2334 Apple Tree Cove	11/16/20XX; 85025—$40.00
Middletown, XT 12345	11/16/20XX; 36415—$15.00
555-466-3422	11/16/20XX; 88142—$35.00
ID # 111-22-3333	Diagnosis: Annual physical examination (V70.0)
Relationship to sponsor: Spouse	Attending Physician: Marilou Lucero, M.D.
Employer: Unemployed	
Sponsor Name: Alan V. Carson; USMC/AD	
Sponsor's Address: APO 47349A, NY, NY, 22222	
Sponsor's DOB: 03/18/1972	
Sponsor's ID # 111010122	

Performance Objective 10-2—CMS-1500 Claim: TRICARE Prime with Other Health Insurance

Conditions: Student will complete a CMS-1500 claim form for a patient with TRICARE Prime and group health insurance (OHI) using the information in Patient Record No. 052556.

Supplies/Equipment: Patient Record No. 052556, CMS-1500 claim form (paper or electronic)

Time Allowed: 50 minutes

Accuracy Needed to Pass: 90%

Procedural Steps	Points Earned	Comments
Evaluator: Note time began: _____		
1. Carefully read and study Patient Record No. 052556		
2. Complete *all* blocks required for a TRICARE claim.		
3. Proofread claim for accuracy.		
Optional: May deduct points for taking more time than allowed.		

Total Points = _____

Student's Score: _____

Evaluator: _____

Comments: _____

_____

_____

_____

_____

Patient/Insurance Information	Billing Information
Wyatt D. Peters	Record No. 052556
DOB: 12/13/2002	11/15/20XX; 99383—$125.00
811 Linden Circle	11/20/20XX; 92506—$110.00
Middletown, XT 12345	11/21/20XX; 99241—$65.00
555-321-5050	Diagnosis: Autism (299.00)
ID # 222-11-4567	Attending Physician: R.L. Jones, M.D.
Sponsor name: David R. Peters	
Sponsor DOB: 04/28/1977	
Sponsor SSN: 202-22-8765	
Sponsor service status: USN	
Relationship to sponsor: Child	
Other insurance: Metropolitan Group Health	
Policy holder: Helen Peters; DOB: 01/01/1980	
Employer: Clinton County School District	
Policy # 655778111; Group # YZ449	

Performance Objective 10-3—CMS-1500 Claim: CHAMPVA Coverage Only

Conditions: Student will complete a CMS-1500 claim form for a patient with CHAMPVA (only) coverage using the information in Patient Record No. 052557.

Supplies/Equipment: Patient Record No. 052557, CMS-1500 claim form (paper or electronic)

Time Allowed: 50 minutes

Accuracy Needed to Pass: 90%

Procedural Steps	Points Earned	Comments
Evaluator: Note time began: _____		
1. Carefully read and study Patient Record No. 052557.		
2. Complete CHAMPVA claim.		
3. Proofread claim for accuracy.		
Optional: May deduct points for taking more time than allowed.		

Total Points = _____

Student's Score: _____

Evaluator: _____

Comments: _____

_____

_____

_____

_____

Patient/Insurance Information	Billing Information
Edward (Eddie) T. Houston	Record No. 052557
DOB: 01/10/1949	11/21/20XX; 80053—$37.00
14 Baluster Road	11/21/20XX; 80061—$48.00
Middletown, XT 12345	11/21/20XX; 85025—$35.00
555-366-1222	11/21/20XX; 84153—$63.00
ID # 009-66-0987	11/21/20XX; 36415—$14.00
Employer: Unemployed	Diagnosis: Hypertension, benign (401.1)
Sponsor name: Self (single)	Diagnosis: Long-term drug use (V58.69)
Sponsor service status: USAF Ret.	Attending Physician: R.L. Jones, M.D.
No secondary insurance	

Performance Objective 10-4—CMS-1500 Claim: Medicare and CHAMPVA

Conditions: Student will complete a CMS-1500 claim form for a patient with Medicare and CHAMPVA coverage using the information in Patient Record No. 052558.

Supplies/Equipment: Patient Record No. 052558, CMS-1500 claim form (paper or electronic)

Time Allowed: 50 minutes

Accuracy Needed to Pass: 90%

Procedural Steps	Points Earned	Comments
Evaluator: Note time began: _____		
1. Carefully read and study Patient Record No. 052558.		
2. Complete *all* blocks required for a Medicare/CHAMPVA claim.		
3. Proofread claim for accuracy.		
Optional: May deduct points for taking more time than allowed.		

Total Points = _____

Student's Score: _____

Evaluator: _____

Comments: _____

_____

_____

_____

Patient/Insurance Information	Billing Information
Dora L. Michaels	Record No. 052558
DOB: 10/23/1941	11/21/20XX; 74400-26—$140.00
29 Orchard Meadows	11/21/20XX; 71020-26—$55.00
Middletown, XT 12345	11/21/20XX; 76770-26—$108.00
555-444-6666	Diagnosis: Bladder neck obstruction (596.0)
ID # 222-11-4567	Diagnosis: Respiratory distress (786.09)
Medicare ID # 222-11-4567B	Attending Physician: R.L. Jones, M.D.
Sponsor name: Alvin Michaels; DOB: 02/18/1937	POS: 22
Sponsor SSN: 220-00-0001	
Sponsor service status: USMC	
Relationship to sponsor: Spouse	
Employer: Unemployed	

Performance Objective 10-5—Posting to the Insurance Record Tracking Form

Post the four military claims completed in Performance Objectives 10-1 through 10-4 to the insurance record tracking form (Fig. 10-1).

Conditions: Student will post the claims generated in Performance Objectives 10-1 through 10-4 to the insurance tracking form (see Fig. 10-1).

Supplies/Equipment: Pen/typewriter, medical insurance record tracking form

Time Allowed: 50 minutes

Accuracy Needed to Pass: 90%

Procedural Steps	Points Earned	Comments
Evaluator: Note time began: _____		
1. Assemble the claims generated in Performance Objectives 10-1 through 10-4		
M. Carson (8)		
W. Peters (8)		
E. Houston (8)		
D. Michaels (8)		
2. Insert correct page heading. (3)		
3. Proofread each entry for accuracy.		
Optional: May deduct points for taking more time than allowed.		

Total Points = 35

Student's Score: _____

Evaluator: _____

Comments: _____

_____

_____

_____

_____

Name: _____

Year: _____ Page: _____

Medical Insurance
Record Tracking Form

Service Provided			Medicare/Medicaid						Private Insurance			Patient Responsibility	
Date of Service	Patient Name & ID Number	CPT Service Codes	Assign-ed Y or N	Amount Billed	Amount Approved	Applied To Deductible	Amount Paid Provider	Amount Paid Patient	Date Sent	Amount Paid Provider	Amount Paid Patient	Amount Patient Paid	Date Paid Check #

Fig. 10-1 Insurance tracking form.

Health Insurance Professional's Notebook

Because this chapter covers TRICARE and CHAMPVA claims, students should have accumulated information that would be helpful for filing military-associated claims when they become employed. The following are some suggestions for inclusion in the Health Insurance Professional's Notebook:

- Sample TRICARE/CHAMPVA ID cards
- Current charts/tables noting what various military plans cover
- Name, address, and telephone number(s) along with specific personnel to contact for:
  - TRICARE claims
  - Current CHAMPVA claims
  - Local military healthcare facilities (if any)

- Templates and completed examples of:
  - TRICARE-only claims
  - TRICARE with OHI
  - CHAMPVA-only claims
  - MEDICARE/CHAMPVA claims

- Representative examples of TRICARE and CHAMPVA EOBs (with explanations)
- Samples of miscellaneous forms affiliated with military claims processing
- Other documents as applicable

"JUST FOR FUN!"

A. Develop a crossword puzzle of chapter terms.

B. Generate a matching exercise using the chapter terms.

Chapter Check List

Student name: _____

Chapter completion date: _____

1.	Record	Your start time and date: _____
2.	Read	The assigned chapter in the text
3.	View	PowerPoint slides (if available)
4.	Complete	Exercises in the Workbook as assigned
5.	Compare	Your answers with the answers posted on the bulletin board/website/handout
6.	Correct	Your answers
7.	Complete	All tests and required activities
8.	Read	Assigned readings (if any)
9.	Complete	Chapter performance objectives (competencies), if any
10.	Evaluate	Chapter performance and submit to your instructor
11.	Record	Your ending time and date: _____
12.	Move on	Begin next chapter as assigned

PERFORMANCE EVALUATION

Evaluate your classroom performance. Complete the self-evaluation, and submit it to your instructor. When your instructor returns this form to you, compare your self-evaluation with the evaluation completed by your instructor.

Skill	Student Self-Evaluation			Instructor Evaluation		
	Good	Average	Poor	Good	Average	Poor
Attendance/punctuality						
Personal appearance						
Applies effort						
Is self-motivated						
Is courteous						
Has positive attitude						
Completes assignments in timely manner						
Works well with others						

Student's Initials: _____

Date: _____

Instructor's Initials: _____

Date: _____

Points Possible: _____

Points Awarded: _____

Chapter Grade: _____

11 Miscellaneous Carriers: Workers' Compensation and Disability Insurance

Up to now, the textbook has been presenting information regarding healthcare insurance for individuals with illness or injuries that are not related to employment. Workers' compensation is different from all the other types of insurance because to be eligible for benefits, the individual's injury or illness must be work related. As we learned from the text, most workers in the United States are covered by the Workers' Compensation Law, and the employer, not the employee, pays the premiums.

Disability insurance, another type of insurance discussed in Chapter 11, differs from regular health insurance and workers' compensation. Disability insurance replaces a portion of an individual's earned income in the event he or she is unable to work because of accident or sickness. An individual might have disability insurance through his or her employer or a private policy unrelated to work. Two well-known federal disability insurance programs are Social Security Disability Insurance (SSDI) and Supplemental Security Income (SSI).

This workbook chapter presents activities and exercises that reinforce the information presented in Chapter 11 of the text and help prepare the health insurance professional for on-the-job tasks associated with workers' compensation and disability claims.

WORKBOOK CHAPTER OBJECTIVES

After completing the workbook activities for Chapter 11, the student should be able to:
- Define the terms used in the chapter.
- Answer the review questions to within the evaluation criteria set by the instructor.
- Demonstrate the ability to process information to find thoughtful solutions to problems, to make judgments or decisions, or to reason.
- Participate in classroom discussions on workers' compensation and disability insurance topics at an informed level.
- Find and explore websites to obtain information needed for successful completion of workbook activities.
- Complete specific forms common to the health insurance professional's role in workers' compensation and disability insurance claims and reports.
- Generate information and collect documents applicable to workers' compensation and disability insurance for inclusion in the student's personal Health Insurance Professional's Notebook.
- Undertake self-analysis/evaluation in completed workbook activities.

DEFINING CHAPTER TERMS

Using the computer (or typewriter), students should key an accurate definition for each of the chapter terms listed. These definitions should be in the students' own words. When finished, students should compare their definitions with those listed in the glossary at the back of the textbook, correcting any inaccuracies.

activities of daily living
Americans with Disabilities Act (ADA)
benefit cap
Black Lung Benefits Act
casual employee
coming and going rule
Disability and Health Team
disability income insurance
earned income
egregious
employment network
exemption
Federal Employment Compensation Act (FECA)
Federal Employment Liability Act (FELA)
financial means test
instrumental activities of daily living
interstate commerce

job deconditioning
Longshore and Harbor Workers' Compensation Act
long-term disability
Merchant Marine Act (Jones Act)
modified own-occupation policy
no fault insurance
occupational therapy
ombudsman
own-occupation policy
permanent and stationary
permanent disability
permanent partial disability
permanent total disability
progress or supplemental report
protected health information
short-term disability
Social Security Disability Insurance (SSDI)

211

Supplemental Security Income (SSI)
temporarily disabled
temporary partial disability
temporary total disability

Ticket to Work Program
treating source
vocational rehabilitation
workers' compensation

ASSESSMENT

Multiple Choice

Directions: In the questions/statements presented, choose the response that **best** answers/completes the stem, and circle the letter that precedes it.

1. Workers' compensation got its start in the 1800s in:
   a. The United States
   b. England
   c. Germany
   d. Japan

2. In workers' compensation insurance, the premiums are paid by:
   a. The employee
   b. The employer
   c. Split equally between employer and employee
   d. There are no premiums with workers' compensation

3. The federal program that establishes workers' compensation for nonmilitary federal government employees is known by the acronym:
   a. OSHA
   b. FEMA
   c. FECA
   d. FELA

4. The federal program that establishes workers' compensation for railroad workers engaged in interstate commerce is known by the acronym:
   a. OSHA
   b. FEMA
   c. FECA
   d. FELA

5. An individual responsible for investigating and resolving workers' complaints against the employer or insurance company that is denying the benefits is called a(n):
   a. Ombudsman
   b. Lead agent
   c. Fiscal intermediary
   d. Claims investigator

6. The time limit for filing a workers' compensation claim is established by:
   a. The employer
   b. The federal government
   c. Individual state statutes
   d. The insurance company that issues the policy

7. An injury or illness that is job related typically must be reported to the employer:

a. Within 24 hours

b. Within 2 days

c. There are no time limits

d. Time limits vary from state to state

8. A patient's inability to perform normal job duties at the previous level of expertise as a result of being absent from work is called:

a. Acquiescing

b. Noncompliance

c. Job deconditioning

d. Job reclassification

9. After the initial attending physician report has been filed, periodic updates must be provided to the employer/insurer, called:

a. Progress reports

b. Supplemental reports

c. Period update reports

d. a and b

10. The type of insurance that replaces a portion of earned income when an individual is unable to perform the requirements of his or her job because of non–job-related injury or illness is called:

a. SSDI

b. Workers' compensation

c. Indemnity insurance

d. Disability insurance

11. The maximum amount of benefits that can be received in a specific time period is called:

a. A benefit cap

b. Liability limit

c. Payment closure

d. A catastrophic cap

12. The federal act established in 1990 that protects the civil rights of individuals with disabilities is called the:

a. Consolidated Omnibus Budget Reconciliation Act (COBRA)

b. Occupational Health and Safety Administration (OSHA) Act

c. Social Security Disability Insurance (SSDI)

d. Americans with Disabilities Act (ADA)

13. The examining body that determines if an applicant qualifies for SSDI is the:

a. State Disability Determination unit

b. Social Security Administration

c. Centers for Medicare and Medicaid Services (CMS)

d. Department of Health and Human Services

14. The method of determining whether or not an individual is eligible for SSI benefits is through a(n):

a. Activities of daily living evaluation

b. Financial means test

c. Spend-down process

d. Patient/provider interview

15. The program that provides greater choice in selecting the providers and rehabilitation services disabled individuals need to help them keep working or return to work is called:

a. SSI

b. SSDI

c. Ticket to Work

d. CDC Disability and Health

True/False

Directions: Place a "T" in the blank preceding the numbered statement if it is true; place an "F" if it is false.

_____ 1. Employers must purchase workers' compensation policies from the state in which their business operates.

_____ 2. In the United States, any employee who is injured on the job or develops an employment-related illness that prevents the individual from working is likely to be eligible to collect workers' compensation benefits.

_____ 3. If an employee is injured on the job, the employer can be penalized if the cause of injury or illness was due to the employer being conspicuously negligent.

_____ 4. Most state workers' compensation laws include coverage for injuries sustained while an employee is commuting to and from work.

_____ 5. If a workers' compensation claim is denied, the worker may file a claim with his or her health insurance carrier only after all workers' compensation appeals have been exhausted.

_____ 6. The first thing an injured employee must do is call his or her family physician.

_____ 7. Workers' compensation claims must be submitted on the universal CMS-1500 claim form.

_____ 8. As long as a workers' compensation claim is pending, the provider cannot bill the patient.

_____ 9. Workers' compensation patients are not required to sign a release of information form for a claim form to be filed.

_____ 10. An individual may receive benefits from only one federal disability program even if he or she meets all the eligibility requirements for several.

_____ 11. The SSI program provides monthly cash payments to low-income aged, blind, and disabled individuals.

_____ 12. The CDC Disability and Health Team's focus is promoting safe workplace procedures.

Short Answer

Directions: Answer each question fully in the space provided.

1. List four work-related incidents in which injury occurs that would be exceptions to the employee drawing workers' compensation benefits.

_____

_____

_____

_____

2. List five classifications of businesses that do not have to provide workers' compensation for their employees.

_____

_____

_____

_____

_____

3. Workers' compensation insurance is **no-fault insurance**. Explain what this means.

_____

4. List the four major benefit components to workers' compensation.

_____

_____

_____

_____

5. List the physician's two distinct roles in workers' compensation claims.

_____

_____

6. List and explain the various classifications of workers' compensation disability cases, as mandated by federal law.

_____

_____

_____

7. List and explain the two major classifications of disability coverage.

_____

_____

8. List five pertinent items the attending physician's statement must include when filing a disability claim.

_____

_____

_____

_____

_____

9. List the nine federal disability programs.

_____

_____

_____

_____

_____

_____

_____

_____

_____

10. Name at least four of the commonly used factors federal programs look at in assessing disability.

_____

_____

_____

_____

11. Name the two criteria an individual must meet to become eligible for SSDI.

_____

_____

12. List the three ways disabled individuals can receive SSDI.

_____

_____

_____

13. Discuss the health insurance professional's role in the disability claims process.

_____

_____

_____

CRITICAL THINKING ACTIVITIES

A. Casey Belmont, a 33-year-old established patient, comes to Broadmoor Medical Clinic for treatment of a back injury. Casey, who is employed by National Parcel Delivery Service, claims he was injured at work while lifting a heavy box onto a conveyor. When Casey's chart arrives in your office for claims processing, you notice that the clinical notes from this visit are added to his ongoing health record. Is this appropriate? Why or why not?

B. You also note from Casey's chart that his employer has not notified Broadmoor Medical Clinic of this alleged work-related injury. How does this affect the case? Can you telephone Casey's employer to confirm or disaffirm this injury without jeopardizing patient confidentiality?

C. On the Patient Information Form, Casey has listed his primary health insurance carrier as Fortune Health through National Parcel. There is no completed "First Report of Injury" form; is it okay to go ahead and file a claim with Fortune Health?

D. During a telephone conversation with the Human Resources Department at National Parcel, they inform you that they do not consider Casey Belmont's claim valid because he did not attend the mandatory safety meetings the company provides periodically, and he did not follow the instructions in the company's safety manual for proper procedure in lifting heavy containers. How does this affect the case?

PROBLEM-SOLVING/COLLABORATIVE (GROUP) ACTIVITIES

Along with the members of your group, study the following scenario. Prepare a short, 3-minute presentation responding to the questions.

You are employed by Broadmoor Medical Clinic as a health insurance professional. Your vacation is coming up, and you are training temporary employee Tessy Banks to take your place while you're gone. Tessy informs you that she was previously employed at Halcyon Health Care Center in Kenobi, MI, for 5 years as a health insurance professional, and she is familiar with the workers' compensation claim filing process from her previous job.

A. Should you be comfortable in assuming that Tessy can handle your job without further training because of her experience in claims processing? Why or why not?

B. What problems might Tessy experience if she has no further instruction?

C. Generate an outline for a suitable training schedule for Tessy.

PROJECTS/DISCUSSION TOPICS

Be prepared to discuss (1) what you, the health insurance professional, should do when you suspect workers' compensation fraud, and (2) how the Health Insurance Portability and Accountability Act's (HIPAA's) confidentiality regulations apply to patients being treated for workers' compensation illnesses and injuries.

217

CASE STUDIES

Determine the amount each workers' compensation patient can be billed in the following scenarios and briefly explain your answer.

1. Brett Swanson, a constructor worker, was treated in your office for a fractured leg sustained in a fall into a footing excavation. Total charges were $1875, and workers' compensation paid $1400.

   Patient can be billed: _____

2. Part-time worker Effie Brockett was treated for a cut above her right eye sustained during an altercation with a fellow worker. Total charges were $256.50. Workers' compensation denied the claim. She has no healthcare coverage.

   Patient can be billed: _____

3. John Stevens underwent surgery for carpal tunnel syndrome caused by repetitive motion from assembly line work. Total charges were $7345. Workers' compensation paid $3500, and his group health insurance paid $2500.

   Patient can be billed: _____

4. Antonio Estabon was treated for a dislocated shoulder sustained while performing his duties as a county roads engineer. Total charges were $3900. Workers' compensation case is pending.

   Patient can be billed: _____

5. Salid Mufazi was treated for an acute case of bronchitis, which he claims was caused by breathing dust while cleaning a grain elevator at his jobsite. Charges totaled $730. Workers' compensation denied the claim, and Mr. Mufazi informs you that he is appealing the decision.

   Patient can be billed: _____

6. Sally Forsythe was treated in the office for injuries sustained in an automobile accident while delivering flowers for Elegant Arrangements. Total charges were $1600. Workers' compensation–allowed charges in your state for the services and procedures provided to Sally are $1195; however, the claim was denied.

   Patient can be billed: _____

INTERNET EXPLORATION

A. Explore the Internet websites on workers' compensation. Determine the following:

   1. Specific rules and regulations for filing claims in your state
   2. Your state's approved claim form

B. Explore the Ticket to Work program website at **http://www.yourtickettowork.com.**

C. Using search words such as "state disability programs," log on to the Internet and see if you can determine what programs, if any, your state provides to disabled workers, and what the eligibility requirements are.

D. Explore the Internet using search words such as "disability" and "HIPAA." Determine how HIPAA affects workers' compensation and disability claims.

Performance Objective 11-1—Workers' Compensation Claim

Using the information in the patient record (#052560), complete a workers' compensation claim using the universal CMS-1500 form. Follow the guidelines given in Table 11-2 in Chapter 11. (A blank CMS-1500 form can be found at the back of this workbook.)

Note: Student should add all claims in the workbook chapter to the ongoing insurance tracking form.

Conditions: Student will complete a workers' compensation claim using the information in Patient Record No. 052560.

Supplies/Equipment: Patient Record No. 052560 (on following page), CMS-1500 claim form (paper or electronic)

Time Allowed: 50 minutes

Accuracy Needed to Pass: 90%

Procedural Steps	Points Earned	Comments
Evaluator: Note time began: _____		
1. Carefully read and study Patient Record No. 052560.		
2. Complete *all* blocks required for a workers' compensation claim.		
3. Proofread claim for accuracy.		
Optional: May deduct points for taking more time than allowed.		

Total Points = _____

Student's Score: _____

Evaluator: _____

Comments: _____

_____

_____

_____

_____

Note: Use the information in the provider block for all CMS-1500 claims in this chapter.

Provider Block	
Broadmoor Medical Clinic 4353 Pine Ridge Drive Milton, XY 12345-0001 Clinic NPI X100XX1000 Telephone: 555-656-7890	Clinic EIN # 42-1898989 Dr. R.L. Jones NPI 1234567890 Dr. Marilou Lucero NPI #2907511822 Date claims 1 day after examination

Patient/Insurance Information	Billing Information
Julia Elenstein	Record No. 052560
DOB: 04/11/1984	Claim # 83104900HJX
1800 Aspen Circle	"First Report of Injury" Date: 11/23/20XX
Milton, XY 12345	11/23/20XX; 99203—$130.00
555-551-1115	11/24/20XX; 73030—$55.00
SSN: 333-33-0000	Diagnosis: 831.00
Employer: Milton Basket Works	Unable to work from 11/23/20XX through 12/21/20XX
Address: 2799 Industrial Complex, Milton, XY 12345	Attending physician: R.L. Jones, M.D.
555-566-9988	
Occupation: Sorter/Packer	
Primary Insurance: BCBS XYZ333330000	
Group # 1414 XL	

Performance Objective 11-2—Completing an Attending Physician's Statement for a Workers' Compensation Claim

Using the information in the Patient Record No. 052561 and the patient's clinical notes in Fig. 11-1, complete the attending physician's statement for a workers' compensation case in Fig. 11-2.

Conditions: Student will complete an attending physician's statement using the information in Patient Record No. 052561 and chart notes in Fig. 11-1.

Supplies/Equipment: Pen/typewriter, Patient Record No. 052561, chart notes, attending physician's statement form

Time Allowed: 50 minutes

Accuracy Needed to Pass: 90%

Procedural Steps	Points Earned	Comments
Evaluator: Note time began: _____		
1. Carefully read and study Patient Record No. 052561.		
2. Complete *all* applicable blanks on the attending physician's form. (30)		
3. Proofread claim for accuracy.		
Optional: May deduct points for taking more time than allowed.		

Total Points = 30

Student's Score: _____

Evaluator: _____

Comments:_____

_____

_____

_____

_____

Patient/Insurance Information	Billing Information
Frank E. Messmer	Record No. 052561
DOB: 01/16/1953	11/23/20XX; 99202—$140.00
601 Butternut Lane	DX: 959.19
Milton, XY 12345	Attending physician: R.L. Jones, M.D.
555-521-2226	
SSN: 321-00-5555	
Employer: Milton Creamery	
555-521-2226	
Occupation: Bottler	

221

```
CHART NOTES                          Record # 052561

11/23/20XX        Frank E. Messmer        DOB: 01/16/1953

HX    This 53-year-old white male presents to the clinic today for
      chief complaint of a sharp pain in the left groin after loading
      a truck at his place of work yesterday.  His work is
      repetitious, and patient recalls lifting something "the wrong
      way" after which he felt "sort of a dull pain." Patient states
      this has never occurred before. He denies bulging in the
      area of the lower abdomen, scrotal swelling, or scrotal pain.
      Patient denies urgency, frequency, or dysuria.
      PAIN ASSESSMENT:  Scale 0-10, 3-4 involving the left
      groin area.
      ALLERGIES: NKA
      CURRENT MEDS: None

PE    NAD.  Ambulatory.  Appears well
      VS:  BP: 116/80   P: 82   R: 18   WT: 193#
      ENT: TMs:  Clear bilaterally without inflammation,
                 bulging, or retraction
      NOSE:      Clear
      SINUS:     Nontender to palpation and percussion
      THROAT:    Clear without tonsillar enlargement,
                 inflammation, or exudates
      NECK:      Supple, not rigid, without adenopathy or
                 thyropathy
      LUNGS:     CTA all fields with good breath sounds heard
      throughout.  No wheezes or rales.  Normal vocal freitus
      without egophony change.  Respiratory excursion is
      symmetric and equal.
      ABDOMEN:  Soft with active bowel sounds in all
      quadrants.  No hepatosplenomegaly or palpable masses.
      No involuntary guarding or rebound tenderness.  Patient
      has a mild palpable pain on the left side of the groin along
      the inguinal ligament.  There is no obvious bulging.
      GU EXAM:   Testes are descended bilaterally, normal
      size, shape, and consistency without nodularity.  Cord
      structure is normal, nontender.  There is no swelling.
      Patient was checked for hernia, and none was noted,
      though there is some mild laxity in the left inguinal ring.
      Penis is without urethral discharge, circumcised, no
      lesions.
IMP.  Left inguinal groin strain with no evidence of hernia
      at this time.
PLAN  Recommended no work for one week.  When he returns to
      work, he should decrease his activity to lifting no greater
      than 10-15 pounds. This decreased activity should
      continue until his return visit in two weeks.  I also
      counseled patient on signs/symptoms of hernias, and if he
      notes any changes, he should return for follow up at that
      time.
      Routine follow up 2 wk.

R. L. Jones
R. L. Jones, MD/xxx
```

Fig. 11-1 Chart notes for Messmer.

ATTENDING PHYSICIAN'S STATEMENT

Patient Information

Name: _Frank E. Messmer_   Social Security #: _321-00-SSSS_   Medical Record # _OS261_
First Name   Middle Name   Last Name

Address: _601 Butternut Lane, Milton   XY   12345_
Street #   Street   City   State   Zip

Current Department: _Bottling_   Agency: _N/A_

I hereby authorize any agency of the State of Michigan insurance company, prepayment organization, employer, hospital, or physician, to release all information with respect to myself or any of my dependents which may have a bearing on the benefits payable under this or any other plan providing benefits or services. I certify that the information furnished by me in support of this claim is true and correct. _Frank E Messmer_

Date _11/23/20XX_   Employee's Signature _Frank E Messmer_

History

When did symptoms first appear or accident happen?   Mo. _____ Day _____ Year _____

Date doctor authorized patient to cease work because of disability?   Mo. _____ Day _____ Year _____

Has patient ever had same or similar condition?   ❏ Yes ❏ No

If yes, state when and describe

Present Condition

Subjective symptoms _____

Is the condition due to injury or sickness arising out of the patient's employment? ❏ Yes ❏ No If "yes" please explain. _____

Objective findings. (Include results of current X-rays, EKGs or any other special tests). _____

Is patient…Ambulatory? ❏ Bed Confined? ❏ House Confined? ❏ Hospital Confined? ❏ Contagious? ❏ On Narcotic Medication? ❏

Restrictions/limitations

Diagnosis

Diagnosis _____ ICD 9 _____

Name Of Hospital _____ Anticipated Length of Hospitalization _____

Surgical Procedure _____ Date of Surgery _____

If Pregnancy, date of LMC _____ EDC Date _____ Delivery Date _____

Treatment

Date of first visit for this period of disability   Month _____ Day _____ Year _____

Frequency of visits   ❏ Weekly   ❏ Monthly   ❏ Other _____

When did you last examine/treat the patient?   Month _____ Day _____ Year _____

Date of next scheduled visit   Month _____ Day _____ Year _____

Progress . . . . Recovered ❏   Improved ❏   Unimproved ❏   Retrogressed ❏

Extent Of Disability

	FOR ANY OCCUPATION	FOR USUAL OCCUPATION
Is patient now totally disabled?	❏ Yes ❏ No	❏ Yes ❏ No
If no, when was patient able to go to work?	Month ____ Day ____ Year ____	Month ____ Day ____ Year ____
If yes, when do you think patient will be able to resume any work?	Month ____ Day ____ Year ____	Month ____ Day ____ Year ____
	Never ❏	Never ❏

If yes, is patient a suitable candidate for a return to work program? ❏ Yes ❏ No   If yes, please complete the appropriate return to work assessment form.

Is the patient competent to endorse the checks and direct the proceeds thereof? ❏ Yes   ❏ No

Print Name _____ Street Address _____ City or Town _____ State _____ Zip Code _____

Signature (Attending Physician/Mental/Health Provider) _____ Date _____ Degree _____ Telephone Number _____

Fig. 11-2 Attending physician's statement for Messmer.

Using the information in Patient Record No. 052572, complete the attending physician's form shown in Fig. 11-3.
Conditions: Student will complete an attending physician's statement using the information in Patient Record No. 052572.
Supplies/Equipment: Pen/typewriter, Patient Record No. 052572, attending physician's statement form
Time Allowed: 50 minutes
Accuracy Needed to Pass: 90%

Procedural Steps	Points Earned	Comments
Evaluator: Note time began: _____		
1. Carefully read and study Patient Record No. 052572.		
2. Complete *all* applicable blanks on the attending physician's form. (30)		
3. Proofread claim for accuracy.		
Optional: May deduct points for taking more time than allowed.		

Total Points = 30

Student's Score: _____

Evaluator: _____

Comments:_____

_____

_____

Patient/Insurance Information	Billing Information
Benjamin R. Shalimar	Record No. 052572 (New Patient)
DOB: 10/06/1950	Date of accident: 11/23/20XX
82 Sylvan Annex	TRF # 00233389XYZ
Milton, XY 12345	S: Pt was knocked unconscious as a result of a fall from a grain bin this a.m. He fell about 8 ft, landing on his R side. He was "out for a spell." Complains of a severe left frontal headache. Cannot walk w/o assistance; R arm/hand numbness; blurred vision.
555-533-6665	O: See emergency department report in patient record.
SSN: 766-55-7777	A: Diagnosis: 959.01
Employer: Farm Ag Resources	P: Referred to the Neurology Clinic for CT scan and/or MRI. See chart for meds. Scheduled follow-up OV 11/25/20XX at 8 a.m. Return to work: unknown
555-511-0087	11/23/20XX; 99283 ER visit—$180.00
Occupation: Livestock Inspector	Attending physician: M. Lucero, M.D.
Policy #8 692G	

224

| ATTENDING PHYSICIAN'S STATEMENT | REFERENCE NUMBER |
| | |

ATTENDING PHYSICIAN'S STATEMENT

REFERENCE NUMBER

POLICY NUMBER (with Prefix)

**THE INSURED IS RESPONSIBLE FOR COMPLETION OF THIS FORM
WITHOUT EXPENSE TO THE COMPANY**

SEX: M OR F   D.O.B.:

PATIENT'S NAME AND ADDRESS ....

....

WHAT IS DISABLING PATIENT? ....

Please give a complete diagnosis of this condition ....

....

....

....

HISTORY:

1. When did patient first receive medical treatment?...

2. (a) Was there a previous history of this or a similar condition? Yes/No...

   (b) If Yes, please state condition and advise when previous treatment was given...

....

....

3. (a) How long have you known the patient?...

   (b) Are you the regular general practitioner? Yes/No.............................   If not, please advise who is...................

....

IF INJURY:

1. When did patient suffer the injury?...

2. What were the circumstances surrounding the injury?...

IF SICKNESS:

1. When was sickness first contracted?...

2. When did symptoms become evident?..

DEGREE OF DISABILITY:

1. Patient's occupation?..

2. When was patient obliged to cease work?..

3. If patient is still disabled, when approximately will the patient be able to resume:

   (a) Some Duties?...

   (b) Full Duties?...

OR

4. If patient has recovered, when was patient able to resume:

   (a) Some Duties?...

   (b) Full Duties?...

Fig. 11-3 Attending physician's statement for Shalimar.

Performance Objective 11-4—Private Disability Claim with Attending Physician's Report

Using the information in Patient Record No. 052573 and the chart notes in Fig. 11-4, complete the employer-sponsored disability claim form shown in Fig. 11-5. For questions that you do not know the answer to, indicate "unknown." When asked for facts/information, indicate that a copy of the patient's medical record is attached. Dr. Jones has been in practice for 22 years and received his education at the University of Xanthia.

Conditions: Student will complete an attending physician's statement using the information in Patient Record No. 052573 and the chart notes in Fig. 11-4.

Supplies/Equipment: Pen/typewriter, Patient Record No. 052573, attending physician's statement form

Time Allowed: 50 minutes

Accuracy Needed to Pass: 90%

Procedural Steps	Points Earned	Comments
Evaluator: Note time began: _____		
1. Carefully read and study Patient Record No. 052573.		
2. Complete *all* applicable blanks on the attending physician's form. (35)		
3. Proofread claim for accuracy.		
Optional: May deduct points for taking more time than allowed.		

Total Points = 35

Student's Score: _____

Evaluator: _____

Comments:_____

_____

_____

_____

_____

Patient/Insurance Information	Billing Information
Shaley Sue Graham	Record No. 052573
DOB: 07/24/1970	TRF # 00087878IJ
1846 Creamery Row	11/23/20XX; 99202-25—$180.00
Milton, XY 12345	11/24/20XX; 20610—$45.00
555-526-6622	11/24/20XX; J3301 × 4—$100.00
SSN: 123-32-2222	Diagnosis: 726.10, 726.2, E927
Employer: Milton Community College	Attending physician: R.L. Jones, M.D.
555-566-3222	
Occupation: Instructor	

226

CHART NOTES

PATIENT NAME: Shaley Sue Graham RECORD NO. 052573

DATE OF VISIT: 11/23/20XX   DATE OF BIRTH 7/24/1970

S: Shaley is a new pt to me. She is here with complaints of shoulder pain. On Nov. 23 she was working at home in the storage area of the garage. When she went to lift down a box of books from a high shelf, she felt a catching sensation in her L shoulder along with pain and pulling sensation in her shoulder. She reports limited ROM from the very beginning. There is severe pain with overhead activity.

ROS: Denies any numbness or tingling in the upper extremity.
PFSH: See Form 811A (in chart)
ALLERGIES: Penicillin and aspirin
PMH: Usual childhood diseases and occasional headaches

O: Vitals are stable. She is alert and oriented x 3 and does not appear to be in acute distress. On exam of the L shoulder, she has no deltoid or parascapular atrophy. No evidence of winging with wall pushup. She has no warmth or erythema of the shoulder. Good grip strength bilaterally and positive radial pulses. She does have positive impingement. No signs of instability. There is pain with empty-can supraspinatus testing, and there is posterior capsular tightness. Pt does have weakness with external rotation with arm at her side secondary to pain. No weakness with internal rotation with the arm at the side. Lift off sign is negative. She does have an intact Napoleon's sign. Spurling's sign for cervical radiculopathy is negative. ROM is 85 degrees abduction, active assist to 120-130 degrees before pain. Active ROM is 105 degrees with pain.

A: Rotator cuff tendonitis/impingement syndrome

P: I went over the MRI with the patient, which we had ordered this morning, and it shows rotator cuff tendonitis and impingement syndrome. I have recommended an intra-articular injection in the L shoulder. Pt consents for injection. I advised no work for the next 2 weeks. She is not to do any overhead activity and is not to lift more than 15 pounds. F/U in two weeks. I recommend PT and Celebrex. Papers for disability were filled out today and given to pt.

PROCEDURE: L shoulder Injection: The pt is in the sitting position on the examining table. The shoulder joint is palpated. Plan is to inject from a posterior portal into the joint itself. The area is sterilely prepped followed by inserting the needle into the shoulder joint itself. 1 cc of Kenalog, 40 mg, and 5 cc of Xylocaine was injected in L joint. Needle is removed and pressure applied. The shoulder is placed through a ROM to disseminate the fluid.

R. L. Jones

R. L. Jones, MD/xxx

CPT: 20610*, 99202-25 & J3301 x 4
DX: 726.10, 726.2, & E927

Fig. 11-4 Chart notes for Graham.

ATTENDING PHYSICIAN'S STATEMENT

PRIVACY NOTICE		
Patient Name (Last, First, Middle)	Social Security Number	TRF Number

Date of Birth (MM/DD/YY)	Marital Status	Sex (circle one)	Phone Number
	Single	Male Female	( ) -

PATIENT HISTORY

How long have you personally known patient?	Date of your first visit with patient for illness claimed to have brought about present condition?
Number of visits?	Date of last visit?

What organ, system, or parts of the body have been affected?

Describe fully the course of the disease—its initial symptoms—history of its progress.

Has patient suffered from any ailments other than those above mentioned? If so, describe each case, and state how long it lasted and if recovery was complete?

Has patient been attended to or prescribed for by any other physician or surgeon within three years? If so, what was the reason? Give name and addresses of all such physicians and surgeons:

Is patient wholly and continuously unable to perform any work, or follow any occupation for compensation or profit?

If so, how long has patient been totally disabled?

Fig. 11-5 Attending physician's statement for Graham.

If not so disabled, is patient wholly and continuously unable to perform the work of a community college instructor?

Is the disability, in your opinion, likely to be temporary; permanent and total; or permanent and partial?

Please give any other facts or information, which in your judgment will aid in the correct solution of the claims presented.

How long have you practiced as a physician and where did you receive your medical education?

Signature of Physician	Printed Name of Physician	Date

Signature of Patient for the release of this information	Printed Name of Patient	Date
Shaley Sue Graham	Shaley Sue Graham	11/23/20XX

Address of Physician	City

State		ZIP	Phone Number
			( ) -

Fig. 11-5, cont'd

Performance Objective 11-5—Supplemental Security Income Claim

Using the information in the patient record (#052530) and the chart notes in Fig. 11-6, complete the application for SSI Disability form in Fig. 11-7. Under No. 8 and No. 10 on the form, indicate that a copy of patient's recent health record is attached.

Conditions: Student will complete an SSI disability application (see Fig. 11-7) using the information in Patient Record No. 052530 and chart notes in Fig. 11-6.

Supplies/Equipment: Pen/typewriter, Patient Record No. 052530, attending physician's statement form

Time Allowed: 50 minutes

Accuracy Needed to Pass: 90%

Procedural Steps	Points Earned	Comments
Evaluator: Note time began: _____		
1. Carefully read and study Patient Record No. 052530.		
2. Complete *all* applicable blanks on the attending physician's form. (35)		
3. Proofread claim for accuracy.		
Optional: May deduct points for taking more time than allowed.		

Total Points = 35

Student's Score: _____

Evaluator: _____

Comments:_____

_____

_____

_____

_____

Patient/Insurance Information	Billing Information
Lynette Kay Burns	Record No. 052530
DOB: 05/06/1961	11/26/20XX; 99455-32—$225.00
156 Castle Courts	Diagnosis: 278.01, 401.1, 112.3, 311
Milton, XY 12345	Attending physician: M. Lucero, M.D.
No telephone	
SSN 456-65-4321	
Employer: Unemployed	
Primary insurance: None	

CHART NOTES

PATIENT NAME: Lynette K. Burns   DOB: 05/06/1961

DATE OF EXAM: 11/26/20XX   RECORD NO.   052530

S: Lynette presents today at the request of the Social Security Administration. She has applied for disability based on her morbid obesity. I have been asked by the SSA to do a physical exam. Lynette is a longtime pt of mine. I have been managing her chronic diseases since 4/6/1995.

    FH: Non-contributory
    SH: Single, does not smoke; drinks 1 or 2 beers a wk
    PMH: HTN, arthritis, morbid obesity, depression
    MEDS: Prozac/HCTZ

O: BP 142/105, P 90, R 19, W 355, H 5'2". Patient appears to not be in distress. On asking her questions she does not show good eye contact; her affect is flat. She seems more depressed today than usual. Abd is obese but soft. Heart RRR, Lungs CTA. Skin: there is a candidiasis infection under her breast. She has a Grade I-II stasis ulcer on her R ankle. Pt has bilateral varicose veins due to poor circulation. Pt becomes SOB when she walks less than 100 yards and she becomes tachycardic. She has chronic complaint of knee, ankle, and back pain. Legs show mild edema. She has arthritis of the knees, and today on exam they show crepitus bilaterally. Patient is unable to bend or stoop. She cannot stand for prolonged periods of time and needs rest in between.

A: Physical exam, requested by State of XY.

    1. Morbid obesity
    2. HTN, elevated
    3. Candidiasis, skin of breast
    4. Depression

P: I have been educating and working with Lynette since 1995, trying to get her motivated for weight loss and exercise program consisting of walking. She has tried a walking program of walking less than 100 yards the first week, then increasing her distance as tolerated week by week. She is encouraged to walk to help increase her tolerance. She has been on an 1800-cal. diet and low salt diet with no success. She is instructed to continue with her Prozac 20mg d, and HCTZ 25mg d for her leg edema and HTN. Rtn 1 mo.

Marilou Lucero
_____
M. Lucero, MD/xx

CPT: 99455-32
DX: 278.01, 401.1, 112.3, 311

Fig. 11-6 Chart notes for Burns.

APPLICATION FOR SSI DISABILITY

MEDICAL PROVIDER'S STATEMENT

1. PATIENT'S NAME: _____ DATE OF BIRTH: _____ / _____ / _____
                        (First)   *(Middle)*   *(Last)*   *MM*   *DD*   *YYYY*

2. CURRENT MEDICAL CONDITION(s):

   PRIMARY DIAGNOSIS: _____ ICD-9 CM CODE: _____

   SECONDARY DIAGNOSIS: _____ ICD-9 CM CODE: _____

3. DATE THAT SYMPTOMS FIRST APPEARED OR ACCIDENT HAPPENED: _____ / _____ / _____
                                                                    (Month) *(Day)* *(Year)*

4. DATE THAT PATIENT FIRST CONSULTED YOU FOR THIS CONDITION: _____ / _____ / _____
                                                                     (Month) *(Day)* *(Year)*

5. DATE YOU LAST TREATED THE PATIENT: _____ / _____ / _____
                                           (Month) *(Day)* *(Year)*

6. IS THIS CONDITION RELATED TO PATIENT'S EMPLOYMENT?   YES ☐   NO ☐

7. WAS PATIENT REFERRED TO YOU BY ANOTHER PRACTITIONER? YES ☐   NO ☐
   (If "yes," please provide the name and address of that practitioner): _____

   _____

8. OBJECTIVE FINDINGS *(Include x-rays, lab results and clinical findings. If pregnancy, also give LMP and EDC):* _____

   _____

   _____

9. HAS PATIENT BEEN HOSPITALIZED? YES ☐   NO ☐ *(if "yes," provide reason, hospital name and dates of confinement):* _____

10. NATURE OF TREATMENT CURRENTLY BEING PROVIDED OR PLANNED: *(Include surgery and medications prescribed if applicable):*

    _____

    _____

11. HAVE YOU REFERRED THE PATIENT TO ANOTHER PRACTITIONER? YES ☐ NO ☐ *(If "yes," please provide the name and address of all applicable physicians or practitioners):* _____

    _____

12. IN YOUR OPINION IS THE PATIENT ABLE TO WORK AT THIS TIME?   YES ☐   NO ☐
    IF "NO," WHEN DO YOU EXPECT THAT THE
    PATIENT WILL BE ABLE TO PERFORM SOME WORK?   _____ / _____ / _____
                                                                     (Month) *(Day)* *(Year)*

13. IS THERE ANY TYPE OF JOB MODIFICATION OR ACCOMMODATION THAT WOULD
    ENABLE THE PATIENT TO WORK AT THIS TIME? YES ☐ NO ☐ *(If "yes," please describe):* _____

Fig. 11-7 Application for Supplemental Security Income benefits (Burns).

14.   BASED ON OBJECTIVE FINDINGS AND YOUR MEDICAL OPINION:

a) THE PATIENT WAS TOTALLY DISABLED FROM: _____ / _____ / _____ THROUGH: _____ / _____ / _____
                                                    (Mo.) (Day) (Year)   (Mo.) (Day) (Year)

b) THE PATIENT WAS PARTIALLY DISABLED FROM: _____ / _____ / _____ THROUGH: _____ / _____ / _____
                                                    (Mo.) (Day) (Year)   (Mo.) (Day) (Year)

15.   LIST ALL CURRENT RESTRICTIONS AND LIMITATIONS YOU HAVE PLACED ON THE
      PATIENT'S WORK AND PERSONAL ACTIVITIES DUE TO HIS OR HER MEDICAL
      CONDITION *(If none, indicate "NONE")*: _____

      _____

      _____

16.   HAS THE PATIENT BEEN RELEASED FROM YOUR CARE? YES ☐ NO ☐

      IF "YES," DATE RELEASED   IF "NO," DATE OF NEXT SCHEDULED
      FROM YOUR CARE: TREATMENT OR EVALUATION:

      _____ / _____ / _____   _____ / _____ / _____
      (MO)   (DAY)   (YEAR)   (MO)   (DAY)   (YEAR)

**ANY PERSON WHO KNOWINGLY AND WITH THE INTENT TO DEFRAUD ANY INSURANCE COMPANY OR OTHER
PERSON FILES AN APPLICATION FOR INSURANCE OR STATEMENT OF CLAIM CONTAINING ANY MATERIALLY FALSE
INFORMATION, OR CONCEALS FOR THE PURPOSE OF MISLEADING, INFORMATION CONCERNING ANY FACT
MATERIAL THERETO, COMMITS A FRAUDULENT INSURANCE ACT, WHICH IS A CRIME AND SUBJECTS
SUCH PERSON TO CRIMINAL AND CIVIL PENALTIES.**

MEDICAL PROVIDER'S DECLARATION AND SIGNATURE

I declare that the answers on this statement are complete and true to the best of my knowledge and belief. I understand that
periodic updates (including providing copies of medical records when requested) will be required in the event of a continuing
claim.

_____   _____   (____) _____
PROVIDER'S NAME/SPECIALTY   TAX ID/SOCIAL SECURITY #   TELEPHONE NUMBER
   (PLEASE PRINT)

_____   _____
STREET ADDRESS   CITY   STATE   ZIP CODE

_____   _____
PROVIDER'S SIGNATURE   DATE SIGNED

Please return completed forms to:

State of XY Services
Attn: Disability Department
PO Box 22333
Crescent City, XY 21112

Fig. 11-7, cont'd

Performance Objective 11-6—Employer-Sponsored Expanded Disability Certification

Patient Benjamin Shalimar returns to the clinic for follow-up. Because his disability continues, students must complete a "Disabled Expanded Certification Verification" form using the information in the patient record (#052572) and the form in Fig. 11-8. (Mother's maiden name is Lutz.)

Conditions: Student will complete an "expanded" disability form using the information in Patient Record No. 052572.
Supplies/Equipment: Pen/typewriter, Patient Record No. 052572, disabled expanded certification verification form (see Fig. 11-8)
Time Allowed: 50 minutes
Accuracy Needed to Pass: 90%

Procedural Steps	Points Earned	Comments
Evaluator: Note time began: _____		
1. Carefully read and study Patient Record No. 052572.		
2. Complete *all* applicable blanks on the attending physician's form. (30)		
3. Proofread claim for accuracy.		
Optional: May deduct points for taking more time than allowed.		

Total Points = 30

Student's Score: _____

Evaluator: _____

Comments:_____

_____

_____

Patient/Insurance Information	Billing Information
Benjamin R. Shalimar	Record No. 052572
DOB: 10/06/1950	Progress report: 12/07/20XX
82 Sylvan Annex	Patient returns to the office today. He continues to have blurred vision and tremors from this farm accident on 11/23/XX. There is still weakness in R hand and leg. He is able to walk with a cane.
Milton, XY 12345	It is my opinion that this patient's head injury significantly restricts his ability to perform his usual job and any related occupation and is likely permanent.
555-533-6665	Continue PT; return 2 wk
SSN: 766-55-7777	Attending physician: M. Lucero, M.D.
Employer: Farm Ag Resources	
555-511-0087	
Occupation: Livestock Inspector	
Policy #8 692G	

234

DISABLED EXPANDED CERTIFICATION VERIFICATION

<u>APPLICANT, SEND COMPLETED FORM TO:</u>

Disabled Certification Department
4526 Central Avenue
Springfield, XY 12345

_____

APPLICANT'S SOCIAL SECURITY
NUMBER (or assigned 9-digit number)

MOTHER'S MAIDEN NAME (enter your mother's maiden name or another name or word that will serve as an additional identifier to make your applicant record unique)

_____

NAME (please print Last Name, First Name)

_____

ADDRESS (please print mailing address, city, state, and zip code)

TELEPHONE NO.

RELEASE OF INFORMATION AUTHORIZATION

I authorize you to release the information requested on this form to the Division of Merit Recruitment and Selection. I understand that this information will be used only to determine my eligibility for the Disabled Expanded Certification Program.

Benjamin R Shalimer _____ 12/07/20XX _____
APPLICANT'S SIGNATURE   DATE

* *

DOES THE PERSON NAMED ABOVE HAVE A PERMANENT PHYSICAL OR MENTAL DISABILITY THAT SUBSTANTIALLY LIMITS THE MAJOR LIFE ACTIVITY OF WORKING? This means that the disability significantly restricts the person's ability to perform a class of jobs or broad range of jobs in different classes when compared to the average person who has comparable training, skills and abilities. **(CHECK ONE)**

YES _____   NO _____

If yes, please identify the disability and describe how it affects the person's ability to work:

_____

_____

_____

NAME (PRINT): _____   DATE: _____

SIGNATURE: _____

TITLE: _____   TELEPHONE NO.: _____

ADDRESS: _____
              STREET   CITY   STATE   ZIP CODE

Fig. 11-8 Expanded benefits form (Shalimar).

James Morrison has returned to the clinic for a follow-up visit. He is being referred to a neurosurgeon for surgical treatment. Student must complete progress form for this patient's continued disability.

Conditions: Student will complete a physician's progress notes for continued disability using the information in Patient Record No. 052576.

Supplies/Equipment: Pen/typewriter, Patient Record No. 052576, progress notes form (Fig. 11-9)

Time Allowed: 50 minutes

Accuracy Needed to Pass: 90%

Procedural Steps	Points Earned	Comments
Evaluator: Note time began: _____		
1. Carefully read and study Patient Record No. 052576.		
2. Complete *all* applicable blanks on the attending physician's form. (20)		
3. Proofread claim for accuracy.		
Optional: May deduct points for taking more time than allowed.		

Total Points = 20

Student's Score: _____

Evaluator: _____

Comments:_____

_____

_____

Patient/Insurance Information	Billing Information
James T. Morrison	Record No. 052576
DOB: 03/18/1951	Progress notes: 11/25/20XX
916 Brown Street	Professor Morrison is in my office again for a follow-up and test results of his acute back injury sustained after a fall from a ladder while cleaning the gutters on his house 2 days ago. He continues his daily PT at Milton Rehab Center.
Milton, XY 12345	MRI shows vertebral dislocation (L4-5). He is referred to Dr. Jonas Palmer, neurosurgeon at this same clinic, for lumbar laminotomy and decompression on 11/30/20XX.
555-566-2047	It is estimated that patient will be unable to work for 6-8 wk after his surgery.
SSN: 110-01-0101	Recommendations: No work until further notice; walking on level ground; PT.
Employer: Harvest College	Diagnosis: 959.19; 839.20
Occupation: Director, Human Resources	Attending physician: M. Lucero, M.D.
Primary Insurance: BCBS XWQ110010101	
Group # HU088	

236

HARVEST COLLEGE CERTIFICATION FORM

Progress Report

Section I:	**To Be Completed by EMPLOYEE**

Employee Name: JAMES T. MORRISON   Harvard I.D. 110-01-0101PHR

Home Address:
916 Brown St.
Milton, XY 12345

Office Address:

Home Telephone: SSS-S66-2047   Office Telephone: SSS-780-1000 EX 8112

Job Title: Dir. H.R.   Work Schedule: _N/A_ days/week _N/A_ hours/day
Salaried

Employment Date: 08-31-1993   Last Day Worked: 11-22-20XX

Employee Signature: *James T. Morrison*   Date: 11/25/20XX

In some cases, it may be necessary to request medical information and records. I agree to release medical information and records related to my current disability, if requested, by the Disability Claims Unit (DCU) of Harvest College within 10 days of the request by the DCU. I understand that I may not receive benefits until the necessary medical information is received and reviewed. I understand that such information will be used solely to determine my eligibility for STD benefits.

Section II:	**To Be Completed by HEALTH CARE PROVIDER**

Date of examination leading to disability determination ___/___/___   Date of onset of disability ___/___/___

Please indicate ICD-9-CM Diagnosis Code: _____

Is surgery expected? If yes, give date: _____   Is illness/injury acute? _____

Is illness chronic? _____ If so, what has led to disability at this time? _____

Is disability related to work activities? _____

Is employee treating with any other physician(s)? _____ If so, please provide name, address and specialty:

Is employee compliant with treatment recommendations? _____

Expected duration of incapacity (Please note that re-certification is required every 60 days):

Is a return to work on a reduced work schedule or modified work duties appropriate at this time? Yes _____ No _____

Will one of those options become appropriate within the next 60 days? Yes _____ No _____

Expected date of return to work ___/___/___

Name of Health Care Provider: Telephone Number:

Name and Address of Practice:

Signature of Health Care Provider: Date

Revised: 7/03

Fig. 11-9 Progress notes for Morrison.

Performance Objective 11-8—Release to Return to Work

Patient Shaley Graham has been released to return to work. Student must complete a Release to Return to Work form.

Conditions: Student will complete a Release to Return to Work form using the information in Patient Record No. 052573 and chart notes in Fig. 11-10.

Supplies/Equipment: Pen/typewriter, Patient Record No. 052573, Release to Return to Work form (Fig. 11-11)

Time Allowed: 50 minutes

Accuracy Needed to Pass: 90%

Procedural Steps	Points Earned	Comments
Evaluator: Note time began: _____		
1. Carefully read and study Patient Record No. 052573.		
2. Complete *all* applicable blanks on the attending physician's form. (25)		
3. Proofread claim for accuracy.		
Optional: May deduct points for taking more time than allowed.		

Total Points = 25

Student's Score: _____

Evaluator: _____

Comments:_____

_____

_____

_____

_____

Patient/Insurance Information	Billing Information
Shaley Sue Graham	Record No. 052573
DOB: 07/24/1970	TRF# 00087878IJ
1846 Creamery Row	12/14/20XX; 99213—$55.00
Milton, XY 12345	Diagnosis: 726.10, 726.2, E927
555-526-6622	Follow-up appt: 2 mo
SSN: 123-32-2222	Attending physician: R.L. Jones, M.D.
Employer: Milton Community College	
555-566-3222	
Occupation: Instructor	

238

```
CHART NOTES

PATIENT NAME:  Shaley Sue Graham        DOB:  07/24/1970

DATE:              12/14/20XX               RECORD NO.  052573

S.     I saw Shaley today in the office for follow up.  Her shoulder pain has diminished
       considerably since I last saw her.  She believes she is well enough to return to
       work.

O.     On examination, abduction,130 degrees w/o pain; forward flexion, 180 degrees;
       extension, 45 degrees; external rotation, 90 degrees; elbow at 90 degrees with
       arm comfortable at side and with arm at 90 degrees abduction.  Internal rotation,
       90 degrees.

A:     Rotator cuff tendonitis/impingement syndrome, resolved.

P.     It is my opinion that Shaley's rotator cuff injury is resolved, and she has been
       released to return to her job without limitations.  I cautioned the patient, however,
       of certain repetitive arm/shoulder motions that could aggravate the rotator cuff
       again, such as lifting weights and certain active sports, such as tennis, golf, and
       archery—all of which she previously engaged in.  Rtn PRN.


R.L. Jones

R. L. Jones, MD/xxx
```

Fig. 11-10 Chart notes for Graham (return visit).

RELEASE TO RETURN TO WORK

Name of worker	Claim number

Please fill out this form and return it to us at the address indicated above.

1. Is the worker   ☐ Yes   Date: _____   (Provide closing information and complete Form 827.)

    medically stationary?   ☐ No   Next scheduled appointment date: _____

2. Worker is released to:

    ☐ full duty without limitations   Date: _____   (Do not complete lines 3 through 11. Sign below.)

    ☐ modified duty from (date) _____ through (date) _____   (specify limitations below)

    ☐ modified hours — specify _____ from (date) _____ through (date) _____

	Hours:	No limitations	1	2	3	4	5	6	7	8
3. In an eight-hour workday, worker can stand/walk a total of		☐	☐	☐	☐	☐	☐	☐	☐	☐
4. At one time, worker can stand/walk		☐	☐	☐	☐	☐	☐	☐	☐	☐
5. In an eight-hour workday, worker can sit a total of		☐	☐	☐	☐	☐	☐	☐	☐	☐
6. At one time, worker can sit		☐	☐	☐	☐	☐	☐	☐	☐	☐

7. The worker is released to return to work in the following range for lifting, carrying, pushing/pulling:

Pounds	<10	10	15	20	25	30	35	40	45	50	55	60	65	70	75	80	85	90	95	100	>100
Occasionally	☐	☐	☐	☐	☐	☐	☐	☐	☐	☐	☐	☐	☐	☐	☐	☐	☐	☐	☐	☐	☐
Frequently	☐	☐	☐	☐	☐	☐	☐	☐	☐	☐	☐	☐	☐	☐	☐	☐	☐	☐	☐	☐	☐

8. Worker can use hands for repetitive: **Right**   **Left**

    a. Fine manipulation   ☐ Yes ☐ No   ☐ Yes ☐ No   Dominant hand

    b. Pushing and pulling   ☐ Yes ☐ No   ☐ Yes ☐ No   ☐ Right ☐ Left

    c. Simple grasping   ☐ Yes ☐ No   ☐ Yes ☐ No

    d. Keyboarding   ☐ Yes ☐ No   ☐ Yes ☐ No

9. Worker can use feet for repetitive raising and pushing (as in operating foot controls):   ☐ Yes   ☐ No

10. Worker is able to:

	Continuous 67-100% of the day	Frequently 34-66% of the day	Occasionally 6-33% of the day	Intermittently 1-5% of the day	Not at all
a. Stoop/bend	☐	☐	☐	☐	☐
b. Crouch	☐	☐	☐	☐	☐
c. Crawl	☐	☐	☐	☐	☐
d. Kneel	☐	☐	☐	☐	☐
e. Twist	☐	☐	☐	☐	☐
f. Climb	☐	☐	☐	☐	☐
g. Balance	☐	☐	☐	☐	☐
h. Reach	☐	☐	☐	☐	☐
i. Push/pull	☐	☐	☐	☐	☐

11. Other functional limitations or modifications necessary in worker's employment:

Additional comments may be written on back of form.

Signature of medical service provider*	Printed name	Date

Fig. 11-11 Return to work form (Graham).

Health Insurance Professional's Notebook

A. Examples of forms and completion instructions for:

1. Workers' compensation claims
2. Employer/private disability claims
3. SSDI and SSI claims
4. Attending physician's statement of disability forms
5. Continued disability forms
6. Release to Return to Work Forms

B. Names of agencies and telephone numbers for workers' compensation and disability claims in your state

Chapter Check List

Student name: _____

Chapter completion date: _____

1.	Record	Your start time and date: _____
2.	Read	The assigned chapter in the text
3.	View	PowerPoint slides (if available)
4.	Complete	Exercises in the Workbook as assigned
5.	Compare	Your answers with the answers posted on the bulletin board/website/handout
6.	Correct	Your answers
7.	Complete	All tests and required activities
8.	Read	Assigned readings (if any)
9.	Complete	Chapter performance objectives (competencies), if any
10.	Evaluate	Chapter performance and submit to your instructor
11.	Record	Your ending time and date: _____
12.	Move on	Begin next chapter as assigned

PERFORMANCE EVALUATION

Evaluate your classroom performance. Complete the self-evaluation, and submit it to your instructor. When your instructor returns this form to you, compare your self-evaluation with the evaluation completed by your instructor.

Skill	Student Self-Evaluation			Instructor Evaluation		
	Good	Average	Poor	Good	Average	Poor
Attendance/punctuality						
Personal appearance						
Applies effort						
Is self-motivated						
Is courteous						
Has positive attitude						
Completes assignments in timely manner						
Works well with others						

Student's Initials: _____

Date: _____

Points Possible: _____

Points Awarded: _____

Chapter Grade: _____

Instructor's Initials: _____

Date: _____

12 Diagnostic Coding

Diagnosis codes started out as a way to track morbidity and mortality. As their use evolved, changes were made to add information, resulting in a coding structure that describes the clinical picture of a patient. ICD-9-CM codes are composed of 3 to 5 digits usually grouped by organ system. Diagnosis codes are found in the *International Classification of Diseases, Ninth Revision, Clinical Modification*, the ICD-9-CM coding manual.

Chapter 12 in the textbook introduced you to the concepts of diagnostic coding and the use of the ICD-9-CM coding manual for outpatient healthcare. The activities in this accompanying workbook chapter are designed to enhance your understanding of ICD-9 coding and its relationship to the total reimbursement process. Completing these exercises provides valuable practice in applying coding conventions, interpreting coding guidelines, and assigning ICD-9-CM diagnostic codes to the highest level of specificity.

WORKBOOK CHAPTER OBJECTIVES

After completing the workbook activities for Chapter 12, the student should be able to:
- Define the terms used in the chapter.
- Answer the review questions to within the evaluation criteria set by the instructor.
- Use problem-solving skills (individually or in a group setting) to determine correct responses and outcomes in case studies and application exercises.
- Identify coding conventions and their meaning.
- Recognize the main terms in a medical diagnosis.
- Apply the correct steps for accurate coding.
- Assign the correct codes to clinical diagnoses (to the greatest specificity).
- Complete performance objectives to the criteria set by the instructor.
- Compile a section in the Health Insurance Professional's Notebook on ICD-9 coding.

DEFINING CHAPTER TERMS

Using the computer, students should key an accurate definition in their own words for each of the chapter terms listed. When finished, students should compare their definitions with those listed in the glossary at the back of the textbook, correcting any inaccuracies.

adjectives
category
code set
coding
combination code
conditions
diagnosis
diseases
E codes
eponyms
essential modifiers
etiology
hypertension
in situ

International Classification of Diseases, Ninth Revision, Clinical Modification (ICD-9-CM)
International Classification of Diseases, Tenth Revision (ICD-10)
main term
manifestation
morbidity
mortality
neoplasm
nonessential modifiers
notes
noun
subcategory
subclassification
V codes

Multiple Choice

Directions: In the questions/statements presented, choose the response that **best** answers/completes the stem, and circle the letter that precedes it.

1. The determination of the nature of a cause of disease, or the art of distinguishing one disease from another, is commonly referred to as:
   a. Assignation
   b. Coding
   c. Diagnosis
   d. Insurance

2. Use of ICD-9 began in the United States when the U.S. National Center for Health Statistics (NCHS) modified the system in:
   a. 1937
   b. 1966
   c. 1977
   d. 1988

3. The transformation of verbal descriptions of a diagnosis into numbers or a combination of alphanumeric characters is called:
   a. Coding
   b. Classifying
   c. Documenting
   d. Modifying

4. The first several pages of the ICD-9 manual constitute:
   a. A list of anatomic sites
   b. An introduction
   c. Conventions and symbols
   d. A guide to clinical procedures

5. An alphabetic listing of diagnoses is contained in:
   a. Volume 1
   b. Volume 2
   c. Appendix A
   d. Appendix B

6. *Italics* are used in Volumes 1 and 2 to:
   a. Identify new codes
   b. Highlight all exclusionary notes
   c. Identify rubrics that should not be listed as primary codes
   d. b and c

7. The largest section in Volume 2, the Index to Diseases, is organized:
   a. By anatomic sites
   b. Alphabetically by main terms
   c. Numerically
   d. By body systems

8. Diseases, procedures, or syndromes named for individuals who discovered or first used them are called:

   a. Eponyms

   b. Main terms

   c. Modifiers

   d. Diagnoses

9. Essential modifiers describe:

   a. Various anatomic sites

   b. The cause or origin of a disease or condition

   c. Clinical types

   d. All of the above

10. Terms in parentheses following main terms are called:

    a. Subterms

    b. Essential modifiers

    c. Nonessential modifiers

    d. Eponyms

11. The codes used to classify environmental events, circumstances, and other conditions that are the cause of injury and other adverse effects are referred to as:

    a. Main terms

    b. V codes

    c. E codes

    d. Modifiers

12. Codes in the Tabular List (Volume 1) are arranged:

    a. Alphabetically

    b. Numerically

    c. Alphanumerically

    d. By anatomic site

13. Codes on health insurance forms must conform to the standards that are published in/on:

    a. *JAMA*

    b. The Centers for Medicare and Medicaid Services (CMS) website

    c. The *Federal Register*

    d. The Health Insurance Portability and Accountability Act (HIPAA) manual

14. If a patient's condition has not been specifically diagnosed, the health insurance professional must code the:

    a. "Suspected" disease(s)

    b. Disease(s) to be "ruled out"

    c. Probable disease(s)

    d. Signs or symptoms

15. When a single code is used to describe conditions that frequently occur together, a(n) _____ code is used:

    a. V

    b. E

    c. Combination

    d. Volume III

16. Under HIPAA, any set of codes used for encoding data elements, such as tables of terms, medical concepts, medical diagnosis codes, or medical procedure codes, is called a:

a. Code set

b. Coding rubric

c. HIPAA cluster

d. Concept set

17. The main term for *acute depressive reaction* is:

a. Acute

b. Depressive

c. Reaction

d. Either a or c

18. The following instruction "*330—Cerebral degenerations usually manifest in childhood: Use additional code to identify associated mental retardation*" indicates to the health insurance professional:

a. A fourth and fifth digit must be assigned to the code

b. An additional code should be used for better clarification

c. a and b are correct

d. There is not enough information to answer correctly

19. V codes show problems or situations that influence a patient's health status but are not a current illness or injury, such as:

a. Family history of cancer

b. Routine physical examination

c. Colonoscopy screening

d. All of the above

20. E codes provide a classification of external causes, such as:

a. How an accident occurred

b. Whether a drug overdose was accidental or purposeful

c. a and b

d. Neither a nor b

True/False

Directions: Place a "T" in the blank preceding each of the following statements if it is true; place an "F" if it is false.

_____ 1. A diagnosis should never be coded from the Alphabetic List alone.

_____ 2. You can show only one diagnosis code in Block 21.

_____ 3. Anatomic sites are often listed as main terms in ICD-9-CM.

_____ 4. Essential modifiers must be a part of the diagnosis documented in the health record.

_____ 5. Nonessential modifiers usually are not a part of the diagnostic statement.

_____ 6. See or see also tells the coder to continue the search under another main term.

_____ 7. V codes are used when circumstances other than a disease or injury are recorded as diagnosis or problem.

_____ 8. V codes can never be used alone on the CMS-1500 claim form.

_____ 9. Italicized type is used for main terms in the Alphabetic Index (Volume 2) and all codes and titles in the tabular list.

_____ 10. Boldface type is used for all exclusion notes and to identify codes that should not be used for describing the primary diagnosis.

_____ 11.   When the notation "code first underlying disease" is seen, the etiology is coded before the manifestation.

_____ 12.   HCPCS Level 3 codes, known as local codes, have mostly been eliminated from use.

_____ 13.   A colon is used in the tabular list after an incomplete term that needs one or more modifiers to make it a complete statement.

_____ 14.   If the healthcare provider inadvertently omits a diagnosis in the patient's health record, an experienced health insurance professional may abstract the correct diagnosis for coding purposes without consulting the physician.

_____ 15.   The abbreviation NOS is the equivalent of "unspecified."

Short Answer/Fill-in-the-Blank

1. Define "diagnosis" in your own words.

   _____

2. A diagnosis code can be _____ to _____ digits.

3. ICD-9-CM stands for _____.

4. The "primary diagnosis" is used by _____; the "principal diagnosis" is used by _____.

5. Name the three volumes of ICD-9-CM and what each contains.

   _____

   _____

   _____

6. Why is it important for the health insurance professional to use the most recent volume of ICD-9-CM?

   _____

7. In the blank following the name of the volume or appendix, list what is contained in that portion of the ICD-9-CM manual.

   Volume 2: _____

   Volume 1: _____

   Appendix A: _____

   Appendix B: _____

   Appendix C: _____

   Appendix D: _____

   Appendix E: _____

8. The first step in diagnostic coding is to identify the _____ _____.

9. List the four ways main terms appear in the Index to Diseases, and give an example of each.

_____

_____

_____

_____

10. Name the tables that appear in the Alphabetic Index to Diseases.

_____

_____

11. Explain the content and purpose of the Table of Drugs and Chemicals.

_____

_____

12. List the seven essential steps to diagnostic coding.

_____

_____

_____

_____

_____

_____

_____

13. List steps for selecting the correct E code.

_____

_____

_____

14. ICD-10 is now being used in some parts of the world. Describe this revised method of coding, and explain some of the differences compared with ICD-9.

_____

_____

_____

A. Underline the main term in each of the following:

    1. breast mass
    2. deviated nasal septum
    3. heel spurs
    4. excessive eye strain
    5. tension headache
    6. bronchial croup
    7. senile cataract
    8. paranoid delusions
    9. acute hemorrhagic otitis media with effusion
  10. coronary insufficiency

B. Explain what an eponym is and give two examples.

C. Underline the main terms in the following diseases/conditions, and assign the correct ICD-9-CM code.

    1. angina pectoris: _____

    2. hemorrhoids: _____

    3. irregular menstruation: _____

    4. Parkinson's disease: _____

    5. Skene's gland abscess: _____

D. Explain each of the following conventions/symbols:

NOS: _____

NEC: _____

[ ]: _____

§: _____

✓5th: _____

E. A diagnostic statement from the physician may contain many medical terms, but there is only one main term that describes the patient's illness or injury. All accompanying words that describe the main term further are called *modifiers*. These are found in the Alphabetic Index following the main terms.
    1. Name the two types of modifiers.
    2. Explain how these two types of modifiers are differentiated, how they are used, and their effect on assigning a correct diagnostic code.

F. Cross-references assist the coder in locating the appropriate code. They are found only in the Alphabetic Index. There are three types of cross-references; name them and explain what each means.

G. There are four kinds of punctuation marks used in the Tabular List, and each punctuation mark has a different meaning. List these four punctuation marks, and explain what each means to the coder.

H. Four symbols appear in Volume 1 (the Tabular List) of ICD-9-CM. List these four symbols, and give a detailed explanation of what each one tells the coder.

I. The following instructional notes appear only in the Tabular List of Diseases. Explain what each means in your own words.

Includes
Excludes
Use additional code
Code first underlying disease
Code, if applicable, any causal condition first
Omit code

J. Other conventions include two different styles of type. Explain where and for what purpose each of these style types are used.

Boldface: _____

Italicized: _____

PROBLEM SOLVING/COLLABORATIVE (GROUP) ACTIVITIES

A. V codes are intended to be used to explain reasons for an office visit when a patient is not currently ill. List four (or more) situations when the use of V codes is appropriate.

B. Give at least five main terms commonly used in V code diagnoses.
Note: Although V codes are acceptable for use, reimbursement for V codes depends on the individual insurance policy.

C. In the following table, underline the main term, find the appropriate ICD-9-CM code, and indicate whether the code should be a primary or secondary diagnosis:

V Code	Primary	Secondary
Routine chest x-ray		
Well-baby examination		
Annual pelvic examination		
Postsurgical follow-up examination		
Dietary counseling for diabetes		

D. Code the following accidents:

Injury caused by train derailment: _____

Injury caused to a passenger in a horse-drawn buggy struck by an automobile: _____

Injury caused by a controlled fire in a private dwelling: _____

E. Code the following acute and chronic conditions. (Some conditions may require two codes.)

Acute and chronic tonsillitis: _____ _____

Subacute and chronic endocarditis: _____ _____

Acute and chronic cholecystitis: _____ _____

Acute and chronic renal failure: _____ _____

F. Code the following diagnoses, which were documented in the health records of various patients. Keep in mind that you must code the symptoms only.

Chest pain (suspected myocardial infarction): _____

Abdominal discomfort: _____

Fatigue (suspected iron deficiency anemia): _____

Head trauma (possible cerebral concussion): _____

G. Two main terms are sometimes joined together by combination terms. With this in mind, code the following diagnoses/conditions:

Acute cholecystitis with bile duct calculus: _____

Influenza with upper respiratory infection: _____

Acute appendicitis with peritoneal abscess: _____

Skull fracture with subdural hemorrhage*: _____

Salmonella meningitis: _____

*If it is not stated in the record, assume it is a closed fracture.

PROJECTS/DISCUSSION TOPICS

A. Make a table of coding conventions with examples for quick reference to use when coding diagnoses.

B. Participate in a class discussion on the history and purpose of ICD-9-CM coding.

C. Discuss HIPAA's impact on ICD-9 coding.

CASE STUDIES

A. Aileen Fortune visited Broadmoor Medical Clinic on 12/29/20XX. On examining her health record, you find the following diagnoses:

Hypertension, essential, benign: _____

Urinary incontinence: _____

Multiple vesicovaginal fistula of bladder: _____

Underline the main terms and assign the correct ICD-9-CM codes to each.

B. Patient Marcus Aberle's chief complaint and diagnoses are documented as follows:

CC: shortness of breath, chest discomfort, nausea, and profuse sweating
DX: (1) probable myocardial infarction; (2) rule out gastroesophageal reflux disease
What would the correct ICD-9-CM code(s) be for this patient?

C. A 51-year-old man is seen at Broadmoor Medical Clinic for an annual health maintenance examination. In addition to the examination, three diagnoses are listed in his health record as follows:
  1. Health maintenance examination, 51-year-old man
  2. Tobacco dependence
  3. Gastroesophageal reflux disease
  4. Arthritis of spine (degenerative)

Underline the main terms for this patient's diagnoses/conditions, and assign the proper codes to each.

D. Archie Simpson, a 14-year-old boy, presents to the clinic with an insect bite to the right hand, etiology unknown. What would this diagnostic code be?

E. Katie Olivier, a 6-year-old girl, comes to the clinic with complaints of fever of 101.5° F, chills, sweats, mild earache, stuffy nose, sinus pain and pressure, an episodic cough (that is worse in the evening), wheezing, and dyspnea that started approximately 5 days ago. The diagnosis documented in Katie's health record is *acute upper respiratory infection with mild sinusitis, possibly allergy related*. How many diagnostic codes would you list on the claim form? What would this/these code(s) be?

F.
  1. David Scott presented to the clinic as a new patient on 08/05/2004. The documentation in his health record states a diagnosis of *ulcer of the midfoot* on this first visit. What is the code for the diagnosis?

  2. Over the next 2 years, Mr. Scott continues to come to the clinic on follow-up visits for treatment of his foot ulcer, which tends to heal and then recur. Would the ICD-9 code be the same for this patient's follow-up visit on 04/09/2006?

  3. If not, what is the correct code for this follow-up visit?

G. Assign the correct diagnosis for a 6-year-old boy who presents to the clinic with a cat bite and associated cellulitis of the right lower leg.

H. Marcie Emmerson, a 22-year-old woman, presents to the clinic with a chief complaint of sore throat, mild discomfort with swallowing, hoarseness in her voice, nasal congestion with a greenish nasal discharge, and slight postnasal drainage. She denies sinus pain and pressure. She has had a minimal cough with no wheezing, shortness of breath, or dyspnea. The patient is afebrile. Impression: Acute pharyngitis.
  1. How many diagnosis codes are needed for this patient's claim form?
  2. State the diagnosis(es).
  3. Assign the correct code(s).

A. The following website contains helpful information and ICD-9-CM coding resources: **http://www.cms.hhs.gov/ICD9ProviderDiagnosticCodes.** Explore this expansive website for additional information on diagnostic coding.

B. On the above-mentioned website, locate and click on the following topics:

- New, Deleted, and Revised ICD-9-CM Codes-Summary Tables
- ICD-9-CM Official Coding Guidelines
- ICD-9-CM Conversion Table (this table shows the date the new code became effective and its previously assigned code equivalent)
- ICD-10-PCS Draft Coding System and Manual

C. The NCHS is dedicated to monitoring health in the United States. Their website, **http://www.cdc.gov/nchs/icd9.htm,** provides information on "What's New" in healthcare. Explore the topic, "Classification of Death and Injury Resulting from Terrorism," which discusses how the events of 9/11 affected coding.

Performance Objective 12-1—Identifying Format Components in Volume 2 of the ICD-9-CM Manual

Conditions: Student will identify the various format components in Volume 2 of the ICD-9-CM Manual.
Supplies/Equipment: Pen/typewriter, current ICD-9-CM manual (with Volume 2), instruction sheet (Fig.12-1)
Time Allowed: 30 minutes
Accuracy Needed to Pass: 90%

Procedural Steps	Points Earned	Comments
Evaluator: Note time began: _____		
1. Carefully read and study the instruction sheet in Fig. 12-1.		
2. Correctly label the format components by writing/keying the correct term that identifies the component in its corresponding numbered blank.		
Item A—5 points		
Item B—6 points		
Item C—4 points		
3. Proofread your answers for accuracy.		
Optional: May deduct points for taking more time than allowed.		

Total Points = 15

Student's Score: _____

Evaluator: _____

Comments: _____

_____

_____

_____

_____

Identifying Format Components in Vol. 2 of the ICD-9-CM Manual

The following are sections taken from Vol. 2 (Index to Diseases) of the ICD-9-CM manual. Identify each component by labeling the corresponding number with the correct name/term of that portion of the disease/condition:

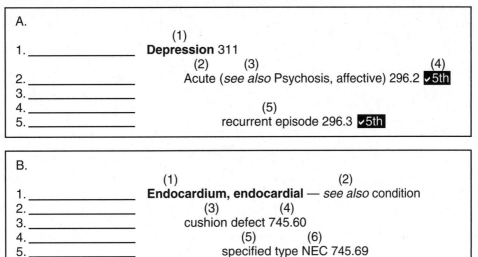

A.

1. _____   **Depression** 311 (1)

2. _____   Acute (*see also* Psychosis, affective) 296.2 ✓5th (2) (3) (4)

3. _____

4. _____

5. _____   recurrent episode 296.3 ✓5th (5)

B.

1. _____   **Endocardium, endocardial** — *see also* condition (1) (2)

2. _____

3. _____   cushion defect 745.60 (3) (4)

4. _____

5. _____   specified type NEC 745.69 (5) (6)

6. _____

C.

1. _____   **Hemorrhage, hemorrhagic** (nontraumatic) 459.0 (1) (2)

2. _____

abdomen 459.0 (3)

3. _____   accidental (antepartum) 641.2 ✓5th

4. _____   affecting fetus or newborn 762.1 (4)

Fig. 12-1 Coding exercise.

Performance Objective 12-2—Assigning Diagnostic Codes

Conditions: Student will study the 10 diseases/conditions listed on the instruction sheet in Fig. 12-2, after which he or she will underline the main term and apply the steps for diagnostic coding to locate the correct ICD-9-CM code (to the greatest level of specificity).

Supplies/Equipment: Pen/typewriter, current ICD-9-CM manual, instruction sheet (see Fig. 12-2)

Time Allowed: 30 minutes

Accuracy Needed to Pass: 90%

Procedural Steps	Points Earned	Comments
Evaluator: Note time began: _____		
1. Carefully read and study the instruction sheet in Fig. 12-2.		
2. Determine and underline the main term for each of the 10 diseases or conditions listed. (10)		
3. Apply the seven steps to accurate diagnostic coding, and assign the correct code (to the greatest specificity) to each of the 10 diagnoses. (20)		
4. Proofread your answers for accuracy.		
Optional: May deduct points for taking more time than allowed.		

Total Points = 30

Student's Score: _____

Evaluator: _____

Comments: _____

_____

_____

_____

_____

Instructions: (1) Determine the main term in each of the following diagnoses and underline it. (2) Using the seven steps to accurate diagnostic coding, code each disease/condition to its greatest specificity.

NOTE: Never code from Volume 2 alone. Find the main term in the Index to Diseases, then turn to the Tabular Section and code to the greatest specificity. Remember: Codes can have up to 5 digits.

1. urinary incontinence   _____

2. multiple vesicovaginal fistula of bladder   _____

3. carcinoma of prostate   _____

4. prepyloric gastric ulcer   _____

5. hypertension, benign essential   _____

6. two infected rectal polyps   _____

7. acute tonsillitis   _____

8. acute cephalgia   _____

9. nasal laceration   _____

10. deviated septum   _____

Fig. 12-2 Coding exercise.

Performance Objective 12-3—Assigning E and V Codes

Conditions: Student will study the 10 health status/injuries listed on the instruction sheet in Fig. 12-3, after which he or she will code each using either an E code or a V Code.

Supplies/Equipment: Pen/typewriter, current ICD-9-CM manual, instruction sheet (Fig. 12-3)

Time Allowed: 30 minutes

Accuracy Needed to Pass: 90%

Procedural Steps	Points Earned	Comments
Evaluator: Note time began: _____		
1. Carefully read and study the instruction sheet in Fig. 12-3.		
2. Review the instructions given for coding health status and injuries.		
3. Using the most current ICD-9-CM manual, identify and underline each main term, then code each of the 10 diagnoses using either an E or a V code. (30)		
4. Proofread your answers for accuracy.		
Optional: May deduct points for taking more time than allowed.		

Total Points = 30

Student's Score: _____

Evaluator: _____

Comments: _____

_____

_____

_____

Instructions: (1) Determine the main term in each of the following diagnoses and <u>underline</u> it. (2) Using the seven steps to accurate diagnostic coding, code each disease/condition to its greatest specificity.

NOTE: Never code from Volume 2 alone. Find the main term in the Index to Diseases, then turn to the Tabular Section and code to the greatest specificity. Remember: Codes can have up to 5 digits.

1. personal history of egg allergy   _____

2. family history of asthma   _____

3. supervision of high risk pregnancy

    with history of infertility   _____

4. routine health check up (18 yo male)   _____

5. dietary counseling   _____

6. follow-up vaginal Pap smear   _____

7. injury sustained by a pedestrian

    hit by a car   _____

8. injury sustained from a fall from a

    snowmobile   _____

9. injury sustained due to being thrown

    from a horse   _____

10. injuries sustained due to tidal wave

    caused by an earthquake   _____

Fig. 12-3 Coding exercise.

Performance Objective 12-4—Assigning Multiple Codes

Conditions: Student will study the diagnoses/conditions on the instruction sheet in Fig. 12-4, after which he or she will code each using the required multiple codes.

Supplies/Equipment: Pen/typewriter, current ICD-9-CM manual, instruction sheet (see Fig. 12-4)

Time Allowed: 30 minutes

Accuracy Needed to Pass: 90%

Procedural Steps	Points Earned	Comments
Evaluator: Note time began: _____		
1. Carefully read and study the instruction sheet in Fig. 12-4.		
2. Using the most current ICD-9-CM manual, underline the main term in each of the five diagnoses. (4 points each; 20 total)		
3. Using the most current ICD-9-CM manual, code each of the five diagnoses using multiple coding. (30)		
4. Proofread your answers for accuracy.		
Optional: May deduct points for taking more time than allowed.		

Total Points = 50

Student's Score: _____

Evaluator: _____

Comments: _____

_____

_____

_____

_____

NOTE: Multiple coding is encouraged when more than one code will fully identify a given condition. The documented statement of diagnosis must mention the presence of all the elements for each code number used. Multiple coding is mandatory when the instructional term "code also" appears in the code being assigned. "Code Also" requires the use of both codes. List the cause as primary and the effect as secondary on the claim. Multiple coding should not be used when a combination code accurately identifies the diagnosis.

Disease/Condition	Primary	Secondary
1. diabetic ulcer, skin	_____	_____
2. viral arthritis	_____	_____
3. malarial fever with hepatitis	_____	_____
4. myocarditis due to tuberculosis	_____	_____
5. endocarditis due to typhoid	_____	_____

Fig. 12-4 Coding exercise.

Health Insurance Professional's Notebook

Create a section in your Health Insurance Professional's Notebook for help with diagnostic coding when you become employed. Include such things as the following:

- Guidelines to accurate diagnostic coding
- Coding examples
- Table of Conventions
- Informative websites
- Resources/references

ADDITIONAL CODING EXERCISES

Using the guidelines given in the text and the most current ICD-9-CM manual, code the following diagnoses/conditions to their greatest level of specificity. (Some may need more than one code.)

Exercise 1

Abdominal discomfort: _____

Abdominal pain, right upper quadrant: _____

Acute conjunctivitis: _____

Acute cephalgia: _____

Acute hemorrhagic otitis media with effusion: _____

Acute otitis media: _____

Acute rheumatoid juvenile arthritis: _____

Acute, obstructed gastric ulcer with hemorrhage and perforation: _____

Alcoholic gastritis: _____

Cardiovascular disease, angina pectoris: _____

Pelvic inflammatory disease: _____

Contact dermatitis: _____

Breast mass: _____

Bronchial croup: _____

Chest pain: _____

Closed fracture of fifth cervical vertebra: _____

Color blindness (congenital): _____

Exercise 2

Compound fracture of right humerus: _____

COPD: _____

Coronary insufficiency: _____

Cystic fibrosis: _____

Deviated septum: _____

Diabetes mellitus: _____

Dietary counseling with dietitian for diabetes: _____

Diverticulitis of duodenum: _____

Exertional dyspnea: _____

Extra thyroid gland: _____

Follow-up examination after surgery: _____

Food poisoning NOS with vomiting: _____

Acute idiopathic pericarditis: _____

Chronic lymphadenitis: _____

Gangrene due to insulin-dependent diabetes: _____

Heartburn: _____

Ileitis, noninfectious: _____

Infected rectal polyps (2): _____

Infection, base of left great toe: _____

Inflammatory cystic lesion of scalp (⅕ cm): _____

Klebsiella pneumonia: _____

Exercise 3

Lumbago due to displacement of intervertebral disc: _____

Lung abscess: _____

Myocardial infarction with hypertension, subsequent episode of care: _____

Nasal laceration: _____

Necrosis of liver: _____

Onychauxis and onychocryptosis: _____

Osteoarthrosis, localized, primary of ankle: _____

Paranoid delusions: _____

Parkinson's disease: _____

Potassium deficiency: _____

Premature ventricular contractions: _____

Pulmonary emphysema: _____

Exposure to rabies: _____

Reflux esophagitis: _____

Right hip fracture, closed: _____

Right otitis media, necrotizing with rupture of eardrum: _____

Ringing in the ears: _____

Routine chest x-ray: _____

Sebaceous cyst: _____

Senile cataract: _____

Exercise 4

Severe onychocryptosis, both margins of left hallux: _____

Shortness of breath: _____

Tension headache: _____

Toxic nodular goiter with crisis: _____

Urinary tract infection due to *Trichomonas:* _____

Varicose veins, lower extremities: _____

Well-baby examination: _____

Yellow jaundice: _____

Actinic keratosis: _____

Common migraine with blurred vision: _____

Urinary tract infection with vaginitis (NOS): _____

Food poisoning (NOS) without vomiting: _____

Colles' fracture: _____

Irritable colon: _____

6-week postpartum checkup: _____

Accidental drowning after fall from motorboat: _____

Measles (no complications documented): _____

Irritable bladder: _____

Kaposi's sarcoma: _____

Adverse reaction to pertussis vaccine: _____

Hypokalemia: _____

Chapter Check List

Student name: _____

Chapter completion date: _____

1.	Record	Your start time and date: _____
2.	Read	The assigned chapter in the text
3.	View	PowerPoint slides (if available)
4.	Complete	Exercises in the Workbook as assigned
5.	Compare	Your answers to the answers posted on the bulletin board/website/handout
6.	Correct	Your answers
7.	Complete	All tests and required activities
8.	Read	Assigned readings (if any)
9.	Complete	Chapter performance objectives (competencies), if any
10.	Evaluate	Chapter performance, and submit to your instructor
11.	Record	Your ending time and date: _____
12.	Move on	Begin next chapter as assigned

PERFORMANCE EVALUATION

Evaluate your classroom performance. Complete the self-evaluation, and submit it to your instructor. When your instructor returns this form to you, compare your self-evaluation with the evaluation completed by your instructor.

Skill	Student Self-Evaluation			Instructor Evaluation		
	Good	Average	Poor	Good	Average	Poor
Attendance/punctuality						
Personal appearance						
Applies effort						
Is self-motivated						
Is courteous						
Has positive attitude						
Completes assignments in timely manner						
Works well with others						

Student's Initials: _____

Date: _____

Instructor's Initials: _____

Date: _____

Points Possible: _____

Points Awarded: _____

Chapter Grade: _____

13 Procedural, Evaluation and Management, and HCPCS Coding

Current Procedural Terminology (CPT) is "a list of descriptive terms and identifying codes for reporting medical services and procedures that physicians perform. The purpose of CPT is to provide a uniform language that accurately describes medical, surgical, and diagnostic services, thereby serving as an effective means for reliable nationwide communication among physicians, patients, and third parties" (American Medical Association [AMA], 1992).

"The only legal way to be paid for a service is to bill using the correct CPT code. The medical facility also must document that the level of service claimed was delivered. Failure to do so may be fraud" (American Academy of Child and Adolescent Psychiatry, 2007).

CPT codes describe medical or psychiatric procedures performed by physicians and other healthcare providers. The codes were developed by the Health Care Financing Administration (HCFA), now known as the Centers for Medicare and Medicaid Services (CMS), to assist in the assignment of reimbursement amounts to providers by Medicare carriers. More and more managed care and other insurance companies now base their reimbursements on the values established by HCFA.

Chapter 13 provides students with the basics of CPT coding. The text identifies and explains the organization and structure of the CPT manual, and how procedures and services provided to patients treated in physicians' offices are transformed into valid procedural codes. After reading Chapter 13, students should have a basic understanding of CPT coding terminology and definitions. This text is not intended to prepare students for CPT certification; rather, it provides a foundation of the procedural coding process. After thoroughly reading and studying the chapter and completing the exercises and activities in the text and the workbook, students should be able to identify and execute the step-by-step process of assigning CPT, Evaluation and Management (E & M), or HCFA's Common Procedure Coding System (HCPCS) codes.

WORKBOOK CHAPTER OBJECTIVES

After completing the workbook activities for Chapter 13, the student should be able to:
- Define the terms used in the chapter.
- Answer the review questions to within the evaluation criteria set by the instructor.
- Identify coding conventions and their meaning.
- Make judgments or arrive at rational solutions to coding scenarios requiring critical thinking.
- Use problem-solving skills (individually or in a group setting) to determine correct responses and outcomes in case studies and application exercises.
- Apply the correct steps for accurate coding.
- Assign the correct CPT and HCPCS codes to procedures and services.
- Identify the correct use of modifiers.

DEFINING CHAPTER TERMS

Using the computer (or typewriter), students should key an accurate definition for each of the chapter terms listed. These definitions should be in the students' own words. When finished, students should compare their definitions with those listed in the glossary at the back of the textbook, correcting any inaccuracies.

category	Evaluation and Management (E & M) codes
Category III codes	face-to-face time
Centers for Medicare and Medicaid Services (CMS)	HCFA's Common Procedure Coding System (HCPCS)
chief complaint (CC)	HCPCS codes
concurrent care	Health Care Financing Administration (HCFA)
consultation	history of present illness (HPI)
counseling	indented code
critical care	inpatient
crosswalk	key components
emergency care	Level I (codes)
established patient	

Level II (codes)
Level III (codes)
modifier
modifying term
neonates
new patient
observation
outpatient
past, family, and social history (PFSH)
Physicians' Current Procedural Terminology, Fourth
    Edition (CPT-4)

Physicians' Current Procedural Terminology, Fifth
    Edition (CPT-5)
review of systems (ROS)
section
see
special report
stand-alone code
subheading
subjective information
subsection
unit/floor time

ASSESSMENT

Multiple Choice

Directions: In the following questions/statements, choose the response that **best** answers/completes the stem, and circle the letter that precedes it.

1. The manual containing codes used in reporting medical services and procedures performed and supplies used by healthcare providers in the care and treatment of patients is the:
   a. HCPCS Level II
   b. ICD-9-CM
   c. CPT-4
   d. All of the above

2. CPT codes were developed by:
   a. The World Health Organization (WHO)
   b. The AMA
   c. HCFA
   d. The Department of Health and Human Services (HHS)

3. The CPT manual is published by:
   a. the AMA
   b. HCFA
   c. the WHO
   d. the HHS

4. A new CPT manual is published:
   a. Annually
   b. Semiannually
   c. Biannually
   d. Every 5 years

5. The first CPT was developed and published in:
   a. 1955
   b. 1966
   c. 1970
   d. 1977

6. The 5-digit coding system replaced the 4-digit system in the CPT edition published in:
   a. 1955
   b. 1966
   c. 1970
   d. 1977

7. The main body of the CPT manual is organized in:
   a. 4 sections
   b. 6 sections
   c. 10 sections
   d. 12 sections

8. The 5-digit CPT codes may be defined further by 2 additional digits to help explain an unusual circumstance associated with a service or procedure, which are called:
   a. Modifiers
   b. Amendments
   c. Appendices
   d. CPT codes cannot have more than 5 digits

9. As with the ICD-9-CM, the CPT index is organized by:
   a. Disease process
   b. Anatomic sites
   c. Main terms
   d. Symptoms

10. A main term can stand alone, or it can be followed by up to _____ modifying term(s).
    a. One
    b. Two
    c. Three
    d. Four

11. To help determine the appropriateness and medical necessity of a service or procedure, a _____ should accompany the claim.
    a. Copy of the patient's health record
    b. Letter of explanation
    c. Special report
    d. Diagram

12. The narrative describing a procedure/service that contains the full description of the procedure without additional explanation is referred to as a(n):
    a. Complete code
    b. Unmodified code
    c. Descriptive code
    d. Stand-alone code

13. Procedures that do not contain the entire written description and refer back to the common portion of the procedure listed in the preceding entry are coded with a(n):
    a. Modified code
    b. Indented code
    c. Unfinished code
    d. Incomplete code

14. CPT uses _____ to separate main and subordinate clauses in the code descriptions.
    a. A bullet
    b. Parentheses
    c. A triangle
    d. A semicolon

15. The reason the patient is seeing the physician—usually stated in the patient's own words—is referred to as the:
    a. Chief complaint (CC)
    b. History of present illness (HPI)
    c. Review of systems (ROS)
    d. Past, family, and social history (PFSH)

16. The series of questions the provider asks the patient to identify what body parts or body systems are involved is referred to as the:
    a. Chief complaint (CC)
    b. History of present illness (HPI)
    c. Review of systems (ROS)
    d. Past, family, and social history (PFSH)

17. The amount of time the physician spends on bedside care of the hospitalized patient and reviewing the health record and writing orders is called:
    a. Face-to-face time
    b. Unit/floor time
    c. Counseling time
    d. Treatment time

18. The classification for a patient who is not sick enough to qualify for acute inpatient status, but requires hospitalization for a brief time, is referred to as:
    a. Outpatient status
    b. Observation status
    c. Unit/floor time
    d. Nonemergency status

19. A procedure by which codes used for data in one database are translated into the codes of another database, allowing information to be shared among databases, is called:
    a. A crosswalk
    b. Database sharing
    c. Intervention
    d. Electronic recognition

20. HCPCS Level II codes are organized into _____ sections.
    a. 5
    b. 8
    c. 12
    d. 17

True/False

Directions: Place a "T" in the blank preceding each of the following statements if it is true; place an "F" if it is false.

_____ 1. Today, most managed care and other insurance companies base their reimbursements on the values established by the CMS.

_____ 2. If the correct CPT code is not known, a narrative description of the procedure/service rendered can be used in Block 24d of the CMS-1500 form.

_____ 3. Modifiers are listed in Appendix A at the back of the CPT manual.

_____ 4. Missing or incorrect modifiers are a common reason for claim denial.

_____ 5. If a Category I code is available and accurately describes the service provided, it should be used instead of a Category III code.

_____ 6. Modifier -99 can be used if the coder cannot find a 5-digit CPT code that adequately describes the procedure performed.

_____ 7. There are two types of CPT codes: stand-alone and indented.

_____ 8. Every office visit, regardless of location, must include at least two of these three components—history, examination, and medical decision making.

_____ 9. The key to reimbursement for office/outpatient visits is being able to prove the level of complexity of the services performed.

_____ 10. Coding E & M services is based on the amount of time spent with the patient or his or her family.

_____ 11. Time is not considered a factor unless 75% of the encounter is spent in counseling.

_____ 12. Time is never a factor for emergency department visits.

_____ 13. All three key components (history, examination, and medical decision making) must be met or exceeded for new patients; only two must be met for established patients.

_____ 14. Hospital Discharge Services codes are used for reporting services provided on the final day of a multiple-day stay.

_____ 15. To qualify for the use of E & M codes 99281 to 99288, the facility must be available for immediate emergency care 24 hours a day for patients on "observation status."

_____ 16. Critical Care Services can be provided only if the facility has an emergency department that operates 24 hours a day.

_____ 17. To use the Critical Care Services codes properly, the physician must be constantly at the patient's bedside.

_____ 18. Time is the controlling factor for assigning the appropriate critical care code.

_____ 19. Modifiers are never used in E & M coding.

_____ 20. HCPCS Level II (national) codes are 5-digit alphanumeric codes consisting of one alphabetic character (a letter between A and V), followed by 3 digits.

_____ 21. If there are CPT and HCPCS Level II codes for the service provided, the CMS requires that the HCPCS Level II code be used.

_____ 22. As with CPT-4, HCPCS Level II code sets contain modifiers; however, modifiers in HCPCS Level II are either alphabetic or alphanumeric.

_____ 23. HIPAA requires that procedure coding be standardized.

_____ 24. With the implementation of HIPAA, the CMS has required medical offices to eliminate any unapproved local procedure or modifier codes (Level III codes).

_____ 25. The AMA is in the process of developing CPT-5, which will totally change the procedural coding process.

Short Answer/Fill-in-the-Blank

1. What is the purpose of CPT coding?

   _____

   _____

   _____

2. List the four things accomplished by the first CPT edition.

   _____

   _____

   _____

   _____

3. List and discuss the three levels of procedural coding.

   _____

   _____

   _____

4. The health record must contain adequate documentation to support the use of _____.

5. Each main section of the CPT is preceded by _____ specific to that section.

6. What is the purpose of Category III codes?

   _____

   _____

7. List the 12 appendices found in CPT and describe what each contains.

   _____

   _____

   _____

   _____

   _____

   _____

   _____

_____

_____

_____

_____

_____

8. Name and give an example of each of the four primary classes of main term entries.

_____

_____

_____

_____

9. What are the three ways a CPT code can be displayed? Include examples of each.

_____

_____

_____

10. If a "special report" accompanies a claim to explain unusual circumstances, list what should be included in this document.

_____

_____

_____

_____

_____

11. Explain the use and importance of a semicolon (;) in assigning a CPT code.

_____

_____

_____

12. Codes in the tabular section of CPT are formatted using four classifications. List and explain each of these.

_____

_____

_____

_____

13. List the six basic steps of CPT coding discussed in the textbook.

_____

_____

_____

_____

_____

_____

14. Distinguish between a "new" patient and an "established" patient.

_____

_____

_____

15. The range of codes for office or other outpatient services is _____ to _____ for new

patients and _____ to _____ for established patients.

16. List the three factors that direct the health insurance professional to the proper category in the E & M coding section of CPT.

_____

_____

_____

17. In addition to determining each of the three factors listed in question 16, the health insurance professional must establish what level of service the patient received. Levels of service are based on three key components, which are:

_____

_____

_____

18. In addition to the three key components listed in question 17, there may be four contributing factors that affect the E & M coding level reported. These contributing factors include:

_____

_____

_____

_____

19. The first element to consider in assigning an E & M code is the level of patient history. Name the four elements of history taking.

_____

_____

_____

_____

20. The second component in determining the correct E & M level is the patient examination. As with history taking, there are four degrees, or detailed intensities, involved in a patient examination. Name these four degrees of patient examination.

_____

_____

_____

_____

21. The last of the three key components is medical decision making. In determining the complexity of decision making, the health insurance professional must consider what three elements?

_____

_____

_____

22. Discuss the importance of thorough and accurate documentation in a health record.

_____

_____

_____

_____

23. Explain the main differences between the 1995 and the 1997 guideline criteria for assigning E & M codes.

_____

_____

_____

_____

24. Explain in what ways, if any, CPT-5 differs from CPT-4.

_____

_____

_____

_____

Matching

Directions: Place the letter identifying the correct symbol in the blank in front of the numbered statements. (**Note:** Not all symbols are used.)

_____ 1. Code is new to the CPT book

_____ 2. Description has been changed/modified

_____ 3. Identifies changes in wording of new or revised codes

_____ 4. Add-on code

_____ 5. Codes that are modifier-exempt

_____ 6. Modifier 51 exempt

a. *
b. ●
c. –
d. ▲
e. +
f. ▶◀
g. ⊘
h. ⊙

CRITICAL THINKING ACTIVITIES

A. In the following scenarios, determine if each patient is "new" or "established."

1. Jessica Sidwell has an appointment at Broadmoor Medical Clinic today. She is new to the area, having recently moved to Milton from another state.

2. Elwood Camp was seen at the hospital for a consultation 2 weeks ago. He is coming to the office today for a follow-up appointment.

3. While Dr. Jones was attending a seminar in another city, Dr. Lucero treated Barbara Farris for acute sinusitis.

4. Robert Fuller, who was seen by Dr. Jones 2 years ago for an eye infection, has an appointment today with Dr. Lucero. Robert has just returned from an 18-month tour of duty in Afghanistan.

5. Martha Gibbs, who has a 10 AM appointment today, saw Dr. Lucero 5 years ago when she was a resident at Columbia University Clinic in Missouri.

6. Jill Bennet has an appointment with Dr. Jones tomorrow for a consultation. She has not been seen at Broadmoor Medical Clinic before, but her primary care provider has forwarded her complete health record.

B. In the following scenarios, determine if the procedure/service would classify as a "consultation" or a "referral."

1. Dr. Jones has been treating Sylvia Potter for a skin condition. He has prescribed several medications, but the problem persists. Dr. Jones instructs Mrs. Potter to make an appointment with Dr. Fontaine, a renowned dermatologist at the University Clinic, for his opinion of the condition.

2. Dr. Lucero has asked you make an appointment for Zebulon Porter with a cardiologist for diagnostic tests to pinpoint the cause of Mr. Porter's cardiac symptoms.

3. Ellen Tyson is being seen at Broadmoor Medical Clinic for gastrointestinal problems that do not respond to treatment. Dr. Lucero asks Dr. Benson, a psychiatrist, to evaluate Ms. Tyson to see if her symptoms might be psychosomatic.

4. The emergency department physician on duty telephones Dr. Jones to evaluate a patient who has sustained a back injury as a result of an automobile accident. After Dr. Jones examines the patient, the patient is rushed to the operating room for immediate surgery.

5. Dr. Lucero's patient, Lucas Bonnet, asks for an appointment with ophthalmologist Vincent Carter for a second opinion before eye surgery.

C. Underline the main terms in the following procedures:

Intertrochanteric femoral fracture (closed treatment)

Removal of gallbladder calculi

Lung, bullae excision

Closed treatment of wrist dislocation

Dilation of cervix

Placement of upper gastrointestinal feeding tube

Radiograph and fluoroscope of chest, four views

Magnetic resonance imaging, lower spine

Darrach procedure

Manual CBC

Electrosurgical removal, five skin tags

PROBLEM SOLVING/COLLABORATIVE (GROUP) ACTIVITIES

A. Underline the main term, and code the following procedures:

Puncture aspiration of breast cyst: _____

Diagnostic bronchoscopy with biopsy: _____

Pacemaker insertion with transvenous electrode, atrial: _____

T & A; 12-year-old boy: _____

Removal of urethral diverticulum from female patient: _____

Therapeutic D&C, nonobstetric: _____

Penicillin injection, IM, 5 mL: _____

Face-to-face psychotherapy (individual), 50 minutes: _____

B. Select the "new" patient office visit E & M codes using the key components listed.

1. Detailed history, detailed examination, low-complexity decision making: _____

2. Problem-focused history, problem-focused examination, straightforward decision making: _____

3. Comprehensive history, comprehensive examination, high-complexity decision making: _____

C. Select the "established" patient office visit E & M codes using the key components listed.

1. Detailed history, detailed examination, low-complexity decision making: _____

2. Comprehensive history, comprehensive examination, moderate-complexity decision making: _____

3. Detailed history, comprehensive examination, high-complexity decision making: _____

D. Explain the guidelines for reporting a "miscellaneous" procedure/service for which there is no listed CPT code.

E. You have received a denial from an insurance carrier because you, in error, used a deleted procedure code on the claim. How could you have prevented this from happening, and how can you find the correct code?

PROJECTS/DISCUSSION TOPICS

A. Your instructor will choose one or more of the following topics to discuss in class or will assign to you as a project. Study Chapter 13 to be prepared for taking an active part in any or all of these issues:

1. Why is it important to use the most recent CPT manual available?
2. What role does CPT coding play in insurance reimbursement?
3. Discuss the importance of adhering to accurate coding/billing guidelines.
4. When are modifiers used, and how do they affect CPT coding?
5. Discuss the proper use of "observation" codes.

B. Can 99218-99220 be reported for each day a patient is in observation? The codes state "per day" in the definition.

CASE STUDIES

In the Critical Thinking Activities for this workbook chapter, six scenarios were presented for which you had to determine whether the patient was new or established. Now, study these same six scenarios and code the procedures/services listed in each.

1. Jessica Sidwell has an appointment at Broadmoor Medical Clinic today. She is new to the area, having recently moved to Milton from another state.

    Initial new patient office visit Level II
    Intramuscular antibiotic injection

2. Elwood Camp was seen at the hospital for a consultation 2 weeks ago. He is coming to the office today for a follow-up appointment.

    Postoperative follow-up visit

3. While Dr. Jones was attending a seminar in another city, Dr. Lucero treated Barbara Farris for acute sinusitis.

    Established patient office visit Level II
    Removal of nasal polyp, simple

4. Robert Fuller, who was seen by Dr. Jones 2 years ago for an eye infection, has an appointment today with Dr. Lucero. Robert has just returned from an 18-month tour of duty in Afghanistan. Because it had been 2 years since Robert had been to the office, Dr. Lucero performed a complete physical examination.

    Established patient office visit Level III
    Comprehensive eye examination
    Removal of foreign body from right eye (external/superficial)

5. Martha Gibbs, who has a 10 AM appointment today, saw Dr. Lucero 5 years ago when she was a resident at Columbia University Clinic in Missouri.

    New patient office visit Level III
    Pap smear
    Lipid panel
    Electrocardiogram (12 leads)
    Occult blood fecal test

6. Jill Bennet has an appointment with Dr. Jones tomorrow for a consultation. She has not been seen at Broadmoor Medical Clinic before, but her primary care provider has forwarded her complete health record. Jill has been experiencing problems with her periods (heavy bleeding, bleeding between periods, and severe cramping).

Initial visit new patient Level III
Transvaginal ultrasound
Vaginal colposcopy with biopsy

INTERNET EXPLORATION

A. Log on to and peruse the AMA website's page on CPT coding at **http://www.ama-assn.org/ama/pub/category/3113.html.**

B. The following are just a few of many websites that provide information for further education if you are interested in becoming a certified coder:

- **http://www.aapc.com**
- **http://www.ahima.org/certification**
- **http://www.physicianswebsites.com/medical-coding-education.htm**
- **http://www.cms.hhs.gov/medlearn/ncci.asp?**

C. Log on to the website **http://www.medicarenhic.com/cal_prov/med_review/coding.htm#one** and read through some of the pertinent questions and answers regarding typical coding questions.

Performance Objective 13-1—Coding Procedures and Services

Conditions: Student will identify the main term in each of 10 procedural events by underlining it and then correctly code these same procedures.

Supplies/Equipment: Pen/typewriter, current CPT manual, list of procedures to code

Time Allowed: 30 minutes

Accuracy Needed to Pass: 90%

Procedural Steps	Points Earned	Comments
Evaluator: Note time began: _____		
Colonoscopy with biopsy		
Chest x-ray, single view, frontal		
Lipid panel		
HDL cholesterol		
Strep test, rapid		
ECG with interpretation		
Simple suture (face), local anesthetic		
Bilateral mammography		
Destruction, flat wart		
Partial splenectomy		

Total Points = 20 (2 points each)

Student's Score: _____

Evaluator: _____

Comments: _____

_____

_____

_____

_____

Performance Objective 13-2—Coding Office Visits (E & M Codes)

Conditions: Student will study the scenarios in Box 13-1 and code each encounter using E & M codes from the CPT manual.

Supplies/Equipment: Pen/typewriter, current CPT manual, instruction sheet in Box 13-1

Time Allowed: 30 minutes

Accuracy Needed to Pass: 90%

Procedural Steps	Points Earned	Comments
Evaluator: Note time began: _____		
1. Carefully read and study the case studies in Box 13-1.		
2. Correctly identify the proper E & M code for each of these scenarios:		
Scenario 1:		
Scenario 2:		
Scenario 3:		
Scenario 4:		
Scenario 5:		
Scenario 6:		
Optional: May deduct points for taking more time than allowed.		

Total Points = 30 (5 points each)

Student's Score: _____

Evaluator: _____

Comments: _____

_____

_____

_____

_____

Box 13-1

1. Heidi Andrews, an 8-year-old girl, presents as a new patient to Broadmoor Medical Clinic with a severe skin rash. History and examination are problem focused; decision making is straightforward.

2. Forrest Gunther, an established patient with a history of chronic sinusitis, presents with sinus drainage, sore throat, severe nasal congestion, cough, and fever of 100.1 °F. History and examination are problem focused; medical decision making is low complexity.

3. Elena Rodriguez presents with a benign lesion on her right leg. Although this patient has not been seen in the clinic before, she says she has had the mole for several years. The problem is low to moderate severity, and Dr. Jones spends 20 minutes face-to-face with Ms. Rodriguez.

4. Loris Hiller, an 82-year-old man, comes to the clinic for a follow-up examination. He is a controlled diabetic, but has other health problems, including diabetic retinopathy, hypertension, glaucoma, and chronic obstructive pulmonary disease. History and examination are detailed with moderate-complexity medical decision making. Dr. Lucero spends 25 minutes with Mr. Hiller.

5. Melinsa Delarosa, a 55-year-old woman, was admitted for observation because of chest pains to Broadmoor Medical Center and discharged the same day. The key components are comprehensive history and examination with moderate-complexity medical decision making.

6. Dr. Jones admits 15-month-old Brittany Lanz to Broadmoor Medical Center. Brittany has been experiencing recurring episodes of respiratory distress with greenish yellow nasal discharge, cough with wheezing, and fever of 103.6 °F. Her mother reports a decrease in appetite and irritability with intermittent ear pulling. A comprehensive history is taken with a complete multisystem examination. Because of multiple diagnosis and management options plus an excessive amount of data to be reviewed in the health record, the medical decision making is high complexity.

Performance Objective 13-3—Locating HCPCS Codes

Conditions: Student will code 10 procedures/services/supplies listed.
Supplies/Equipment: Pen/typewriter, current HCPCS (CPT Level II codes) manual
Time Allowed: 30 minutes
Accuracy Needed to Pass: 90%

Procedural Steps	Points Earned	Comments
Evaluator: Note time began: _____		
2-mL sterile syringe with needle		
Nonemergency transport (taxi)		
Diaphragm for contraceptive use		
Depo-Provera injection		
Standard wheelchair with footrests		
Ampicillin injection, 500 mg		
Ostomy pouch, closed with barrier and filter		
Thoracic rib belt		
Spenco molded foot insert, removable		
Cephalin flocculation test		
1. Proofread your answers for accuracy.		
Optional: May deduct points for taking more time than allowed.		

Total Points = 20 (2 points each)

Student's Score: _____

Evaluator: _____

Comments: _____

_____

_____

_____

_____

Performance Objective 13-4—Choosing Modifiers

Conditions: Student will identify the correct modifier to use in each of the scenarios given in Box 13-2.
Supplies/Equipment: Pen/typewriter, current CPT manual, scenarios listed in Box 13-2
Time Allowed: 30 minutes
Accuracy Needed to Pass: 90%

Procedural Steps	Points Earned	Comments
Evaluator: Note time began: _____		
1. Carefully read and study the scenarios in Box 13-2.		
2. Correctly identify the proper modifier to use for each of these scenarios:		
Scenario 1:		
Scenario 2:		
Scenario 3:		
Scenario 4:		
Scenario 5:		
Scenario 6:		
3. Proofread your answers for accuracy.		
Optional: May deduct points for taking more time than allowed.		

Total Points = 30 (5 points each)

Student's Score: _____

Evaluator: _____

Comments: _____

_____

_____

_____

_____

Box 13-2

1. When Teresa Hardy underwent her hysterectomy, complications occurred during the surgical procedure. Typically, the procedure lasts about 1½ hours; however, Teresa's lasted nearly 3 hours.

2. Performing a cystoscopy on an adult normally would not require general anesthesia; however, for 3-year-old Benjamin Field, Dr. Lucero determined that a general anesthetic would be best.

3. Dr. Jones removed a ruptured appendix from a patient and provided a general anesthetic for the procedure. Listing separate charges for each of the services would be appropriate; the health insurance professional would code as follows: 44960—appendectomy, ruptured appendix. The code for a surgeon administering his or her own anesthetic for the procedure (44960) would require a modifier.

4. The bilateral modifier is restricted to surgical procedures only (CPT codes 10040-69990). It is not required for radiology procedure codes or diagnostic procedure codes. Procedures now are assumed to be unilateral, unless they are always performed bilaterally or are otherwise noted in CPT. The most commonly accepted method of reporting bilateral procedures is to list the procedure twice and add the correct modifier.

5. Certain complex surgical procedures require the skills of more than two surgeons. A good example is the surgical team that implants an artificial heart. The physicians performing the surgery usually have different skills or specialties. Each member of the team would add a modifier to the procedures he or she performed as part of the surgical team.

6. A patient is brought to the hospital with internal hemorrhaging that is repaired surgically. Three days after surgery, the patient begins hemorrhaging again, and the surgeon must perform the same repair again. If a different physician had performed the second repair, he or she would use a different modifier.

Health Insurance Professional's Notebook

Create a section in your Health Insurance Professional's Notebook for help with procedural coding when you become employed. Include such things as the following:

- Guidelines to accurate procedural coding
- Coding examples
- List of CPT manual appendices and their contents
- CPT manual sections and their code ranges
- Informative websites
- Resources/references

ADDITIONAL CODING EXERCISES

Using the guidelines given in the text and the most current CPT manual, code the following procedures/services/supplies.

Exercise 1

Procedure: Surgery Section

_____ Removal of 25 skin tags

_____ Partial removal of the spleen

_____ Radical cervical lymphadenectomy

_____ Excision of benign tumor of the mediastinum

_____ Incision and drainage of a simple lymph node abscess

_____ Flexible sigmoidoscopy with three biopsies

_____ Colonoscopy with removal of polyp by a snare

_____ Exploratory laparotomy with cholecystectomy

_____ Repair of an initial incarcerated inguinal hernia in a 5½-year-old

_____ Complete vasectomy

_____ Reversal of urethral anastomosis

_____ Anterior segment of the left eyes, emboli removal

_____ Removal of left eye, muscles attached to implant

_____ Destruction of 0.4-cm malignant lesion of the neck

_____ Suture of sciatic nerve

Exercise 2

Procedure: Radiology, Pathology, and Laboratory Sections

_____ Bilateral mammography

_____ Radiologic examination of mastoids, two views

_____ Chest x-ray single view, frontal

_____ Complete hip x-ray study, two views

_____ Ultrasound of the chest using B-scan

_____ Fetal profile, biophysical

_____ Teletherapy, isodose plan, simple

_____ Automated urinalysis without microscopy

_____ Gases, blood pH only

Code the following using one of the six surgical pathology codes in the CPT manual:

_____ The specimen is a uterus, tubes, and ovaries. The procedure was an abdominal hysterectomy for ovarian cancer.

_____ The specimen is a portion of the lung. The procedure was a left lower lobe wedge resection (Level VI).

_____ The specimen is the prostate. The procedure was a transurethral resection of the prostate (Level IV).

Exercise 3

Procedure: Medicine Section

_____ Routine electrocardiogram with 12 leads, with interpretation and report

_____ Cardiac catheterization on the right side of the heart

_____ Pulmonary stress test, simple

_____ Direct nasal mucous membrane test

_____ Awake and drowsy electroencephalogram and photic stimulation in clinic

_____ Range of motion measurement and report on both legs

_____ Chemotherapy administered subcutaneously

_____ Initial psychiatric interview examination

_____ Acid reflux test of the esophagus with nasal catheter pH electrode placement, recording, analysis, and interpretation

_____ Fitting of contact lens for treatment of cataract, including the lens

_____ Nasopharyngoscopy with evaluation

_____ Hemodialysis with a single physician evaluation

_____ Oral polio vaccine

Exercise 4

Procedure: Integumentary System

_____ Destruction, flat wart

_____ Layer closure of skin wound, >30 cm, trunk

_____ Repair nail bed

_____ Mastectomy, partial

Procedure: Musculoskeletal System

_____ Injection, ganglion cyst

_____ Treatment of closed patella dislocation without anesthesia

_____ Injection of small joint bursa

_____ Biopsy, bone, trocar, or needle superficial

Procedure: Hemic/Lymphatic/Diaphragm (38100-39599)

_____ Repair, esophageal/diaphragmatic hernia

_____ Partial splenectomy

_____ Excision, two deep cervical nodes

Procedure: Radiology/Pathology

_____ Upper gastrointestinal x-ray study with films and KUB

_____ Ultrasound, pregnant uterus after first trimester

_____ Routine urinalysis with microscopy

_____ Colorimetric hemoglobin

Chapter Check List

Student name: _____

Chapter completion date: _____

1.	Record	Your start time and date: _____
2.	Read	The assigned chapter in the text
3.	View	PowerPoint slides (if available)
4.	Complete	Exercises in the Workbook as assigned
5.	Compare	Your answers to the answers posted on the bulletin board/website/handout
6.	Correct	Your answers
7.	Complete	All tests and required activities
8.	Read	Assigned readings (if any)
9.	Complete	Chapter performance objectives (competencies), if any
10.	Evaluate	Chapter performance, and submit to your instructor
11.	Record	Your ending time and date: _____
12.	Move on	Begin next chapter as assigned

PERFORMANCE EVALUATION

Evaluate your classroom performance. Complete the self-evaluation and submit it to your instructor. When your instructor returns this form to you, compare your self-evaluation with the evaluation completed by your instructor.

Skill	Student Self-Evaluation			Instructor Evaluation		
	Good	Average	Poor	Good	Average	Poor
Attendance/punctuality						
Personal appearance						
Applies effort						
Is self-motivated						
Is courteous						
Has positive attitude						
Completes assignments in timely manner						
Works well with others						

Student's Initials: _____   **Instructor's Initials:** _____

Date: _____   **Date:** _____

Points Possible: _____

Points Awarded: _____

Chapter Grade: _____

14 The Patient

In Chapter 14, we learned about the importance of patient needs and expectations. Patients need to be recognized and treated as individuals by all members of the healthcare team. Patients want to be continuously informed about their illness and condition. An atmosphere of respect for the individual patient focuses on quality of life, involves the patient in medical decisions, treats the patient with dignity, and respects a patient's autonomy. Patients have indicated that they feel vulnerable and powerless in the face of illness, and proper treatment and coordination of their care help to ease those feelings.

Chapter 14 also looked at future trends in patient care, specifically that patients are "consumers" of healthcare, and as consumers, they have a right to expect quality care. Patient advocacy begins with the relationship between the patient and the physician.

A wide scope of patient topics was presented in Chapter 14, including billing policies and practices. The activities and exercises in this accompanying workbook chapter will expand your knowledge of the important relationship between the patient and the healthcare team, and help develop a better understanding of the topics presented in Chapter 14.

WORKBOOK CHAPTER OBJECTIVES

After completing the workbook activities for Chapter 14, the student should be able to:
- Define the terms used in the chapter.
- Answer the review questions to within the evaluation criteria set by the instructor.
- Use problem-solving skills (individually or in a group setting) to determine correct responses and outcomes in case studies and application exercises.
- Work in a group setting to resolve scenarios dealing with credit and collection policies.
- Generate suitable collection techniques (e.g., telephone conversations and letters).
- Create a table of pertinent laws and acts that apply to collection and credit.
- Explore the Internet to learn more about the topics addressed in Chapter 14.

DEFINING CHAPTER TERMS

Using the computer (or typewriter), students should key an accurate definition for each of the chapter terms listed. These definitions should be in the students' own words. When finished, students should compare their definitions with those listed in the glossary at the back of the textbook, correcting any inaccuracies.

accounts receivable
alternate billing cycle
assignment of benefits
billing cycle
collection agency
collection ratio
daily journal
defendant
de-identified
disbursements journal
Equal Credit Opportunity Act
Fair Credit Billing Act
Fair Credit Reporting Act
Fair Debt Collection Practices Act

general journal
general ledger
HIPAA-covered entities
identifiable health information
"one-write" systems
patient information form
patient ledger
payroll journal
plaintiff
self-pay patient
small claims litigation
surrogates
Truth in Lending Act

295

Multiple Choice

Directions: In the questions/statements presented, choose the response that **best** answers/completes the stem by circling the letter that precedes it.

1. Creating a good patient-staff relationship begins when:
   a. The patient arrives at the medical facility
   b. The patient is in the examination room
   c. The patient telephones for an appointment
   d. The patient encounter has been completed

2. The healthcare staff can find out what their patients' expectations are by:
   a. Writing a letter
   b. Asking questions
   c. Having them fill out forms
   d. Taking a survey

3. The services offered by a medical facility usually cannot be felt or seen, which means they:
   a. Are intangible
   b. Are not important
   c. Cannot be documented
   d. Cannot be billed

4. Most physicians prefer to leave the subject of fees up to their:
   a. Nurse
   b. Accountant
   c. Reception staff
   d. Health insurance professional

5. Experts predict that over the next 30 years, the number of Americans older than age 65 will:
   a. Double
   b. Triple
   c. Quadruple
   d. Decrease by about 20%

6. Data that are explicitly linked to a particular individual (including data items that reasonably could be expected to allow individual identification) are referred to as:
   a. Protected health information
   b. HIPAA-explicit information
   c. Individually identifiable health information
   d. a and c are correct

7. An arrangement by which a patient requests that his or her health insurance benefit payments be made directly to a physician or hospital is called a(n):
   a. Release of information
   b. Discharge of authority
   c. Power of attorney
   d. Assignment of benefits

8. Although healthcare practitioners are dedicated to the health and well-being of their patients, their ultimate goal is:
   a. Research
   b. Making a profit
   c. Keeping up on new medical technologies
   d. Publishing articles in prestigious journals

9. The total amount of fees collected divided by the total amount charged provides the practice with a(n):
   a. Profit
   b. Billing ratio
   c. Collection ratio
   d. Accounts receivable balance

10. A patient's name, age, address, telephone number, Social Security number, and employer information are generally referred to as:
    a. Demographics
    b. Vital statistics
    c. "De-identified" data
    d. All of the above

11. When a medical facility uses patient billing software, it is *crucial* to:
    a. Input data correctly
    b. Keep the equipment clean
    c. Make weekly backups
    d. Use state-of-the-art electronic equipment

12. Most medical offices send out statements periodically, which is referred to as a:
    a. Collection practice
    b. Statement control
    c. Billing cycle
    d. Mailing

13. Patients who have inadequate health insurance coverage or no insurance at all are called:
    a. Self-pay patients
    b. Deadbeats
    c. Indigent
    d. Red-flaggers

14. When no insurance is listed on a patient information form, the health insurance professional should:
    a. Alert the physician
    b. Ask the patient to leave
    c. Ask the patient to pay up front
    d. Inquire as to why no insurance is listed

15. An installment payment plan of more than four payments falls under:
    a. HIPAA regulations
    b. The Fair Credit Billing Act
    c. The Equal Credit Opportunity Act
    d. The Federal Truth in Lending Act of 1968, Regulation Z

16. The act that deals primarily with credit reports issued by credit reporting agencies is called:
    a. The Fair Credit Reporting Act
    b. The Fair Credit Billing Act
    c. The Equal Credit Opportunity Act
    d. The Federal Truth in Lending Act of 1968, Regulation Z

17. An organization that obtains or arranges for payment of money owed to a third party is referred to as a:
    a. Legal aid society
    b. Small claims association
    c. Collection agency
    d. Certified public account (CPA) group

18. The process available to individuals or businesses to recover legitimate debts without using expensive legal advisors is known as:
    a. Adjudication
    b. Small claims litigation
    c. Appellate court
    d. Grievance

19. In a small claims suit, the party initiating the action is referred to as the:
    a. Plaintiff
    b. Defendant
    c. Bailiff
    d. Attorney

20. The party being sued is the:
    a. Plaintiff
    b. Defendant
    c. Bailiff
    d. Attorney

True/False

Directions: Place a "T" in the blank preceding each of the following statements if it is true; place an "F" if it is false.

_____ 1.   Patient expectations are the same from office to office.

_____ 2.   Besides being brief and of high quality, paperwork in a medical office should be relevant to the reason the patient is there.

_____ 3.   Patients need to be tolerant of long waits because the physician's time is worth more than their own.

_____ 4.   If the reception area is empty when the patient enters, he or she may think the healthcare provider is second-rate.

_____ 5.   Patients must realize and accept the fact that partition walls are thin in many medical facilities, and private conversations can be overheard.

_____ 6.   Most patients typically have no idea what their medical care and treatment should cost before they make an appointment.

_____ 7.   Today's healthcare consumers expect the cost of their healthcare to be addressed up-front.

_____ 8.   It is a trend in today's fast-paced world for people to believe that their time is just as valuable as their healthcare provider's time.

_____ 9. Members of the healthcare team should discuss their personal lives with patients to promote good provider-patient relationships.

_____ 10. Identifiable medical information includes medical records, medical billing records, any clinical or research databases, and tissue bank samples.

_____ 11. "Covered entities" can transfer protected health information to noncovered entities (those who do not come under HIPAA rules) without violating HIPAA.

_____ 12. HIPAA gives patients the right to access their medical information and to know to whom the covered entity has disclosed this information.

_____ 13. Patients have the right to obtain copies of their protected health information from their physicians or health plans, unless the information is likely to endanger their lives or the lives of other people.

_____ 14. Patients have the right to correct or amend their medical records.

_____ 15. Covered entities can release "de-identified" health information without patient authorization.

_____ 16. Most patients appreciate having fee and billing information presented clearly and matter-of-factly, but in a pleasant and courteous manner.

_____ 17. Experts consider the most effective payment policy is for the front desk staff to request payment when the patient/provider encounter is concluded.

_____ 18. Computerized patient billing software typically includes accounts receivable, insurance billing, and practice management modules.

_____ 19. The most effective way to collect money is to establish a formal financial policy that is clear to patients and the medical staff and to enforce it.

_____ 20. By law, medical facilities are not allowed to extend credit.

_____ 21. Under most state laws, full payment for medical services is due and payable at the time the service is provided.

_____ 22. Regarding collection and credit, it is mandatory that every patient be treated equally.

_____ 23. It is often not cost-effective to use small claims litigation for past due accounts that are less than $30.

_____ 24. To use the small claims process, the practice must retain an attorney.

_____ 25. Professional collection agencies typically retain 50% of collected fees.

Short Answer/Fill-in-the-Blank

1. The text discussed "surrogates" that patients look for in a medical office. List at least four of these common surrogates.

_____

_____

_____

_____

2. List some successful online patient-centered topics.

_____

_____

_____

3. It is the trend for patients to be viewed as "consumers" in today's healthcare world. Explain this phenomenon.

_____

_____

_____

_____

_____

4. The text lists five consumer essentials that experts believe should be mandatory for any medical facility wishing to provide patient-centered service. These are:

_____

_____

_____

_____

_____

5. HIPAA states that specific "covered entities" must comply with HIPAA rules for any health or medical information of identifiable individuals. Identify these covered entities.

_____

_____

_____

6. List the elements that a HIPAA-compliant release of information must include.

_____

_____

_____

_____

_____

Matching

Directions: Place the letter identifying the correct choice in the blank in front of the numbered statements. (**Note:** Not all choices are used.)

_____ 1. A chronological record of all patient transactions, including previous balances, charges, payments, and current daily balances

_____ 2. A listing of all expenses paid out to vendors, such as building rent, office supplies, and salaries

_____ 3. A separate record some offices keep for wages and salaries

_____ 4. A chronological listing of all transactions, considered the most basic of all office records

_____ 5. The "core" of a practice's financial records

_____ 6. A chronological accounting of activities of a particular patient (or family), including all charges and payments

_____ 7. The entire grouping of patient ledgers

a. accounts receivable

b. general ledger

c. patient ledger

d. payroll journal

e. accounts payable

f. general journal

g. disbursements journal

h. chronological journal

i. core journal

j. activities journal

k. daily journal

CRITICAL THINKING ACTIVITIES

A. This statement recently appeared in the *Health Day News:* "Patients who have good relationships with their physicians tend to be more satisfied with their care and have better results." Write a critical thinking paragraph discussing whether or not you agree with this statement, and why or why not.

_____

_____

_____

_____

_____

_____

B. Lindell Holmes, a former patient at Broadmoor Medical Clinic, has not made a payment on his outstanding account for more than 90 days. His account was turned over to the Milton County Collection Agency on 10/07/20XX. Two weeks later, Mr. Holmes comes to the Clinic and pays his bill in full with money order #003665UPS. Assuming that the collection agency keeps 50% of all collections, correctly post this payment on the ledger card in Fig. 14-1.

DOB: 03/22/51
Self-pay

STATEMENT

BROADMOOR MEDICAL CLINIC
4353 Pine Ridge Drive
Milton, XY 12345-0001
Telephone: 555-656-7890

LINDELL R. HOLMES
4216 WEST PINE AV
MILTON, XY 12345

DATE 20XX	PROFESSIONAL SERVICE DESCRIPTION	CHARGE	CREDITS PAYMENTS	ADJUSTMENTS	CURRENT BALANCE
6/09	99203 New Pt Exam	135 00			135 00
6/10	94620 ROA-CASH	185 00	132 00		188 00
7/10	Phone call				
8/10	Col. Letter-cert				

Due and payable within 10 days.   **Pay last amount in balance column** ⇧

Fig. 14-1 Ledger card.

C. Assume that Broadmoor Medical Clinic does not use a collection agency for delinquent accounts, but instead files small claims suits at the local county courthouse on 10/07/20XX. The filing fee is $30, and the Milton County Sheriff's Department charges $25 for serving the papers to Mr. Holmes on 10/09. Using the ledger card in Fig. 14-2, post these charges to Mr. Holmes' account.

DOB: 03/22/51
Self-pay

STATEMENT

BROADMOOR MEDICAL CLINIC
4353 Pine Ridge Drive
Milton, XY 12345-0001
Telephone: 555-656-7890

LINDELL R. HOLMES
4216 WEST PINE AV
MILTON, XY 12345

DATE 20XX	PROFESSIONAL SERVICE DESCRIPTION	CHARGE	CREDITS PAYMENTS	CREDITS ADJUSTMENTS	CURRENT BALANCE
6/09	99203 New Pt Exam	135 00			135 00
6/10	94620 ROA-CASH	185 00	132 00		188 00
7/10	Phone call				
8/10	Col. Letter-cert				

Due and payable within 10 days.   Pay last amount in balance column ⇧

Fig. 14-2 Ledger card.

PROBLEM SOLVING/COLLABORATIVE (GROUP) ACTIVITIES

A. Create a page for Broadmoor Medical Clinic's Policy Manual outlining a payment and collection policy.

B. Compose an outline for a conversation you would use for collecting delinquent accounts using the telephone. Follow the policy you generated in the previous exercise, and remember to be courteous but firm. Also, make sure you do not violate any collection laws or consumers' rights.

C. Set up a payment plan for a self-pay patient who owes $850. Make certain that you follow the policy you generated in Exercise A and the rules outlined in the Federal Truth in Lending Act of 1968, Regulation Z.

PROJECTS/DISCUSSION TOPICS

A. Generate a table of all of the pertinent laws and acts discussed in Chapter 14 that address credit and collection, along with the date they were enacted and a brief description of what each addresses. Use library references and the Internet to complete this assignment, if necessary.

B. Patient "identifiers."
   1. Generate a comprehensive list of potential identifiers that can link information to a particular individual.

   2. Explain how a patient's health record can be "de-identified."

C. The textbook mentions a topic that has long been controversial—patient ownership of the medical record. Research this topic (using the library or Internet or both), and write a 1-page essay of your findings. You should take into consideration the new HIPAA rules when writing your paper.

D. Research your area to discover if billing services are available and what assistance they offer to medical facilities such as Broadmoor Medical Clinic.

CASE STUDIES

A. When Emily Fortune's appointment is concluded on February 7, 20XX, you hand her an encounter form listing the fees, which total $265. Mrs. Fortune does have insurance, but her policy has a $2500 deductible; her carrier will pay nothing toward the fees generated on this date. She advises you that because her condition restricts her ability to perform her job, she cannot pay the entire bill right now, but she can pay $50 a month. Review the credit policy you created for Broadmoor's Policy Manual. Is Mrs. Fortune's monthly payment in line with this policy? If not, how should the payment plan be revised so that it meets the stipulations outlined in the Policy Manual?

B. LaDon Williams is a self-pay patient at Broadmoor. He has not paid on his outstanding balance ($300) for 2 months. During a telephone conversation, Mr. Williams agrees to come to the Clinic and discuss a credit plan. He informs the reception staff that he can afford to pay only $10 a month on his delinquent account. The reception staff refuses to accept the payment, informing Mr. Williams that the entire bill must be paid at once, or his account will be turned over for collection. Can this situation possibly create a problem for Broadmoor Medical Clinic? If so, explain.

304

INTERNET EXPLORATION

A. Log on to the Internet. Using "find doctors," or similar search words, find how much information is available on the Web for today's healthcare consumers.

B. Using search words, such as "patients as consumers," explore the Internet in search of information and thoughts on this subject.

C. To learn more about how to maximize patient collections, search the Internet using the appropriate search words.

D. Search the Internet on information on how to file a small claims suit.

Performance Objective 14-1—Compose a Patient Termination Letter

Conditions: Student will compose a letter terminating a patient's care because of nonpayment of fees, as discussed in the scenario in Box 14-1.

Supplies/Equipment: Pen/typewriter/computer, textbook, paper, information in Box 14-1

Time Allowed: 30 minutes

Accuracy Needed to Pass: 90%

Procedural Steps	Points Earned	Comments
Evaluator: Note time began: _____		
Read the scenario in Box 14-1, and compose a letter of termination; remember to follow all of the legal requirements discussed in the text.		
1. Format (15)		
Date and Inside Address		
Subject Line		
Salutation		
Body		
Complimentary Close and Signature		
References and Enclosure Lines		
Special Notations		
2. Content (brief, but contains all necessary information; courteous; and offers alternative care). (25)		

Total Points = 40

Student's Score: _____

Evaluator: _____

Comments: _____

_____

_____

_____

_____

Box 14-1

Patricia Henderson, 1111 Spruce Avenue, Milton, XY 12345, owes Broadmoor Medical Clinic $465 for professional services rendered beginning in April 2004 through June 2006. Mrs. Henderson has not made any payments since September 2004, and all letters and telephone calls have proved unsuccessful in collecting this account. Dr. Jones has instructed you to send Mrs. Henderson a letter informing her that he no longer can treat her for her chronic asthma because of her refusal to pay her bill.

Performance Objective 14-2—Composing a Generic Collection Form Letter

Conditions: Student will compose a series of three "generic" form letters to keep on file as a template for sending to patients who are delinquent on their payments. Refer to the examples in the textbook for assistance in this exercise.

Supplies/Equipment: Pen/typewriter/computer, textbook, paper

Time Allowed: 30 minutes

Accuracy Needed to Pass: 90%

Procedural Steps	Points Earned	Comments
Evaluator: Note time began: _____		
Compose a "generic" collection form letter.		
1. Format (15 points × 3)		
Date and Inside Address		
Subject Line		
Salutation		
Body		
Complimentary Close and Signature		
References and Enclosure Lines		
Special Notations		
2. Content (20 points × 3)		
Opening paragraph		
Main content paragraph		
Closing paragraph with expectations		

Total Points = 105

Student's Score: _____

Evaluator: _____

Comments: _____

_____

_____

_____

_____

Health Insurance Professional's Notebook

Generate a section in your notebook for resources to aid in patient services and collections, such as the following:

- Informative websites
- Pertinent HIPAA information
- List of laws (and their explanation) that apply to credit and collection
- Samples of letters dealing with:
  ○ Collections
  ○ Termination of patients
- Information on billing services and collection agencies

Chapter Check List

Student name:_____

Chapter completion date: _____

1.	Record	Your start time and date: _____
2.	Read	The assigned chapter in the text
3.	View	PowerPoint slides (if available)
4.	Complete	Exercises in the Workbook as assigned
5.	Compare	Your answers with the answers posted on the bulletin board/website/handout
6.	Correct	Your answers
7.	Complete	All tests and required activities
8.	Read	Assigned readings (if any)
9.	Complete	Chapter performance objectives (competencies), if any
10.	Evaluate	Chapter performance and submit to your instructor
11.	Record	Your ending time and date: _____
12.	Move on	Begin next chapter as assigned

Evaluate your classroom performance. Complete the self-evaluation, and submit it to your instructor. When your instructor returns this form to you, compare your self-evaluation with the evaluation completed by your instructor.

Skill	Student Self-Evaluation			Instructor Evaluation		
	Good	Average	Poor	Good	Average	Poor
Attendance/punctuality						
Personal appearance						
Applies effort						
Is self-motivated						
Is courteous						
Has positive attitude						
Completes assignments in timely manner						
Works well with others						

Student's Initials: _____

Date: _____

Points Possible: _____

Points Awarded: _____

Chapter Grade: _____

Instructor's Initials: _____

Date: _____

15 The Claim

Processing health insurance claims can be a tedious task. When Medicare and Medicaid are involved, the Department of Health and Human Services mandates that most claims be settled in a timely manner—typically within 28 days. To keep the claims process humming, health insurance professionals must know and keep up-to-date on the guidelines of many different third-party payers with the goal being to file "clean claims" and filter out the bad claims before they enter the system. The exercises and activities in this workbook chapter will help to hone your knowledge and ability to complete claims forms accurately and efficiently.

The steps for correctly filling out the 33 blocks of the CMS-1500 were presented in Chapter 5. Reviewing this chapter will refresh your memory and provide assistance in completing the following exercises.

WORKBOOK CHAPTER OBJECTIVES

After completing the workbook activities for Chapter 15, the student should be able to:
- Define the terms used in the chapter.
- Answer the review questions to within the evaluation criteria set by the instructor.
- Use problem-solving skills (individually or in a group setting) to determine correct responses and outcomes in case studies and application exercises.
- Work in a group setting to resolve scenarios dealing with office functions and duties of the health insurance professional.
- Interpret the information contained on an explanation of benefits (EOB).
- Determine why insurers deny payment of specific medical procedures.
- Establish the primary carrier for patients with dual coverage.
- Compose applicable appeal letters for patients.

DEFINING CHAPTER TERMS

Using the computer (or typewriter), students should key an accurate definition for each of the chapter terms listed. These definitions should be in the students' own words. When finished, students should compare their definitions with those listed in the glossary at the back of the textbook, correcting any inaccuracies.

adjudication
birthday rule
clean claim
coordination of benefits
correct code initiative
downcoding
employer identification number (EIN)

hearing on record
insurance claims register (log)
Medicare Secondary Payer claims
personal hearing
secondary claim
suspension file
telephone hearing

ASSESSMENT

Multiple Choice

Directions: In the questions/statements presented, choose the response that **best** answers/completes the stem and circle the letter that precedes it.

1. The claims process begins when:
   a. The patient/provider encounter is concluded
   b. The CMS-1500 form has been completed and submitted
   c. The patient first contacts the office for an appointment
   d. The patient's record is placed on the health insurance professional's desk

2. The health insurance professional should reverify patient information:
   a. Monthly
   b. At least once a year
   c. Each time the patient visits the office
   d. It is not necessary to reverify patient information

3. In the case of a minor child of a divorced couple who is covered under both parents' group health care plans, the health insurance professional should:
   a. Determine which carrier is primary
   b. Have the patient fill out two patient information forms
   c. Submit CMS-1500 forms to both carriers simultaneously
   d. Check with the office manager to avoid submitting a "dirty" claim

4. Many medical practices include a section (often positioned at the bottom of the form) for the patient to sign an:
   a. Authorization to release information
   b. Agreement to pay the bill in full
   c. Authorization to pay with a credit card
   d. Authorization to use a personal check

5. Services that typically require preauthorization or precertification include:
   a. Laboratory tests
   b. Emergency department services
   c. Routine "wellness" examinations
   d. Inpatient hospitalization

6. After a claim is completed, to help reduce claims rejection and delay, it is good practice *first* to have the claim:
   a. Signed
   b. Proofread
   c. Photocopied
   d. Recorded on the insurance claim log

7. The most important document in the medical insurance process is the:
   a. Patient information form
   b. Insurance claim form
   c. Encounter form
   d. The ledger card

8. The number that is assigned by the Internal Revenue Service (IRS) and used as the employer identifier standard for all electronic healthcare transactions is the:
   a. Group number
   b. Social Security number (SSN)
   c. Provider identification number (PIN)
   d. Employer identification number (EIN)

9. After the claim has been received by a third-party payer, it is reviewed, and the carrier makes payment decisions. This process is referred to as:
   a. Adjudication
   b. Judgment ruling
   c. Claims processing
   d. Decision making

10. When the insurance carrier receives a paper claim, it is dated, and the claim is processed through a(n):
    a. Visual imaging tomographer (VIT)
    b. Optical character recognition (OCR) scanner
    c. Character verification regulator (CVR)
    d. Computerized claim optimizer (CCO)

11. A series of files set up chronologically and labeled according to the number of days since a claim was submitted is referred to as a(n):
    a. Tracking file
    b. Insurance claims register
    c. General ledger file
    d. Suspension file

12. A columnar form on which insurance claims are tracked is a(n):
    a. Tracking file
    b. Suspension file
    c. General ledger file
    d. Insurance claims register

13. The document sent by the insurance carrier to the provider/patient explaining how the claim was adjudicated is called a(n):
    a. Insurance claims register
    b. Adjudication document
    c. EOB
    d. Payment tracking form

14. The key to knowing how much of the claim was paid, how much was not, and why is the:
    a. EOB
    b. EIN
    c. ROA
    d. PIN

15. When a carrier assigns a substitute code because a claim was submitted with outdated, deleted, or nonexistent CPT codes, it is called:
    a. Fraud
    b. Upcoding
    c. Downcoding
    d. Crosswalking

16. *Ideally*, insurance claims should be submitted to the insurance carrier within:
    a. 30 days
    b. 60 days
    c. 90 days
    d. 1 year

17. If there is any question as to time limits for filing claims, the health insurance professional should contact the:
    a. Department of Health and Human Services (HHS)
    b. Office manager
    c. Physician
    d. Carrier

18. The insurance company who pays after the primary carrier is referred to as the:
    a. Subsequent payer
    b. Secondary insurer
    c. Preferred provider
    d. Health maintenance organization

19. In the case of dual coverage, if it is not immediately obvious which payer is primary, the health insurance professional first should ask:
    a. The patient
    b. The employer
    c. The office manager
    d. The insurance carrier

20. If there is a second insurance policy, it is important to check "yes" in:
    a. Block 1a
    b. Block 9
    c. Block 11d
    d. Block 27

21. When a patient and spouse (or parent) are covered under two separate group policies, it results in what is commonly referred to as:
    a. Double coverage
    b. Coordination of benefits
    c. Primary versus secondary coverage
    d. A patient cannot be covered under two separate group policies

22. Claims that are submitted to another insurance company *before* they are submitted to Medicare are called:
    a. Medicare Secondary Payer (MSP) claims
    b. Coordination of benefits claims
    c. Payer of last resort claims
    d. Crossover claims

23. The process of calling for a review of a decision made by a third-party carrier is referred to as a(n):
    a. Appeal
    b. Claims review
    c. Adjudication
    d. Correct coding edit

24. The Medicare appeal process begins when:
    a. The patient/provider encounter is concluded
    b. The Medicare claim is rejected
    c. Disagreement arises with the carrier's payment determination
    d. The patient telephones the provider with a complaint

25. A Medicare review request for Part B appeals must come within:
    a. 30 days
    b. 60 days
    c. 120 days
    d. 1 year

26. After the Medicare appeal has gone through the first step, the provider/beneficiary may file a(n):

 a. Corrected claim

 b. Small claims suit

 c. Request for hearing

 d. Administrative law judge review

True/False

Directions: Place a "T" in the blank preceding each of the following statements if it is true; place an "F" if it is false.

_____ 1. Ultimately, it is the patient's responsibility to know when and how to notify the insurance company for preauthorization or precertification.

_____ 2. Medicare (fee-for-service) does not need prior authorization to provide covered services.

_____ 3. It is the health insurance professional's responsibility to document the appropriate health-related comments in the patient's health record.

_____ 4. It is poor judgment for the health insurance professional to double-check the codes the healthcare provider puts on the encounter form.

_____ 5. All major government payers have the same guidelines for completing the CMS-1500 claim form.

_____ 6. The medical practice should have a mechanism in place for tracking claims.

_____ 7. Claims follow-up does not warrant high priority in a busy medical office.

_____ 8. When dealing with Medicare and Medicaid, claims inquiries should be in writing.

_____ 9. The third-party payer sends an EOB only if a payment accompanies the document.

_____ 10. EOBs can be in electronic or paper format.

_____ 11. When an insurance claim is denied, the health insurance professional cannot pursue the claim further.

_____ 12. Often, if a claim is reduced or rejected, the problem lies with the provider's office.

_____ 13. Coding accurately and knowing which coding systems payers use helps avoid payment errors on claims.

_____ 14. If the claims adjuster changes a valid procedure code that was submitted on the claim, the health insurance professional must accept the change.

_____ 15. Correct code initiative edits are intended to reduce overpayments that result from improper coding.

_____ 16. All participating (PAR) providers are allowed to bill the patient for any balance the insurance carrier does not pay.

_____ 17. The provider cannot waive Medicare copayments unless financial hardship has been established and documented.

_____ 18. All third-party payers have a 30-day time limit for claims to be submitted if they are to be considered for payment.

_____ 19. All government payers (e.g., Medicare, Medicaid, TRICARE/CHAMPVA) have the same time limit for submitting claims.

_____ 20. The time limit for filing appeals varies from carrier to carrier.

_____ 21. When a patient has other insurance coverage primary to Medicare, the other insurer's payment information must be included on the Medicare claim.

_____ 22. When a patient is dual eligible (Medicare/Medicaid), there is an automatic crossover from Medicaid to Medicare.

_____ 23. Only the provider has the right to appeal a rejected insurance claim.

_____ 24. Many payers have a set time limit for claim appeals.

_____ 25. If after all levels of appeal are exhausted the claim remains unpaid, there are no other options.

Short Answer/Fill-in-the-Blank

1. List the six keys to successful claims processing.

_____

_____

_____

_____

_____

_____

2. Explain the rationale for photocopying the front and the back of a patient's health insurance identification card.

_____

3. If any attachments accompany a claim, list the information that should appear on each document.

_____

_____

_____

4. Explain in detail what the health insurance professional should do when a claims error is discovered that could result, or already has resulted, in inaccurate reimbursement.

_____

_____

_____

5. List six items typically found on an EOB (remittance advice [RA]).

_____

_____

_____

_____

_____

_____

6. List six things that influence how often medical facilities submit insurance claims.

_____

_____

_____

_____

_____

_____

7. List two important things the health insurance professional should do when a coordination of benefits situation exists.

_____

_____

8. List and explain the basic rules for appealing a claim.

_____

_____

_____

9. List and explain the five different levels of the Medicare appeals process.

_____

_____

_____

_____

_____

10. List the six informational items that a Medicare appeal request must contain.

_____

_____

_____

_____

_____

_____

CRITICAL THINKING ACTIVITIES

A. A major U.S. university conducted an experiment where patients went online and answered a series of questions about their health history before their medical encounter. The purpose of this study was to "assess the feasibility and reliability of a Web-based, self-administered, patient assessment system as compared to a standard, interviewer-administered approach." Discuss the pros and cons of such a system.

B. What is the difference, if any, between preauthorization and precertification?

C. Write a short paragraph on the importance of documentation in a patient's health record.

PROBLEM SOLVING/COLLABORATIVE (GROUP) ACTIVITIES

A. Create a flow chart diagramming the steps a paper claim goes through from the time the patient concludes his or her healthcare encounter until the payment is posted to the individual's ledger card.

B. Generate a page for Broadmoor Medical Clinic's office policy manual for a nonautomated tracking system for healthcare claims. You may use either the suspension file system or the log system.

C. Fig. 15-1 shows a sample EOB. The blank boxes are numbered 1 through 10. Write a complete description of what each box explains.

1. _____

2. _____

3. _____

4. _____

5. _____

6. _____

7. _____

8. _____

9. _____

10. _____

New Explanation of Benefits Form

This is a sample of our new Explanation of Benefits form, along with descriptions of various sections. This will help plan members and providers understand how benefits are paid.

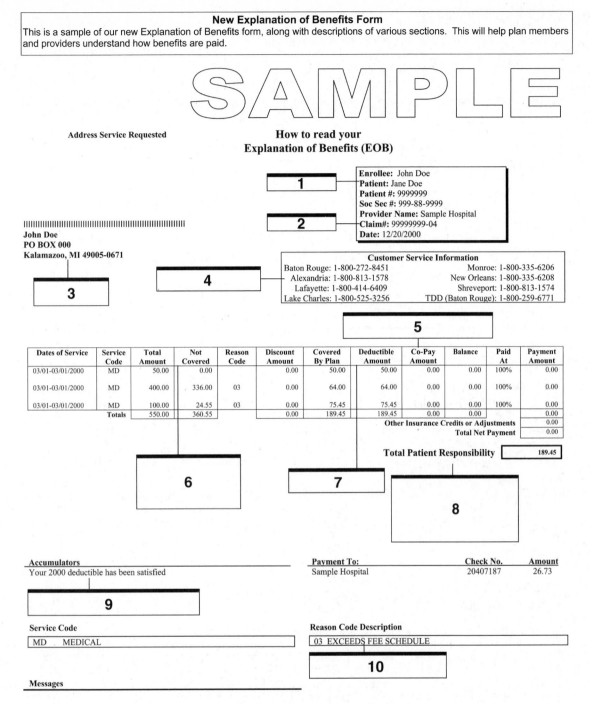

SAMPLE

Address Service Requested

How to read your
Explanation of Benefits (EOB)

| 1 |

Enrollee: John Doe
Patient: Jane Doe
Patient #: 9999999
Soc Sec #: 999-88-9999
Provider Name: Sample Hospital
Claim#: 99999999-04
Date: 12/20/2000

| 2 |

John Doe
PO BOX 000
Kalamazoo, MI 49005-0671

| 3 |

| 4 |

Customer Service Information

Baton Rouge: 1-800-272-8451	Monroe: 1-800-335-6206
Alexandria: 1-800-813-1578	New Orleans: 1-800-335-6208
Lafayette: 1-800-414-6409	Shreveport: 1-800-813-1574
Lake Charles: 1-800-525-3256	TDD (Baton Rouge): 1-800-259-6771

| 5 |

Dates of Service	Service Code	Total Amount	Not Covered	Reason Code	Discount Amount	Covered By Plan	Deductible Amount	Co-Pay Amount	Balance	Paid At	Payment Amount
03/01-03/01/2000	MD	50.00	0.00		0.00	50.00	50.00	0.00	0.00	100%	0.00
03/01-03/01/2000	MD	400.00	336.00	03	0.00	64.00	64.00	0.00	0.00	100%	0.00
03/01-03/01/2000	MD	100.00	24.55	03	0.00	75.45	75.45	0.00	0.00	100%	0.00
Totals		550.00	360.55		0.00	189.45	189.45	0.00	0.00		0.00

Other Insurance Credits or Adjustments   0.00
Total Net Payment   0.00

Total Patient Responsibility | 189.45 |

| 6 |

| 7 |

| 8 |

Accumulators
Your 2000 deductible has been satisfied

| 9 |

Payment To:	Check No.	Amount
Sample Hospital	20407187	26.73

Service Code

| MD | MEDICAL |

Reason Code Description

| 03 EXCEEDS FEE SCHEDULE |

| 10 |

Messages

Fig. 15-1 Sample explanation of benefits form.

Chapter **15** **The Claim**

PROJECTS/DISCUSSION TOPICS

Assign one or more of the following projects/topics as time permits.

A. Join a class discussion on what can be done to avoid errors on CMS-1500 forms.

B. Share experiences with the class regarding errors in claims or billing that you, or family members, may have experienced, and how they were resolved.

C. Reread the "Imagine This" scenario about Mr. Benson and Dr. Peters on p. 341 in the textbook. Discuss how Dr. Peters' health insurance professional might have helped Mr. Benson resolve this problem.

D. Compile a table listing the major payers along with their time limits for submitting claims.

CASE STUDIES

A. Fig. 15-2 shows an insurance ID card. After studying the card, answer the following questions.

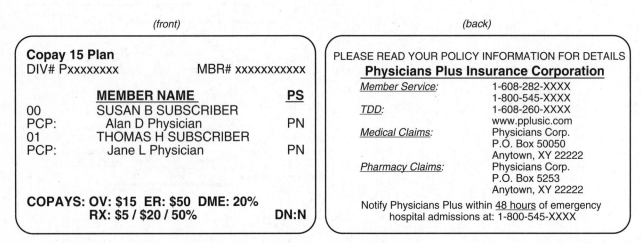

Fig. 15-2 Insurance ID card for S. Subscriber.

1. Who is the subscriber?

2. Do the subscriber and the dependent have the same primary care provider (PCP)?

3. If yes, what is their PCP's name? If no, list the subscriber and the dependent along with the name of each member's PCP.

4. If Thomas had an office visit for which he was charged $75, how much should he pay at the time of the service?

5. Susan was in an accident and was treated in the emergency department and released on the same day. The charges for this encounter totaled $2354. What was Susan's share?

6. Susan was confined to a wheelchair for 6 weeks after her accident. The cost of the wheelchair was $896. How much of this charge did Physicians Plus Insurance Corp. pay?

7. Susan was given a prescription for a pain medication. If the pharmacist gave her the generic form of the drug, the cost would be $26.50; the cost of the brand name would be $67. What would Susan's savings be if she accepted the generic drug?

8. Susan's accident occurred at 7:43 PM on 10/14/20XX, and she was treated in the emergency department on the same date (she was not admitted as an inpatient from the emergency department). She did not report the accident to Physicians Plus until 4 PM on 10/17/20XX. Will Physicians Plus pay this claim?

B. Wanda Fortune's ledger card is shown in Fig. 15-3. Fig. 15-4 shows an EOB from her insurance carrier (TRICARE). Post the information from the EOB onto Ms. Fortune's ledger card. (Assume that the TRICARE payment was received on 8/01/20XX.)

Note: Ms. Fortune's cost share is 25% of the TRICARE approved amount.

TRICARE
SPONSOR: George M.
SS# 321-44-5555
DOB 4/16/77

STATEMENT

BROADMOOR MEDICAL CLINIC
4353 Pine Ridge Drive
Milton, XY 12345-0001
Telephone: 555-656-7890

BENEFICIARY:
Wanda Mae
SS# 321-44-6600
DOB 11/02/80

GEORGE M. FORTUNE
566 LONGMEADOW
MILTON, XY 12345

DATE 20XX	PROFESSIONAL SERVICE DESCRIPTION	CHARGE		CREDITS		CURRENT BALANCE	
				PAYMENTS	ADJUSTMENTS		
7/08	OV EST (99213)	45	00			45	00
"	Comp Met Pane (88054)	20	00			65	00
"	Auto Hemo (85025)	12	00			77	00
7/09	TRICARE Submitted						

Due and payable within 10 days.   **Pay last amount in balance column** ⇧

Fig. 15-3 Ledger ID for Wanda (George) Fortune.

TRICARE EXPLANATION OF BENEFITS

This is a statement of the action taken on your TRICARE Claim.
Keep this notice for your records.

Prime Contractor

Date of Notice:	August 02, 2000
Sponsor SSN:	321-44-5555
Sponsor Name:	George M. Fortune
Beneficiary Name:	Wanda Mae Fortune

Benefits were payable to:

Wanda Mae Fortune
566 Longmeadow
Milton, XY 12345

BROADMOOR MEDICAL CLINIC
4353 PINE RIDGE DRIVE
MILTON XY 12345-0001

Claim Number: 919533693-00-00

Services Provided By Date of Services		Services Provided		Amount Billed	TRICARE Approved	See Remarks
PROVIDER OF MEDICAL CARE						
07/08/20XX	1	Office/outpatient visit, est	(99213)	$ 45.00	$ 38.92	1
07/08/20XX	1	Comprehen metabolic panel	(88054)	20.00	19.33	1
07/08/20XX	1	Automated hemogram	(85025)	12.00	12.00	1
Totals:				**$ 77.00**	**$ 70.25**	

Claim Summary		Beneficiary Liability Summary		Benefit Period Summary		

Fiscal Year Beginning:
October 01, 20XX

Amount billed:	77.00	Deductible	0.00
TRICARE Approved:	70.25	Copayment:	0.00
Non-Covered: 14*	6.75	Cost Share	17.56
Paid by Beneficiary:	0.00		
Other Insurance:	0.00		
Paid to Provider:	52.69		
Paid to Beneficiary:	0.00		
Check Number:			

	Individual	Family
Deductible:	150.00	150.00

Catastrophic Cap:

Enrollment Year Beginning:
December 01, 20XX

	Individual	Family
POS Deductible:	300.00	600.00
Prime Cap:		856.32

Fig. 15-4 TRICARE explanation of benefits for Fortune.

C. Joann Carlyle was seen by Todd Hamblin, a dermatologist at Broadmoor Medical Clinic, for removal of an xanthoma growth beneath each of her eyes. After the procedure, Dr. Hamblin instructed Evelyn Tanner, his health insurance professional, to bill the procedures as follows:

Excision lesion, right cheek	11442	$430
Intermediate repair, right cheek	12051	$360
Excision lesion, left cheek	11442	$430
Intermediate repair, left cheek	12051	$360
TOTAL		$1580

Fig. 15-5 illustrates how Evelyn completed Block 24 of the CMS-1500 form. Assume that Ms. Carlyle had met her deductible for the year, and Dr. Hamblin is a PAR provider for Ms. Carlyle's insurance carrier. Her coinsurance was 90/10 for outpatient hospital surgical procedures; however, the insurance carrier paid only $711 (90% of one excision and 90% of one repair) and denied the second procedure and repair.

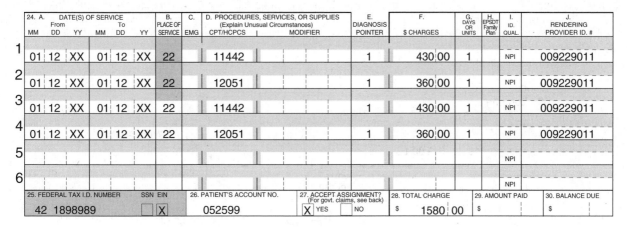

Fig. 15-5 Block 24 of CMS-1500 form for Ms. Carlyle.

1. Why were the second excision and repair denied?
2. What, if anything, can Evelyn do to collect the insurance payment for the second procedure and repair?
3. If Evelyn submits a corrected claim, how should Block 24 be filled out?
4. If Evelyn does nothing and sends a statement to Ms. Carlyle for the balance, what recourse, if any, does Ms. Carlyle have?

INTERNET EXPLORATION

A. Log on to the Internet, and using the search words "Understanding an EOB" (or similar words), explore various websites that offer information on how to interpret and understand an EOB.

B. Log on to the Internet at **http://www.ama-assn.org/amednews/2000/12/25/bisa1225.htm** and read the article, "Downcoding, denial of claims by insurers are facts of life for many doctors: An American Medical Association survey finds that most physicians have had these kinds of troubles with their claims from insurance companies," by Cheryl Jackson, *AMNews* staff, Dec. 25, 2000. If you cannot find this article, use the search word "downcoding" to find alternative articles on this topic.

C. The Internet has a wealth of information for filing appeals—especially appeals for Medicare claims. Search the Web (using the **medicare.gov** and the Centers for Medicare and Medicaid Services websites or search words such as "filing a Medicare appeal") to learn more about this process.

PERFORMANCE OBJECTIVES

Note to Instructors: The elements (time allowed, percent of proficiency required to pass, and points awarded) listed in the following performance objectives are meant to be used as guidelines only. Instructors should feel free to adjust these elements as necessary to fit the particular needs of their class.

Performance Objective 15-1—Determining Primary Coverage

Conditions: Student will study the information in Fig. 15-6, determine the primary carrier, and complete a claim using the information in Patient Record No. 052567.

Supplies/Equipment: Pen/typewriter, Patient Record No. 052567, CMS-1500 claim form (paper or electronic)

Time Allowed: 50 minutes

Accuracy Needed to Pass: 90%

Procedural Steps	Points Earned	Comments
Evaluator: Note time began: _____		
1. Carefully read and study Patient Record No. 052567 in Fig. 15-6.		
2. Determine the primary carrier. (10)		
3. Correctly complete *all* blocks required for the appropriate claim. (65)		
4. Proofread the claim for accuracy.		
Optional: May deduct points for taking more time than allowed.		

Total Points = 75

Student's Score: _____

Evaluator: _____

Comments: _____

_____

_____

_____

_____

Performance Objective 15-1 – Determine Primary Insurer; Complete Claim	
Broadmoor Medical Clinic	Clinic EIN# 42-1898989
4353 Pine Ridge Drive	Dr. R. L. Jones NPI 1234567890
Milton, XY 12345-0001	Dr. Marilou Lucero ID NPI 2907511822
Clinic NPI X100XX1000	
Telephone: 555-656-7890	Date claims one day after encounter

Patient/Insurance Information

Truman Ross Beckler   DOB: 08/29/1946
430 Cedar Drive
Middletown, XT 12345   PH 555-672-4207
555-452-0334   SS # 321-44-5511

Medicare   321445511X
Unix Benefits Inc.   198442000LJ

Vera T. Beckler   DOB 05/02/1950
Employer: ALCAT Industries

Billing Information

Record No. 052567

07/08/20XX	99213	$145.00
07/08/20XX	93000	60.00
07/08/20XX	85025	22.00

Diagnosis: Abdominal Pain (789.06)

Attending Physician: R. L. Jones, MD

Notes: Mr. Beckler is retired and has both Medicare Parts A and B. He also has full health care coverage under his wife's employer group health plan (Unix Benefits Inc.)

Notes: Assume the date of current onset of illness was the same day of the encounter. Date the primary claim one day after the encounter, and date the secondary claim one day after the primary payer's EOB is received.

Fig. 15-6 Patient record information for Beckler.

Performance Objective 15-2—Interpret EOB, Post Payment to Ledger Card, and File Secondary Claim

Conditions: Student will interpret the EOB in Fig. 15-7, post the payment to the ledger card in Fig. 15-8, and file a secondary CMS-1500 claim.

Supplies/Equipment: Patient Record No. 052567, EOB (see Fig. 15-7), ledger card (see Fig. 15-8), CMS-1500 claim form (paper or electronic)

Time Allowed: 50 minutes

Accuracy Needed to Pass: 90%

Procedural Steps	Points Earned	Comments
Evaluator: Note time began: _____		
1. Carefully study the UNIX EOB.		
2. Determine the correct payment to post to patient's ledger card. (15)		
3. Prepare a claim for the secondary carrier. Complete *all* blocks required for secondary claims. (65)		
4. Proofread the claim for accuracy.		
5. Note name of document that must accompany secondary claims. (5)		
Optional: May deduct points for taking more time than allowed.		

Total Points = 85

Student's Score: _____

Evaluator: _____

Comments: _____

_____

_____

_____

_____

EXPLANATION OF BENEFITS

UNIX Benefits Inc.
1000 Alameda Blvd.
San Jose CA 98877
800-222-33-4444
800-222-33-4545 (FAX)

Insured's Name: Vera T. Beckler
UNIX Member # 198442000LJ

Date: 07/20/20XX

Patient Name: Truman R. Beckler
430 Cedar Drive
Middletown XT 12345

Provider: Broadmoor Medical Clinic
R. L. Jones NPI 1234567890
Claim No. 98885050333-XX
Check No. UNIX2034422

(1) Date of Service	(2) CPT Code	(3) Total Charges	(4) Allowable Charges	(5) Applied to Deductible	(6) Co-Pay	(7) Total Benefit	(8) Reason Code(s)
07/08/20XX	99213	145.00	120.00	50.00	10.00	60.00	01A/01C
07/08/20XX	93000	60.00	45.00	--	--	45.00	02B
07/08/20XX	85025	22.00	18.50	--	--	18.50	02B
TOTALS		**227.00**	**183.50**	**50.00**	**10.00**	**123.50**	

Reason Code(S) Description:

01A – Amount in Column 3 exceeds UNIX fee schedule
01C – Amount in Column 5 has been applied to annual deductible
02B – UNIX pays this procedure/service at 100%

NOTES:

Payment has been sent directly to your provider
Annual deductible has been satisfied for year 20XX

THIS IS NOT A BILL – SAVE THIS COPY FOR YOUR RECORDS

Fig. 15-7 Explanation of benefits for Beckler.

Truman DOB 08/29/1946
Medicare 321445511X

Vera DOB 05/02/1950
Emp: AL-CAT Industries
UNIX Benefits Inc.
198442000LJ

STATEMENT

BROADMOOR MEDICAL CLINIC
4353 Pine Ridge Drive
Milton, XY 12345-0001
Telephone: 555-656-7890

PH 555-672-4207

TRUMAN ROSS BECKLER
430 CEDAR DRIVE
MIDDLETOWN XT 12345

DATE 20XX	PROFESSIONAL SERVICE DESCRIPTION	CHARGE		CREDITS PAYMENTS		ADJUSTMENTS		CURRENT BALANCE	
3/16	Vera OV 99212	125	00	12	50			112	50
3/17	Unix Claim								
3/30	Unix CK 2031944	100	00			12	50	Ø	
7/08	Truman 99213	145	00					145	00
"	Truman 93000	60	00					205	00
"	Truman 88025	22	00					227	00
7/09	Unix Claim								

Due and payable within 10 days.   **Pay last amount in balance column** ⇧

Fig. 15-8 Ledger card for Beckler.

Performance Objective 15-3—Composing an Appeal Letter

Scenario

Plastic surgeon Everett Bartholomew performed a bilateral blepharoplasty on 66-year-old Janine Frieze on April 27, 20XX. Before the procedure, you (his health insurance professional) telephoned National Mutual Health Care, Ms. Frieze's insurance carrier, for preauthorization. Susan Peterson of National Mutual provided authorization number 303885030 for Ms. Frieze's blepharoplasty; however, when the EOB was received for this claim (#767678000CG), benefits were denied because the insurance carrier determined the procedure to be "not medically necessary." In his documentation in the health record, Dr. Bartholomew states that the eyelids were "obstructing the patient's vision."

Note: National Mutual's address is PO Box 45446A, Princeton, XY 23456. Address it to the attention of Susan Peterson, Claims Department. Ms. Frieze's date of birth is 09/26/1947, and her SSN is 444-00-1199.

Conditions: Using the information in the scenario, compose a letter to National Mutual Health Care, appealing their decision to not pay for Janine Frieze's blepharoplasty. Explain why you think the procedure should be covered. Note any documentation supporting your case.

Supplies/Equipment: Pen/typewriter/computer/paper

Time Allowed: 50 minutes

Accuracy Needed to Pass: 90%

Procedural Steps	Points Earned	Comments
Evaluator: Note time began: _____		
1. Carefully read the scenario.		
2. Compose a letter appealing National Mutual's decision.		
3. Letter Format (12)		
Date and Inside Address		
Attention line		
Subject line		
Salutation		
Complimentary Close and Signature		
Reference and Enclosure lines		
4. Content (30)		
Opening paragraph		
Main content paragraph		
Closing paragraph		
5. Proofread the letter for accuracy.		
Optional: May deduct points for taking more time than allowed.		

Total Points = 42

Student's Score: _____

Evaluator: _____

Comments: _____

_____

_____

Medicare also has denied the claim for Janine Frieze's blepharoplasty, citing the procedure as being "not medically necessary." Complete the first step of the Medicare appeal process, filing Form CMS-1965 (Fig. 15-9). Explain your reasons in narrative in #3. Note in #4 that you have additional evidence to submit, and you are attaching supporting documentation. Ms. Frieze does not wish to appear in person. You will act as claimant's representative, using the Clinic's address and telephone number. Patient's Medicare ID number is 444001199B. The carrier's name and address is Medicare Part B Carrier, PO Box 91233, Fort Collins, CO, 77888. Patient's address is 2600 Linden Street, Milton, XY 12345, and telephone number is 555-655-8811. Date the form 1 month after the procedure was performed.

REQUEST FOR HEARING
PART B MEDICARE CLAIM
Medical Insurance Benefits - Social Security Act
NOTICE—Anyone who misrepresents or falsifies essential information requested by this form may upon conviction be subject to fine and imprisonment under Federal Law.

CARRIER'S NAME AND ADDRESS

1 NAME OF PATIENT

2 HEALTH INSURANCE CLAIM NUMBER

3 I disagree with the review determination on my claim, and request a hearing before a hearing officer of the insurance carrier named above.
MY REASONS ARE: (Attach a copy of the Review Notice. NOTE: If the review decision was made more than 6 months ago, include your reason for not making this request earlier.)

4 CHECK ONE OF THE FOLLOWING

☐ I have additional evidence to submit.
(Attach such evidence to this form or forward it to the carrier with in 10days.)

☐ I do not have additional evidence.

CHECK **ONLY ONE** OF THE STATEMENTS BELOW:

☐ I wish to appear in person before the Hearing Officer.

☐ I do not wish to appear and here by request a decision on the evidence before the Hearing Officer.

5 EITHER THE CLAIMANT OR REPRESENTATIVE SHOULD SIGN IN THE APPROPRIATE SPACE BELOW

SIGNATURE OR NAME OF CLAIMANT'S REPRESENTATIVE

CLAIMANT'S SIGNATURE

ADDRESS

ADDRESS

CITY, STATE, AND ZIP CODE

CITY, STATE, AND ZIP CODE

TELEPHONE NUMBER | DATE

TELEPHONE NUMBER | DATE

(Claimant should not write below this line)

ACKNOWLEDGMENT OF REQUEST FOR HEARING

Your request for a hearing was received on _____ . You will be notified of the time and place of the hearing at least 10 days before the date of the hearing.

SIGNED | DATE

Fig. 15-9 Form CMS-1965.

Performance Objective 15-4—Completing the First Step of the Medicare Appeal Process—Form 1965

Conditions: Student will complete Form CMS-1965 (see Fig. 15-9) in the first step of the Medicare appeal process.
Supplies/Equipment: Pen/typewriter/computer/paper, blank form CMS-1965
Time Allowed: 50 minutes
Accuracy Needed to Pass: 90%

Procedural Steps	Points Earned	Comments
Evaluator: Note time began: _____		
1. Carefully study Form CMS-1965.		
2. Complete the following sections correctly:		
#1 (2)		
#2 (2)		
#3 (10)		
#4 (2)		
#5 (4)		
3. Proofread the letter for accuracy.		
Optional: May deduct points for taking more time than allowed.		

Total Points = 20

Student's Score: _____

Evaluator: _____

Comments: _____

_____

_____

_____

_____

Health Insurance Professional's Notebook

Assemble information and example forms for the Health Insurance Professional's Notebook regarding claims, such as the following:

- Sample EOBs and RAs along with explanations for interpretation
- Templates for filing secondary claims
- Flow charts showing how claims proceed through the adjudication process
- Sample appeal letters/forms
- Chart of major payers and their time limits for submitting claims
- Steps for submitting Medicare appeals
- Forms for submitting Medicare appeals

Chapter Check List

Student name: _____

Chapter completion date: _____

1.	Record	Your start time and date: _____
2.	Read	The assigned chapter in the text
3.	View	PowerPoint slides (if available)
4.	Complete	Exercises in the Workbook as assigned
5.	Compare	Your answers to the answers posted on the bulletin board/website/handout
6.	Correct	Your answers
7.	Complete	All tests and required activities
8.	Read	Assigned readings (if any)
9.	Complete	Chapter performance objectives (competencies), if any
10.	Evaluate	Chapter performance, and submit to your instructor
11.	Record	Your ending time and date: _____
12.	Move on	Begin next chapter as assigned

Evaluate your classroom performance. Complete the self-evaluation, and submit it to your instructor. When your instructor returns this form to you, compare your self-evaluation with the evaluation completed by your instructor.

Skill	Student Self-Evaluation			Instructor Evaluation		
	Good	Average	Poor	Good	Average	Poor
Attendance/punctuality						
Personal appearance						
Applies effort						
Is self-motivated						
Is courteous						
Has positive attitude						
Completes assignments in timely manner						
Works well with others						

Student's initials: _____   **Instructor's initials:** _____

Date: _____   **Date:** _____

Points Possible: _____

Points Awarded: _____

Chapter Grade: _____

16 The Role of Computers in Health Insurance

Chapter 16 discussed how the 21st century has brought the power of automation and the Internet to the medical office—specifically through electronic billing and insurance claims processing. The electronic claims process may sound complicated, but it is relatively simple. Instead of sending insurance claims to third-party carriers through the mail, the same information is transmitted electronically (in a matter of minutes) by computer over telephone lines. First, the information is input into a computer using special software. Next, the computer transmits the insurance information in the form of a claim to the third-party carrier directly or via a clearinghouse. The clearinghouse checks the data for errors and arranges it in a particular format required by the insurance carrier. The carrier processes the claim and mails the provider a reimbursement check or an EOB or both. The electronic claims submission process is faster than the paper method. Reimbursement often is received in the provider's office within 7 to 14 days as opposed to the 30 to 60 days it takes for payment of a paper claim processing. According to the American Medical Association, electronic claim processing has been shown to reduce claim rejection rates from 30% to 2%.

WORKBOOK CHAPTER OBJECTIVES

After completing the workbook activities for Chapter 16, the student should be able to:
* Define the terms used in the chapter.
* Answer the review questions to within the evaluation criteria set by the instructor.
* Attain logical conclusions (or answers) by analyzing and evaluating given information/scenarios.
* Use problem-solving skills (individually or in a group setting) to determine valid responses and outcomes in case studies and application exercises.
* Actively participate in group discussions.
* Interpret and resolve situations presented in case studies.
* Complete performance objectives to within the criteria determined by the instructor.
* Perform the necessary steps for unbiased self-evaluation and understanding of material presented in the workbook.

DEFINING CHAPTER TERMS

Using the computer (or typewriter), students should key an accurate definition for each of the chapter terms listed. These definitions should be in the students' own words. When finished, students should compare their definitions with those listed in the glossary at the back of the textbook, correcting any inaccuracies.

Administrative Simplification and Compliance Act (ASCA)
billing services
code sets
direct data entry (DDE) claims
electronic claims clearinghouse
electronic data interchange (EDI)
electronic funds transfer (EFT)
electronic medical claim (EMC)
electronic medical record (EMR)

electronic remittance advice (ERA)
enrollment process
identifiers
privacy standards
security standards
small provider of services
small supplier
telecommunication
unusual circumstances

Multiple Choice

Directions: In the questions/statements presented, choose the response that **best** answers/completes the stem, and circle the letter that precedes it.

1. Electronic transmissions began during the:
   a. 1950s
   b. 1960s
   c. 1970s
   d. 1980s

2. The organization created to reform health insurance and simplify the healthcare administrative processes is known as:
   a. CMS
   b. HCFA
   c. HIPAA
   d. DHS

3. The electronic transfer of information in a standard format between two entities is known as:
   a. EDI
   b. PHI
   c. DHS
   d. ICD

4. Transmitting free-format, textual electronic messages from one individual to another is commonly known as:
   a. Faxing
   b. Carding
   c. Mailboxing
   d. E-mailing

5. To send claims electronically, the medical practice needs:
   a. A computer
   b. A modem
   c. HIPAA-compliant software
   d. All of the above

6. If a medical practice chooses to submit claims electronically to an insurance carrier, it must go through a(n):
   a. Internal audit
   b. Background check
   c. Enrollment process
   d. Appeals process

7. A business entity that receives claims from several medical facilities, consolidates these claims, and transmits them to various insurance carriers is called a(n):
   a. Electronic data interchange (EDI) transmitter
   b. Claims clearinghouse
   c. Fiscal intermediary (FI)
   d. Claims consolidation firm

8. The system wherein data representing money are moved electronically between accounts or organizations is called:

   a. Direct data entry (DDE)

   b. Electronic funds transfer (EFT)

   c. Electronic medical record (EMR)

   d. Electronic remittance advice (ERA)

9. An electronic file wherein patients' health information is stored in a computer system is called:

   a. Direct data entry (DDE)

   b. Electronic funds transfer (EFT)

   c. Electronic medical record (EMR)

   d. Electronic remittance advice (ERA)

10. One of the most significant activities of the healthcare industry is:

    a. Information management

    b. Inventory management

    c. Office management

    d. Drug management

11. The basic concern of EMRs is:

    a. Cost

    b. Privacy

    c. Training staff

    d. Keeping hardware/software up-to-date

12. Submitting claims directly to an insurance carrier is referred to as:

    a. Direct data entry (DDE)

    b. Electronic funds transfer (EFT)

    c. Electronic medical record (EMR)

    d. Electronic remittance advice (ERA)

13. If the practice submits claims primarily to one carrier, it may advisable to use:

    a. A clearinghouse

    b. An FI

    c. DDE

    d. ERA

14. The most common form of submitting claims electronically, which involves transmitting claim information over phone lines using a computer and a modem, is called:

    a. E-mail

    b. Facsimile (fax)

    c. Telecommunication

    d. Electronic ANSII transfer

15. The acronym for the organization enacted by Congress to improve the administration of Medicare by taking advantage of the efficiencies gained through electronic claim submission is:

    a. CMS (formerly HCFA)

    b. HIPAA

    c. ASCA

    d. HHS

337

True/False

Directions: Place a "T" in the blank preceding each of the following statements if it is true; place an "F" if it is false.

_____ 1. Federal regulations now mandate that all healthcare information that is electronically transmitted follow specific rules and guidelines to provide security and protection for PHI.

_____ 2. The Administrative Simplification and Compliance Act (ASCA) requires health plans and healthcare clearinghouses to use certain standard transaction formats and code sets for the electronic transmission of health information.

_____ 3. ASCA made it compulsory for all Medicare claims to be submitted electronically effective October 16, 2003, without exception.

_____ 4. ASCA's "rule" does not require any other transactions (changes, adjustments, or appeals to the initial claim) to be submitted electronically.

_____ 5. Claims submitted via DDE are considered to be electronic claims for purposes of the "rule."

_____ 6. The biggest obstacle to getting set up for electronic claims processing is the time that it takes for approval from various federal and state agencies.

_____ 7. The move from paper to electronic submissions will result in significant savings for all medical providers.

_____ 8. The Medicare Program is not considered a covered entity subject to HIPAA regulations because it does not fall within the definition of a "health plan."

_____ 9. ERA payments can be posted automatically to patient accounts.

_____ 10. The EMR of the future will rely on the Internet.

_____ 11. Only the "administrative" staff needs to participate in the preparation and training involved in the conversion from a paper to a computerized office.

_____ 12. A _small provider of services_ is a medical facility (e.g., a hospital or skilled nursing facility) with less than 25 full-time equivalent employees (FTEs).

_____ 13. A _small supplier_ is a physician, practitioner, facility, or supplier with less than 10 FTEs.

_____ 14. ASCA states that no payment may be made under Parts A or B of the Medicare Program for claims submitted in nonelectronic form, _without exception_.

_____ 15. EMR is a system wherein data representing money are moved electronically between accounts or organizations.

Short Answer/Fill-in-the-Blank

1. Name four ways computers are commonly used in today's medical office.

_____

_____

_____

_____

2. List and explain the five specific areas of administrative simplification addressed by HIPAA.

_____

_____

_____

_____

_____

3. Explain the process of EDI in your own words.

_____

_____

_____

4. List the four essential elements of EDI.

_____

_____

_____

_____

5. Discuss the benefits of EDI.

_____

_____

_____

6. There are essentially two ways to submit claims electronically. Name them and briefly explain each process.

_____

_____

7. Explain how a clearinghouse works.

_____

_____

_____

8. Discuss the pros and cons of DDE compared with using an electronic claims clearinghouse.

_____

_____

_____

9. There are several ways to obtain electronic claims capability. List and explain at least two of them.

_____

_____

10. Compile a list of equipment typically necessary for getting set up to submit EDI claims.

_____

_____

_____

11. List and discuss the exceptions to the electronic claims submission requirement under ASCA's "rule."

_____

_____

_____

12. List the various components typically contained in an EMR.

_____

_____

_____

CRITICAL THINKING ACTIVITIES

A. Write a paragraph (250 to 300 words) on the impact of computers on health insurance.

B. The textbook discusses EDI. In its most basic definition, EDI is the replacement of paper-based patient health records with electronic equivalents. How does HIPAA fit into this picture as far as the benefits of EDI are concerned?

C. Some experts say that EMRs will cut healthcare costs. Do you agree? Why or why not?

D. In your own opinion, what do you think the future holds for EMRs?

PROBLEM SOLVING/COLLABORATIVE (GROUP) ACTIVITIES

A. Broadmoor Medical Clinic is planning to computerize its office, and the office manager has asked you to research necessary hardware to switch from paper to electronic claim submission. Generate a list of state-of-the-art hardware necessary for this conversion. The hardware components should have expansion capabilities for anticipated clinic growth. Also, decide whether the clinic should use a clearinghouse or direct claims submission. (**Note:** The clinic submits claims to all major carriers.)

B. Along with the hardware necessary for computerization, Broadmoor Medical Clinic will need a high-quality patient accounting software program. Currently, the patient load at Broadmoor is 1000 patients and 10 physicians. Research possible software that would be suitable for the clinic. Use the Internet or interview local medical facility personnel.

PROJECTS/DISCUSSION TOPICS

A. Join a class discussion on:
- Advantages and disadvantages of EMRs
- Privacy concerns of EMRs

B. Looking at both sides:
1. A study found that approximately 25% of patient charts are unavailable when patients come to a medical office for an appointment. That means the healthcare provider does not have the patient's medical history or treatment regimen available during the patient visit, and information from the encounter will have to be entered into the chart later—if ever.

2. EMRs are one of the most promising developments in medical cost control, patient care, and patient privacy. Ironically, their inability to eliminate the need for supplemental paper charts has been one reason that less than 5% of physicians use them.

C. What kinds of adjustments would health insurance professionals have to make when converting from paper records to EMRs?

D. Compose a page for Broadmoor's Policy Manual for the steps necessary to submit claims electronically. You can choose the clearinghouse method or DDE.

CASE STUDIES

A. Study the sample remittance advice (RA) in Fig. 16-1 and answer the following questions:

1. How many claims are on this RA?
2. What was the total amount billed to Medicare?
3. Of the amount on Benny Fischer's second claim, how much did Medicare pay?
4. By what method were these claims paid?
5. What was the total amount of the payment?
6. Were there any crossover claims?
7. If so, which patients had their claim crossed over?
8. What was the total amount applied to patients' deductible?
9. What does the code "PR" mean?
10. How much of I. M. Hurt's charge is he responsible for?

Provider Block	
Broadmoor Medical Clinic	Clinic EIN # 42-1898989
4353 Pine Ridge Drive	Dr. R.L. Jones NPI 1234567890
Milton, XY 12345-0001	Dr. Marilou Lucero NPI 2907511822
Clinic NPI X100XX1000	Date claims 1 day after examination
Telephone: 555-656-7890	
Fax: 555-656-7899	Number of computers in clinic: 15
E-mail: broadmoorFP@milton.org	

```
PROVIDENCE MEDICARE SERVICES                              MEDICARE REMITTANCE NOTICE
600 EAST PARK DRIVE
SOUTHPARK, YZ 17111-2777

BROADMOOR MEDICAL CLINIC                                  PROVIDER #: 1234567890
4353 PINE RIDGE DRIVE                                     PAGE #: 1 OF 1
MILTON, XY 12345-0001                                     DATE: 04/28/05
555-656-7890                                             CHECK/EFT #: 0003300442

***********************************************************************************************************
***********************************************************************************************************

PERF  PROV  SERV  DATE  POS  NOS  PROC  MODS   BILLED  ALLOWED  DEDUCT   COINS GRP/RC  AMT  PROV  PD

NAME  FISCHER, BENNY        HIC 222665555A   ACNT   FISC 6123133-01    ICN 0202199306840      ASG Y  MOA MA01
123456ABC  0225  022505  11      1 99213     66.00    49.83   0.34      9.97  CO-42  16.17         39.52
PT RESP  10.31              CLAIM TOTALS     66.00    49.83   0.34      9.97         16.17
                                                                              NET          39.52

NAME  FISCHER, BENNY        HIC 222665555A   ACNT   FISC 6123133-01    ICN 0202199306850 ASG Y MOA MA01 MA07
123456ABC  0117  011705  11      1 99213     66.00    49.83   0.00      9.97  CO-42  16.17         39.86
PT RESP  9.97               CLAIM TOTALS     66.00    49.83   0.00      9.97         16.17         39.86
CLAIM INFORMATION FORWARDED TO:  STATE OF XY MEDICAID                           NET   39.86

NAME  HURT, I.M.            HIC 512357683A   ACNT   HURT5-329     ICN 0202199306860      ASG Y  MOA MA01
123456ABC  0117  011705  11      1 90659     25.00     3.32   0.00      0.00  CO-42  21.68          3.32
123456ABC  0117  011705  11      1 G0008     10.00     4.46   0.00      0.00  CO-42   5.54          4.46
PT RESP  0.00               CLAIM TOTALS     35.00     7.78   0.00      0.00         27.22          7.78
                                                                              NET           7.78

NAME  MARLOWE, PHILIP       HIC 033448165A   ACNT   MARLO861-316-   ICN 0202199306870 ASG Y MOA MA01 MA07
123456ABC  0209  020905  11      1 99213     66.00    49.83   0.00      9.97  CO-42  16.17         39.86
PT RESP  9.97               CLAIM TOTALS     66.00    49.83   0.00      9.97         16.17         39.86
CLAIM INFORMATION FORWARDED TO:  STATE OF XY MEDICAID                           NET   39.86

NAME  RAP, JACK             HIC 113778916A   ACNT   RAP33-721       ICN 0202199306880 ASG Y MOA MA01 MA07
123456ABC  0314  031405  11      1 99213     66.00    49.83   0.00      9.97  CO-42  16.17         39.86
123456ABC  0314  031405  11      1 82962     10.00     4.37   0.00      0.00  CO-42   5.63          4.37

123456ABC  0314  031405  11      1 94760     12.00     0.00   0.00      0.00  CO-B15 12.00          0.00
REM: M80
PT RESP  9.97               CLAIM TOTALS     88.00    54.20   0.00      9.97         33.80         44.23
                                                                              NET          44.23

TOTALS:     # of      BILLED    ALLOWED    DEDUCT    COINS    TOTAL   PROV PD    PROV     CHECK
            CLAIMS    AMT       AMT        AMT       RC AMT.  AMT     ADJ AMT    AMT      AMT
            5         321.00    211.47     0.34      39.88    109.53  171.25     .00      171.25

GROUP CODES:
PR          Patient Responsibility
CO          Contractual Obligation
OA          Other Adjustment

PT RESP     Patient responsibility is the unpaid amount for which the patient is liable and includes the patient responsibility for all
            of the details.
CLAIM TOTALS:  The total billed amount.
BILLED AMT
ALLOWED AMT    The total allowed amount.
DEDUCTIBLE     The total amount applied to the deductible.
COINSURANCE    The total amount of coinsurance.
GRP/RC AMT     The GRP/RC amount is the difference between the billed amount and the allowed amount.
PROV PD        The actual payment amount paid to the provider for the service.
```

Fig. 16-1 Providence Medicare remittance advice.

B. Fig. 16-2 is a printout of an electronic page from a company that offers direct claims submission. Using the information from the Broadmoor Medical Clinic provider block (p. 342), complete the questionnaire. In the "Information Requested" box, provide a detailed description of the information desired.

Electronic Contact:
To contact **Direct Technology** electronically, simply fill out the form below and click *submit*.

* = Required field

Name: [_____] *

Company: [_____]

Address: [_____]

City: [_____]

State: [N/A ▾]

ZIP: [_____]

Phone: [_____]

Fax: [_____]

E-mail Address: [_____] *

Specialty: [--Select From List-- ▾] *

Product of interest: [--Select From List-- ▾] *

How did you hear about us: [--Select From List-- ▾] *

Other: specify [_____]

Timeframe for Purchase [-Please Select- ▾]

# of Providers in Practice [_____] *   # of Computers in Practice [_____] *

How do you prefer to be contacted [Select ▾] * Best time to call [_____]

Information requested:

[ ]

[Submit] [Reset]

Address Contact:
Direct Technology
1110 Sylvan Heights
Harper, XY 11233
directtech@support.com

Phone Contact:
Phone: (555) 488-8100
Toll-Free: (800) 233-0321
FAX: (555) 488-7737

Fig. 16-2 Printout of electronic contact form.

INTERNET EXPLORATION

A. Log on to the Internet, and, using the search words "electronic medical records," research what the "experts" have to say about the subject.

B. Log on to the Internet and, using the search words "articles electronic medical records," find pertinent articles that discuss what experts have to say about this topic.

PERFORMANCE OBJECTIVES

Performance Objective 16-1—Composing an E-Mail Message

Conditions: Student will compose an e-mail to Dr. Beatrice Fisher requesting the health records for patient Miriam P. Cover (BD 09/18/1956), who has recently moved to Milton. Mrs. Cover has an appointment on March 7, 20XX, with Dr. Jones for continued treatment of her diabetes. Dr. Fisher's e-mail address is bfisher@uihospclinic.net. Mrs. Cover should get a copy of the message at mpcover@hotmail.com.

Supplies/Equipment: Pen/typewriter/computer/paper, e-mail screen duplicated in Fig. 16-3
Time Allowed: 20 minutes
Accuracy Needed to Pass: 90%

Procedural Steps	Points Earned	Comments
Evaluator: Note time began: _____		
1. Carefully read the instructions given for Performance Objective 16-1.		
2. Enter the e-mail address of Dr. Fisher in the correct space. (5)		
3. Enter the e-mail address of Mrs. Cover in the correct space. (5)		
4. Enter the applicable subject for the message. (5)		
5. Compose a brief message as outlined in the instructions. (10)		
6. Close with your name and the clinic's name, address, and a phone number. (5)		
Optional: May deduct points for taking more time than allowed.		

Total Points = 30

Student's Score: _____

Evaluator: _____

Comments: _____

_____

_____

_____

_____

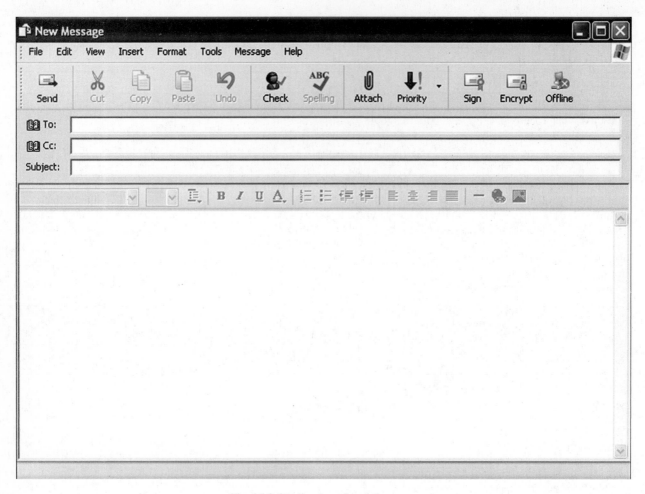

Fig. 16-3 Duplication of e-mail screen.

Performance Objective 16-2—Completing an ETF/ERA Enrollment Form

Conditions: Student will complete the EFT/ERA enrollment form shown in Fig. 16-4 using Broadmoor Clinic's information. Direct Technology is the practice management vendor; Curt Jones is the vendor contact name. ClaimConnect is the clearinghouse you'll be using with user ID # 292927444. EFT will be to a checking account at the Milton National Bank.

Supplies/Equipment: Pen/typewriter/computer/paper, EFT/ERA enrollment form (see Fig. 16-4)

Time Allowed: 30 minutes

Accuracy Needed to Pass: 90%

Procedural Steps	Points Earned	Comments
Evaluator: Note time began: _____		
1. Carefully read the instructions given for Performance Objective 16-2.		
2. Complete the applicable blanks on the EFT/ERA enrollment form using the information provided. (25).		
Optional: May deduct points for taking more time than allowed.		

Total Points = 25

Student's Score: _____

Evaluator: _____

Comments: _____

_____

_____

_____

_____

Electronic Funds Transfer / Electronic Remittance Advice Enrollment Form

Please read all information carefully. Check the appropriate box for this request.
ENROLL IN: ☐ *EFT* ☐ *ERA* *Note: you may enroll in EFT and / or ERA*

Complete the following information, please type or print:

Practice Name _____ Practice Tax ID (TIN)_____

Practice Address _____

Practice Management Vendor _____

Vendor Contact Name_____ Vendor Phone _____

Vendor E-mail Address_____ Approved Vendor/ Clearinghouse _____

Authorized Signature / Date _____

---

1. Electronic Fund Transfer (EFT) – New Enrollment

_____Enroll in EFT   Effective date (Internal Use Only) _____

Do you require payments to be deposited into multiple bank accounts? Yes____ No_____

Do you require payments to be deposited into checking and/or savings account?   Checking_____ Savings_____

New EFT enrollment or changes to existing EFT banking information will trigger a new EFT pre-note validation period. The EFT pre-note validation period will run for 10 days from the effective date. You will be notified of banking issues; otherwise, production will start on day 11.

Request cancellation of EFT as of: _____

NOTE:
You must include a voided check or savings account deposit slip with this enrollment form for your request to be considered. Providers are responsible for notifying Elipse if the above banking information changes.

---

2. Electronic Remittance Advice (ERA) – New Enrollments (only available when registered with Dentalxchange via ClaimConnect). Enrollment in ERA will also eliminate production of paper Explanation of Benefit (EOB) within 60 days of activation.

Enroll in ERA _____   Effective Date (Internal Use Only) _____

ClaimConnect User ID _____   Request Cancellation of ERA as of: _____

ELIPSE INSURANCE CO.
1446 Fortune Lane
Morning Sun, XY 23456
Phone 555-333-4444

Fig. 16-4 Electronic funds transfer form.

Performance Objective 16-3—Completing a Direct Deposit Authorization Form

Conditions: Student will complete the direct deposit authorization form for Broadmoor Medical Clinic shown in Fig. 16-5 using the clinic information acquired to date. Banking information is provided in Box 16-1.

Supplies/Equipment: Pen/typewriter/computer/paper, instructions (see Box 16-1)

Time Allowed: 50 minutes

Accuracy Needed to Pass: 90%

Procedural Steps	Points Earned	Comments
Evaluator: Note time began: _____		
1. Carefully read the instructions given for Performance Objective 16-3.		
2. Complete the applicable blanks on the direct deposit enrollment form using the information provided in Box 16-1. (35)		
Optional: May deduct points for taking more time than allowed.		

Total Points = 35

Student's Score: _____

Evaluator: _____

Comments: _____

_____

_____

_____

_____

_____

Box 16-1

Bank Name: Milton National Bank
Address: 8610 Park Plaza, Milton, XY 12345
Routing No.: 00898870-5216-14
Account No.: 606-445-1
Account Type: Checking

Authorization for Direct Deposit
Enrollment, Change, and Cancellation Authorization

Please read all of the information on this form carefully.
Authorization Information. Check the appropriate box for this authorization.

☐ ENROLL in Direct Deposit   ☐ CHANGE to Direct Deposit   ☐ CANCEL previous authorization

Provider Information
Please print. Complete all of the information below, including your tax identification number (TIN).

PROVIDER INFORMATION

Name(s) _____   Required for Processing: TIN ___ ___ - ___ ___ ___ ___ ___ ___ ___

Street _____   City _____   State _____   Zip _____

Business Telephone Number (   ) _____

E-Mail Address: _____

Account Information
Complete this section for direct payments to either your checking or savings account.

BANK NAME: _____   ADDRESS: _____
BANK ID (first 8 digits of the routing number): ___ ___ ___ ___ ___ ___ ___ ___
BANK SCD (self-checking digit–the last digit of the routing number): ___
ACCOUNT NUMBER: _____   ACCOUNT TYPE: Savings ☐ or Checking ☐

TO BE COMPLETED for each additional bank account

BANK NAME: _____   ADDRESS: _____
BANK ID (first 8 digits of the routing number): ___ ___ ___ ___ ___ ___ ___ ___
BANK SCD (self-checking digit–the last digit of the routing number): ___
ACCOUNT NUMBER: _____   ACCOUNT TYPE: Savings ☐ or Checking ☐

TO BE COMPLETED for each additional bank account

BANK NAME: _____   ADDRESS: _____
BANK ID (first 8 digits of the routing number): ___ ___ ___ ___ ___ ___ ___ ___
BANK SCD (self-checking digit–the last digit of the routing number): ___
ACCOUNT NUMBER: _____   ACCOUNT TYPE: Savings ☐ or Checking ☐

Authorization Agreement for Direct Deposit of Benefits Payments. Read the authorization and sign your name below.

I hereby authorize the Company to initiate credit entries to the account(s) at the bank(s) listed above for all benefits payments. This agreement will remain in effect untill notify Company of the desire to cancel or change this service or until Company notifies me that this service has been terminated. I understand that I must allow reasonable time for my instructions to be executed. If Company credits more money than the correct benefit amount to the account due to duplicate electronic funds transfers (where "duplicate" is defined as multiple electronic funds transfers received for the same services rendered, the same membership, and the same dates of service) or erroneous electronic funds transfers (where erroneus is defined as complete electronic funds transfers received in error), I authorize Company to withdraw the over payment. I authorize and request the bank listed above to accept any credit entries by Aetna to such account and to credit the same to such account.

Please Print Name _____   **Date** _____

Authorized Signature _____

Provider Network Authorization _____   **Date** _____

Fig. 16-5 Direct deposit form.

Health Insurance Professional's Notebook

- Websites and resources for information on EDI and DDE
- Examples of forms and completion instructions for EFT and RMA enrollment
- Names and telephone numbers of reputable hardware/software dealers
- Informational brochures on patient accounting software
- Sample ERAs and instructions on how to interpret each
- Information/resources/websites on EMRs

Chapter Check List

Student name: _____

Chapter completion date: _____

1.	Record	Your start time and date: _____
2.	Read	The assigned chapter in the text
3.	View	PowerPoint slides (if available)
4.	Complete	Exercises in the Workbook as assigned
5.	Compare	Your answers to the answers posted on the bulletin board/website/handout
6.	Correct	Your answers
7.	Complete	All tests and required activities
8.	Read	Assigned readings (if any)
9.	Complete	Chapter performance objectives (competencies), if any
10.	Evaluate	Chapter performance, and submit to your instructor
11.	Record	Your ending time and date: _____
12.	Move on	Begin next chapter as assigned

PERFORMANCE EVALUATION

Evaluate your classroom performance. Complete the self-evaluation and submit it to your instructor. When your instructor returns this form to you, compare your self-evaluation with the evaluation completed by your instructor.

Skill	Student Self-Evaluation			Instructor Evaluation		
	Good	Average	Poor	Good	Average	Poor
Attendance/punctuality						
Personal appearance						
Applies effort						
Is self-motivated						
Is courteous						
Has positive attitude						
Completes assignments in timely manner						
Works well with others						

Student's initials: _____   **Instructor's initials:** _____

Date: _____   **Date:** _____

Points Possible: _____

Points Awarded: _____

Chapter Grade: _____

17 Reimbursement Procedures: Getting Paid

In this chapter, you were introduced to topics that are considered more advanced. Your instructor may or may not include this chapter in the course curriculum because it delves more into the area of health information management as opposed to that of health insurance professionals. Some of the subject matter presented may prove to be confusing and, at best, challenging, but do not become discouraged. Chapter 17 is intended to give students an overview of what a career path to becoming a health information technician (HIT) or a health information management (HIM) specialist involves. These are considered more advanced careers for which students may become certified and typically involve up to 4 years of college. Usually, an HIT or an HIM specialist is employed by hospitals, rather than physician offices or clinics, and employment responsibilities differ greatly from those of a health insurance professional in a medical office. If the information presented in Chapter 17 piques your interest, and you think you may want to pursue a career in HIM, discuss this with your instructor or your student advisor.

WORKBOOK CHAPTER OBJECTIVES

After completing the workbook activities for Chapter 17, the student should be able to:
- Define the terms used in the chapter.
- Answer the review questions to within the evaluation criteria set by the instructor.
- Use problem-solving skills (individually or in a group setting) to determine correct responses and outcomes in case studies and application exercises.
- Interpret a variety of aging reports.
- Research the Internet to locate information to understand given topics better.
- Complete performance objectives to within the criteria determined by the instructor.
- Perform the necessary steps for unbiased self-evaluation and understanding of material presented in the workbook.

DEFINING CHAPTER TERMS

Using the computer (or typewriter), students should key an accurate definition for each of the chapter terms listed. These definitions should be in the students' own words. When finished, students should compare their definitions with those listed in the glossary at the back of the textbook, correcting any inaccuracies.

accounts receivable aging report
activities of daily living
ambulatory payment classifications (APCs)
average length of stay (ALOS)
balance billing
business associate
capitation
comorbidity
contractual write-off
cost outliers
covered entity
diagnosis-related groups (DRGs)
discounted fee-for-service
disproportionate share
DRG grouper
fee-for-service
geographic practice cost index (GPCI)
home health prospective payment system
  (HH PPS)

inpatient rehabilitation facility prospective payment
  system (IRF PPS)
labor component
long-term care hospital prospective payment system
  (LTCH PPS)
managed care organizations
nonlabor component
peer review organization (PRO)
principal diagnosis
prospective payment system (PPS)
reimbursement
relative value scale (RVS)
residential healthcare facility
resource utilization groups (RUGs)
resource-based relative value scale (RBRVS)
short-stay outlier
skilled nursing facility
standardized amount
Tax Equity and Fiscal Responsibility Act (TEFRA)

Multiple Choice

Directions: In the questions/statements presented, choose the response that **best** answers/completes the stem, and circle the letter that precedes it.

1. Payment to the insured (or his or her provider) for a covered expense or loss experienced by or on behalf of the insured is referred to as:
   a. Coverage
   b. Copayment
   c. Deductible(s)
   d. Reimbursement

2. A system of payment whereby the provider charges a specific fee for each service rendered and is paid that fee by the patient or by the patient's insurance carrier is called:
   a. Capitation
   b. Fee-for-service
   c. Discounted fee-for-service
   d. Prospective payment system (PPS)

3. Medicare's system for reimbursing Part A inpatient hospital costs is called:
   a. Capitation
   b. Fee-for-service
   c. Discounted fee-for-service
   d. PPS

4. The amount of payment in the PPS is determined by the assigned:
   a. Capitation amount
   b. Diagnosis-related group (DRG)
   c. Usual, customary, and reasonable (UCR) fee
   d. Either b or c

5. A common method of paying physicians in health maintenance organizations is:
   a. UCR
   b. PPG
   c. Capitation
   d. Fee-for-service

6. PPS for acute hospital care for Medicare patients was mandated by:
   a. Centers for Medicare and Medicaid Services (CMS) in 1980
   b. Department of Health and Human Services (HHS) in 1981
   c. Social Security Amendments of 1983
   d. All of the above

7. Primary authority for implementing the PPS was given to the:
   a. Individual states
   b. HHS
   c. Social Security Administration (SSA)
   d. CMS

8. The method of determining Medicare's reimbursement for services based on establishing a standard unit value for medical and surgical procedures is:

   a. PPS

   b. RVS

   c. DRG

   d. APC

9. The Omnibus Budget Reconciliation Act of 1989 (OBRA89) legislated a system to replace the UCR structure called the:

   a. HCPCS system

   b. Fee-for-service system

   c. Relative value scale (RVS)

   d. Resource-based relative value scale (RBRVS)

10. The key piece of information in determining the DRG classification is the patient's:

    a. Chief complaint

    b. Primary diagnosis

    c. Principal diagnosis

    d. Underlying symptoms

11. The presence of more than one disease or disorder that occurs in an individual at the same time is referred to as a:

    a. Comorbidity

    b. Complication

    c. Dual diagnosis

    d. Medical history

12. A computer software program that takes the coded information and identifies the patient's DRG category is a(n):

    a. Unscrambler

    b. Digitalized coder

    c. DRG identifier

    d. DRG grouper

13. A service classification system designed to explain the amount and type of resources used in an outpatient encounter is:

    a. DRGs

    b. ALOS

    c. APCs

    d. PPS

14. The key data in determining the ambulatory payment classification (APC) payment rate are the coding and classification of services provided to the patient based on the:

    a. ICD-9 coding system

    b. CPT coding system

    c. HCPCS coding system

    d. All of the above

15. The basic idea of the resource utilization groups (RUGs) is to calculate payments according to severity and level of care in:

    a. Outpatient clinics

    b. Acute care hospitals

    c. Skilled nursing facilities

    d. Long-term care facilities

16. A factor used by Medicare to adjust for variance in operating costs of medical practices located in different parts of the United States is the:

    a. GPCI

    b. ANSII

    c. RBRVS

    d. Both a and c

17. Medicare reimburses hospitals for providing inpatient care to beneficiaries with a payment system known as:

    a. HCPCS

    b. ICD-9

    c. IPPS

    d. CPT

18. Under Medicare's PPS, long-term care hospitals (LTCHs) generally treat patients who require hospital-level care for an average of:

    a. 10 days

    b. 15 days

    c. 25 days

    d. There is no limit with long-term care

19. An adjustment to the federal payment rate for LTCH stays that are considerably shorter than the average length of stay for an LTC-DRG is called a(n):

    a. Minimum-stay adjuster

    b. Short-stay outlier

    c. GPCI

    d. ALOS

20. Determination of payment in the home health prospective payment system depends on:

    a. GPSI

    b. ALOS

    c. OASIS

    d. CMS

21. An organization, typically composed of physicians and other healthcare professionals, paid by the federal government to evaluate the services provided by other practitioners and to monitor the quality of patient care is called:

    a. PPS

    b. HIPAA

    c. PRO

    d. CMS

22. When an agreement exists between the provider and an insurance carrier whereby the provider agrees to accept the payer's allowed fee as payment in full for a particular service or procedure, the process is called:

a. Contractual write-offs

b. Prospective payment

c. Balance billing

d. Patient equity

True/False

Directions: Place a "T" in the blank preceding the numbered statement if it is true; place an "F" if it is false.

_____ 1. Medicare patients are not included in the PPS system.

_____ 2. Prospective payment rates are set at a level intended to cover operating costs for treating a typical inpatient in a given DRG.

_____ 3. Under Medicare's PPS, hospitals are paid a set fee for treating patients in a single DRG category, regardless of the actual cost of care for the individual.

_____ 4. The established payment rate for all services that a patient in an acute care hospital receives during an entire stay is based on a predetermined payment level that is selected on the basis of averages.

_____ 5. The biggest challenge in developing an RVS-based payment schedule was patient diversity.

_____ 6. The RBRVS system includes the elimination of balance billing.

_____ 7. DRGs are used for reimbursement in the PPS of the Medicare and Medicaid healthcare insurance systems.

_____ 8. DRGs adopted by CMS are defined by diagnosis and procedure codes used in the ICD-9.

_____ 9. A patient's DRG categorization depends on the coding and classification of the patient's medical information using the CPT coding system.

_____ 10. Each DRG is assigned a relative weight (RW) and an average length of stay (ALOS).

_____ 11. When patients are admitted to either a residential healthcare facility or a nursing home, physicians are required to prepare a written plan of care for treatment.

_____ 12. Activities of daily living are behaviors related strictly to mental health.

_____ 13. Medicare payment rules are established by Congress.

_____ 14. The Medicare program is administered mainly at the local and regional level by private insurance companies that contract with CMS to handle day-to-day billing and payment matters.

_____ 15. DRG payments are adjusted annually to reflect changes in hospital costs and changes in technology.

_____ 16. In the Balanced Budget Act of 1997, Congress mandated that CMS implement a PPS for inpatient rehabilitation (IRF PPS).

_____ 17. Reimbursement in the IRF PPS is based on the length of hospital stay.

_____ 18. Not all peer review organizations (PROs) deal with healthcare.

_____ 19. The cost of a medical billing software system generally has no direct correlation with its capabilities or customer satisfaction ratings.

_____ 20. Contractual write-offs and bad-debt write-offs are basically the same.

_____ 21. As of 2003, HIPAA demanded that all medical facilities be computerized without exception.

_____ 22. The HHS mandates that all medical facilities use the same format for submitting electronic health transactions.

_____ 23. HIPAA has certain transaction standards for all electronic transactions.

_____ 24.   When selecting a hardware/software vendor, it is important to ensure their products comply with the HIPAA Privacy Rule.

_____ 25.   If a medical practice contracts with a "business associate," the practice should ensure that the agreement includes certain protections defined by HIPAA.

Short Answer

Directions: Answer the question fully in the space provided. If more space is needed, use a blank sheet of paper.

1. List and explain Medicare's three primary reimbursement systems.

_____

_____

_____

2. List and discuss Congress' four chief objectives in creating the PPS.

_____

_____

_____

_____

3. List the factors on which the DRG inpatient classification system is based.

_____

_____

_____

4. Explain, in your own words, what a "cost outlier" is.

_____

_____

5. List the three components that make up a relative value unit (RVU).

_____

_____

_____

6. List the three components of the RBRVS system.

_____

_____

_____

7. When calculating DRG payment, the DRG "weight" is multiplied by the "standardized amount," which is the sum of what two factors?

_____

_____

8. Explain how payment is calculated for a CPT code under the RVU system.

_____

_____

9. Explain what a PRO is, and discuss its basic responsibilities.

_____

_____

10. Congress required the HHS to contract with PROs to monitor specific healthcare functions. List these functions.

_____

_____

_____

11. List at least five of the seven system functions that today's patient accounting systems are capable of performing.

_____

_____

_____

_____

_____

12. If a practice is upgrading an existing patient accounting software package for a medical facility, what are some important considerations?

_____

_____

_____

13. What questions should you ask of a potential software/hardware vendor?

_____

_____

_____

14. List at least five capabilities that medical billing software systems typically have built into them.

_____

_____

_____

_____

_____

15. Name the typical reporting capabilities that are built in to most medical accounting software.

_____

_____

16. Explain the purpose of a practice analysis report.

_____

_____

_____

17. What types of firms come under the umbrella of "covered entity"?

_____

_____

_____

CRITICAL THINKING ACTIVITIES

A. Abby Silverton works as a health insurance professional in a small, rural clinic. In addition to Abby, the medical team includes a physician's assistant, a part-time nurse, and a medical assistant. The average yearly patient load is roughly 70 local patients—mostly elderly. The clinic is currently using the "pegboard" system of patient accounting. Prepare an outline for Abby to present at the next staff meeting discussing the advantages and disadvantages of switching to a computerized patient accounting system.

B. The Flexner Report is said by some to be the most important event in the history of American medical education. Research this topic, and write a critical thinking essay on the focus points of this document and its impact on a health insurance professional.

C. Enough cannot be said about the importance of documentation in medical records. There is a common saying, "If it isn't documented, it didn't happen." Generate a 1-page essay on this subject and how it impacts a health insurance professional.

A. The general formula for calculating the Medicare fee schedule amount for a given service in a given fee schedule area can be expressed as:

Payment = [(RVU work × GPCI work) +
(RVU practice expense × GPCI practice expense) +
(RVU malpractice × GPCI malpractice)] × Conversion factor

Using the information from Table 17-3 and accompanying "Imagine This" example on pp. 380 and 381 of the textbook, calculate the amount that Medicare will reimburse a physician with a practice located in your area for a Diagnostic Colonoscopy (CPT/HCPCS 45378-53).

B. Convene a "brainstorming" session in which each group member participates in developing a "wish list" of features and functions of the "ideal" patient billing system for Broadmoor Medical Clinic.

C. Assemble a "fact-finding" group or partnership and investigate educational opportunities in the field of health information technology.

CASE STUDIES

A. One of the standard reports generated by most patient accounting software programs is the accounts receivable aging report. Study the example in Table 17-1, and answer the following questions.

Table 17-1 Aging Report

Broadmoor Medical Clinic Accounts Receivable Aging Report					
Name	**Current**	**>30 Days**	**>60 Days**	**>90 Days**	**>120 Days**
Abel, Paul		419.50			
Allen, Tricia			860.25		
Asner, Robert			90.00		
Benson, Ted			155.50		
Boles, Frieda					334.19
Bumgardner, Leona				11.60	
Callison, Tanner		120.00			
Colby, Ruth		85.00			
Cullen, Vincent			456.30		
Dawson, Cynthia	190.00				
Daymeri, Tao	211.90				
Ditmer, Pauline				142.35	
Dolby, Nelda				96.80	
Dunison, Arthur					1211.42
Edwards, Lois	77.00				
Efflinger, Dorothy		62.50			
Ekdale, Wesley		175.22			
Eversmeier, Theo				200.00	
Page Totals	*478.90*	*862.22*	*1562.05*	*450.75*	*1545.61*

363

1. What percent of the total dollar amounts on this page are current?
2. What percent of the total dollar amounts on this page are more than 30 days old?
3. What percent of the total dollar amounts on this page are more than 60 days old?
4. What percent of the total dollar amounts on this page are more than 120 days old?

Note: Round up to the nearest whole percentage.

B. Fig. 17-1 is a sample page from an insurance claims aging report. Study it, and then on a separate piece of paper list the information that can be abstracted from this report.

BROADMOOR MEDICAL CLINIC
4353 PINE RIDGE DRIVE
MILTON XY 12345-0001

INSURANCE AGING SUMMARY

Date of Service	Procedure	Current 0 - 30	Past 31 - 60	Past 61 - 90	Past 91 - 120	Past 121 ⟶	Total Balance
Aetna (AET00)						Erik (602)333-3333	
SIMTA000 **Tanus J Simpson**						SSN:	
Claim: 1 *Initial Billing Date: 12/3/2002*			*Last Billing Date: 10/30/2003*	*Policy: GG93-GXTA*	*Group: 99999*		
12/3/2002	43220	275.00					275.00
12/3/2002	71040	50.00					50.00
12/3/2002	81000	11.00					11.00
12/3/2002	99213	50.00					50.00
	Claim Totals:	386.00	0.00	0.00	0.00	0.00	386.00
Claim: 15 *Initial Billing Date: 10/30/2003*			*Last Billing Date: 10/30/2003*	*Policy: GG93-GXTA*	*Group: 99999*		
10/25/2003	99213	60.00					60.00
10/25/2003	90707	10.00					10.00
	Claim Totals:	70.00	0.00	0.00	0.00	0.00	70.00
	Insurance Totals:	456.00	0.00	0.00	0.00	0.00	456.00
Cigna (CIG00)						Bill S. Preston 234-5678	
BRIJA000 **Jay Brimley**						SSN:	
Claim: 16 *Initial Billing Date: 10/26/2003*			*Last Billing Date: 10/26/2003*	*Policy: 98547377*	*Group: 12d*		
3/25/2002	99214	55.00					55.00
3/25/2002	97260	30.00					30.00
	Claim Totals:	85.00	0.00	0.00	0.00	0.00	85.00
	Insurance Totals:	85.00	0.00	0.00	0.00	0.00	85.00
U.S. Tricare (US000)							
YOUMI000 **Michael C Youngblood**						SSN:	
Claim: 17 *Initial Billing Date: 10/26/2003*			*Last Billing Date: 10/26/2003*	*Policy: USAA236678*	*Group: 25BB*		
8/22/2002	99213	60.00					60.00
8/22/2002	97128	15.00					15.00
8/22/2002	97010	10.00					10.00
	Claim Totals:	85.00	0.00	0.00	0.00	0.00	85.00
	Insurance Totals:	85.00	0.00	0.00	0.00	0.00	85.00
	Report Aging Totals	$626.00	$0.00	$0.00	$0.00	$0.00	$626.00
	Percent of Aging Total	100.0%	0.0%	0.0%	0.0%	0.0%	100.0%

Printed on 11/01/2003 1:59 pm

This report is being aged by the last billing date

Fig. 17-1 Insurance aging summary.

C. Table 17-2 is an example of an insurance aging report from a different software program. What does this report tell you?

Table 17-2 Insurance Company Aging Summary					
	Current	**30-59 Days**	**60-89 Days**	**90-119 Days**	**≥120 Days**
Personal	$27,806.24	$24,820.84	$16,045.36	$9647.64	$21,824.05
American	$898.00	$0.00	$125.00	$0.00	$0.00
Anthrose	$4637.00	$812.00	$1250.00	$333.00	$45.00
BayShore	$80.00	$0.00	$0.00	$0.00	$0.00
Bayshore Life	$2414.00	$212.00	$40.00	$865.00	$40.00
Catalina	$3604.00	$1546.00	$889.00	$282.00	$26.40
CIGNA	$68.00	$0.00	$60.00	$40.00	$0.00
Central Benefits	$12,647.00	$3103.00	$1100.54	$743.20	$1105.40
Dover Med	$87.00	$0.00	$0.00	$0.00	$90.00
Empire	$135.00	$0.00	$0.00	$0.00	$0.00
MetLife	$110.00	$0.00	$0.00	$0.00	$0.00
Provident	$0.00	$0.00	$32.00	$0.00	$0.00
Salem Health	$4242.70	$2099.70	$638.00	$416.00	$1010.10
United HC	$6237.00	$1087.68	$666.44	$65.00	$77.00
Total	$86,328.84	$45,782.81	$27,276.03	$23,198.23	$36,155.51

D. Table 17-3 is an insurance report summary that provides still another type of information. How does this report differ from the one in Figure 17-1? How does this report differ from the one in Table 17-2? Write your answers in the space below or on a separate piece of paper.

Table 17-3 Insurance Company Reimbursement Report: Summary

Insurance Company Reimbursement Report: Summary Page: 1			
From: 01/01/96	To: 12/31/96		Generated on 01/11/96
Code	Procedure/Group Name	Units	Charged
99213	Office Visit Expanded Focus	11,956	$616,720
99212	Office Visit Problem Focused	1613	$49,662
99054	Office Visit Sundays and Holidays	889	$8890
[many lines deleted]			
	Office Visits	15,496	$702,368
99392	Well Child 1–4 years	2744	$150,920
99391	Well Child less than 1 year	2386	$124,072
99393	Well Child 5–11 years	1042	$61,435
[many lines deleted]			
	Well Child Visits	7516	$428,389

INTERNET EXPLORATION

A. Log on to the Internet and research the Tax Equity and Fiscal Responsibility Act (TEFRA).

B. Research the Internet using the search words "find articles" to locate information and updates on the following systems:
- Medicare's IPPS
- APCs
- OPPS

C. Read the article, "Selecting the Correct Computer System for Your Practice: Points to Consider Before Spending Your Time and Money," by Marsha Summers, which appeared in an issue of *San Francisco Medicine,* the official newsletter of the San Francisco Medical Society, at **http://www.sfms.org/AM/Template.cfm?Section=Home&template= /CM/HTMLDisplay.cfm&ContentID=1868**.

PERFORMANCE OBJECTIVES

The Performance Objectives in Chapter 17 are designed to provide you with additional learning opportunities and reinforcement in the knowledge and understanding of the various types of reimbursement systems used in physicians' offices; clinics; and healthcare facilities such as hospitals, skilled nursing facilities, rehabilitation facilities and other institutional-type care facilities.

Performance Objective 17-1—Explaining Common Reimbursement Types

Conditions: Student will write a short paragraph explaining the following reimbursement types: fee-for-service, discounted fee-for-service, PPS, capitation, and per diem.

Supplies/Equipment: Computer with word processing software, printer, paper

Time Allowed: 30 minutes

Accuracy Needed to Pass: 90%

Procedural Steps	Points Earned	Comments
Evaluator: Note time began: _____		
1. Student explained the FFS payment system satisfactorily. (20)		
2. Student explained the discounted FFS payment system satisfactorily. (20)		
3. Student explained the PPS satisfactorily. (20)		
4. Student explained the capitation payment system satisfactorily. (20)		
5. Student explained the per diem payment system satisfactorily. (20)		

Total Points = 100

Student's Score: _____

Evaluator: _____

Comments: _____

_____

_____

_____

_____

Performance Objective 17-2—Defining DRGs, APCs, and RUGs

Conditions: Student will state what each of the above-listed acronyms stands for, write a brief definition of each, and explain where and how they are used in healthcare facilities.

Supplies/Equipment: Computer with word processing software, printer, paper

Time Allowed: 30 minutes

Accuracy Needed to Pass: 85%

Procedural Steps	Points Earned	Comments
Evaluator: Note time began: _____		
1. Student provided an accurate and adequate explanation of DRGs. (20)		
2. Student provided an accurate and adequate explanation of APCs. (20)		
3. Student provided an accurate and adequate explanation of RUGs. (20)		

Total Points = 60

Student's Score: _____

Evaluator: _____

Comments: _____

_____

_____

_____

_____

Chapter **17**   **Reimbursement Procedures: Getting Paid**

Performance Objective 17-3—Understanding Computerized Patient Accounting Systems

Conditions: Describe a typical computerized patient accounting system, including the seven basic functions that this type of software is capable of performing.

Supplies/Equipment: Computer with word processing software, printer, paper

Time Allowed: 30 minutes

Accuracy Needed to Pass: 85%

Procedural Steps	Points Earned	Comments
Evaluator: Note time began: _____		
1. Student provided an accurate/satisfactory description of a patient accounting system. (20)		
2. Student correctly identified the seven basic functions of this type of software. (20)		
3. Students demonstrated proficiency in writing/ grammar skills. (20)		

Total Points = 60

Student's Score: _____

Evaluator: _____

Comments: _____

_____

_____

_____

_____

APPLICATION EXERCISES

Health Insurance Professional's Notebook

1. Collect pertinent examples of documents discussed in this chapter, such as
   - Electronic remittance advices
   - Aging and other practice reports

2. Include websites for information on
   - Continuing education for health insurance professionals
   - Certification possibilities
   - Keeping current

Chapter Check List

Student name: _____

Chapter completion date: _____

1.	Record	Your start time and date: _____
2.	Read	The assigned chapter in the text
3.	View	PowerPoint slides (if available)
4.	Complete	Exercises in the Workbook as assigned
5.	Compare	Your answers to the answers posted on the bulletin board/website/handout
6.	Correct	Your answers
7.	Complete	All tests and required activities
8.	Read	Assigned readings (if any)
9.	Complete	Chapter performance objectives (competencies), if any
10.	Evaluate	Chapter performance, and submit to your instructor
11.	Record	Your ending time and date: _____
12.	Move on	Begin next chapter as assigned

PERFORMANCE EVALUATION

Evaluate your classroom performance. Complete the self-evaluation and submit it to your instructor. When your instructor returns this form to you, compare your self-evaluation with the evaluation completed by your instructor.

Skill	Student Self-Evaluation			Instructor Evaluation		
	Good	Average	Poor	Good	Average	Poor
Attendance/punctuality						
Personal appearance						
Applies effort						
Is self-motivated						
Is courteous						
Has positive attitude						
Completes assignments in timely manner						
Works well with others						

Student's Initials: _____   **Instructor's Initials:** _____

Date: _____   **Date:** _____

Points Possible: _____

Points Awarded: _____

Chapter Grade: _____

18 Hospital Billing and the UB-04

In this chapter, we left the physician's office and branched out into institutional healthcare—the hospital. As the title indicates, Unit Five presents an alternate step, and the general trend of the material takes the student to a more challenging level. As mentioned in the text, it would take an entire volume to include all of the information necessary to cover every aspect of hospital billing adequately. Just basic information is included to give students a "taste" of what this area of healthcare entails. If it piques the student's interest, he or she might want to explore opportunities for enrollment in a health information technology or health information management program.

The UB-04 is the universal form used for submitting hospital claims, and some students may find it more challenging to complete than the CMS-1500. The UB-04 has 81 "form locators" where various types of data are inserted, whereas the CMS-1500 has 33 blocks for data entry. Additionally, there are two types of patient claims—inpatient and outpatient— each with its own guidelines. As with the CMS-1500, an updated universal billing form for inpatient care, the UB-04, became effective for claims submission in March 2007. Hospitals could use either the previous form UB-92 or the UB-04 until May 22, 2007; since that date, only the UB-04 has been accepted by payers.

The activities in this workbook chapter have been developed to supplement the material presented in the text in hopes of providing students with an opportunity for a better grasp of what is involved in hospital billing.

WORKBOOK CHAPTER OBJECTIVES

After completing the workbook activities for Chapter 18, the student should be able to:
- Define the terms used in the chapter.
- Answer the review questions to within the evaluation criteria set by the instructor.
- Use problem-solving skills (individually or in a group setting) to determine correct responses and outcomes in case studies and application exercises.
- Identify the correct diagnostic codes from a series of case studies.
- Engage in critical thinking techniques to solve case studies.
- Research the Internet to locate information to understand given topics better.
- Complete performance objectives to within the criteria determined by the instructor.
- Perform the necessary steps for unbiased self-evaluation and understanding of material presented in the workbook.

DEFINING CHAPTER TERMS

Using the computer (or typewriter), students should key an accurate definition for each of the chapter terms listed. These definitions should be in the students' own words. When finished, students should compare their definitions with those listed in the glossary at the back of the textbook, correcting any inaccuracies.

accreditation
Accreditation Association for Ambulatory Health Care
  (AAAHC)
activities of daily living
acute care
acute care facility
acute condition
ambulatory payment classifications (APCs)
ambulatory surgery centers (ACSs)
American Osteopathic Association (AOA) Commission
  on Osteopathic College Accreditation
benefit period
billing compliance
Blue Cross and Blue Shield member hospitals
carriers
case mix
cost sharing
covered entity

crosswalk
Defense Enrollment Eligibility Reporting System
diagnosis-related groups (DRGs)
electronic claims submission (ECS)
electronic medical records (EMRs)
electronic remittance notice (ERN)
Emergency Medical Treatment and Labor Act
  (EMTLA)
emergent medical condition
fiscal intermediaries
form locators
for-profit hospitals
general hospital
governance
hospice
hospital outpatient prospective payment system
  (HOPPS)
informed consent

intermediaries
The Joint Commission
licensed independent practitioners
long-term care facilities
medical ethics
Medicare Severity Adjusted (MS-DRG) System
National Committee for Quality Assurance (NCQA)
National Correct Coding Initiative
National Uniform Billing Committee (NUBC)
nonavailability statement (NAS)
outliers
pass-throughs
peer review organizations
per diems
principal diagnosis

prospective payment system (PPS)
quality improvement organizations
registered health information technicians (RHITs)
respite care
routine charges
rubric
skilled nursing facility (SNF)
subacute care unit
surrogate
swing bed
UB-04
UB-92
Utilization Review Accreditation Commission (URAC)
vertically integrated hospitals

ASSESSMENT

Multiple Choice

Directions: In the questions/statements presented, choose the response that **best** answers/completes the stem by circling the letter that precedes it.

1. The construction of today's modern hospital is regulated by:
   a. Federal and state laws
   b. State health department policies
   c. City ordinances
   d. All of the above

2. Today's hospitals typically offer:
   a. Private and semiprivate rooms
   b. Four-bed room options
   c. Wards with up to 30 beds
   d. All of the above

3. Hospitals that provide all levels of care are referred to as:
   a. Mega-complexes
   b. Total care facilities
   c. Inpatient/outpatient centers
   d. Vertically integrated hospitals

4. A popular designation given to today's healthcare patients is:
   a. Users
   b. Clients
   c. Customers
   d. Consumers

5. A single building or campus, typically having a large number of beds, specialized facilities for various medical care types, and an emergency department, is called a:
   a. Clinic
   b. General hospital
   c. Preferred provider organization
   d. Health maintenance organization (HMO)

6. A medical facility smaller than a hospital is typically referred to as a(n):
   a. Clinic
   b. General hospital
   c. For-profit facility
   d. Outpatient facility

7. A healthcare facility that is equipped and staffed to respond immediately to critical situations and provide continuous care to patients with "worst-case" scenarios is a(n):
   a. Acute care facility
   b. Extended care facility
   c. Designated trauma center
   d. Community emergency center

8. A facility designed for patients who have had acute events as a result of an illness, injury, or exacerbation of a disease process is a(n):
   a. Acute care hospital
   b. Subacute care facility
   c. Skilled nursing facility (SNF)
   d. Long-term care facility

9. The type of facility in which patients have the advantage of constant access to nursing care as they move toward recovery and return to their home is a(n):
   a. Acute care hospital
   b. Subacute care facility
   c. SNF
   d. Long-term care facility

10. A facility that is licensed or approved under state or local law that is primarily engaged in providing experienced nursing care and related services is a(n):
    a. Acute care hospital
    b. Subacute care facility
    c. SNF
    d. Long-term care facility

11. Temporary relief for an individual providing healthcare to a family member is commonly called:
    a. Hospice
    b. Respite care
    c. Interval relief
    d. Adult daycare

12. The type of care provided for adults who are chronically ill or disabled and are no longer able to manage in independent living situations is referred to as:
    a. Hospice
    b. Respite care
    c. Activities of daily living care
    d. Long-term care

13. The acronym for the federal act that ensures public access to emergency services regardless of ability to pay is:
    a. NUBC
    b. COBRA
    c. EMTLA
    d. AAAHC

14. The voluntary process through which an organization is able to measure the quality of its services and performance against nationally recognized standards is called:

    a. Accreditation

    b. Certification

    c. Credentialing

    d. Validation

15. The independent, nonprofit organization that performs quality-oriented accreditation reviews on HMOs and similar types of managed care plans is:

    a. NCQA

    b. NUBC

    c. AAAHC

    d. AOA/COCA

16. The acronym for the organization (formed in 1979) to assist ambulatory healthcare organizations improve the quality of care provided to patients is the:

    a. NCQA

    b. URAC

    c. AAAHC

    d. AOA/COCA

17. The independent, nonprofit organization that promotes continuous improvement in the quality and efficiency of healthcare delivery through the establishment of standards, education, and communication is the:

    a. NCQA

    b. URAC

    c. AAAHC

    d. NUBC

18. How any organization is run is, in its simplest definition, referred to as:

    a. Accreditation

    b. Governance

    c. Compliance

    d. Ethics

19. Moral principles that govern the practice of medicine by physicians and other healthcare practitioners are commonly referred to as medical:

    a. Ethics

    b. Etiquette

    c. Protocol

    d. Courtesy

20. Medicare hospital claims are processed by contracted nongovernment organizations or agencies that commonly are referred to as:

    a. Member organizations

    b. Fiscal intermediaries or carriers

    c. Qualifying contracting agents

    d. All of the above

21. Medicare Part A pays toward:

    a. Hospital charges

    b. Physician charges

    c. Long-term healthcare

    d. All of the above

378

22. Medicare's acute care payment system is called the:

    a. Prospective payment system (PPS)

    b. Cost share system

    c. Per-diem system

    d. DEERS

23. An inpatient hospital coding system that groups related diagnoses and their associated medical/surgical treatment is referred to as:

    a. APCs

    b. DRGs

    c. DEERS

    d. CMS

24. Many Medicaid programs adjust payments to reflect such things as patient demographics, diagnostic and treatment information, and total charges, referred to as:

    a. A per-diem structure

    b. A swing-bed configuration

    c. A case mix

    d. Cost-sharing

25. If a military treatment facility is unavailable, TRICARE patients, in many cases, must obtain a:

    a. Military waiver

    b. Preauthorization statement

    c. Statement of authenticity

    d. Nonavailability statement (NAS)

26. Most third-party payers typically change their reimbursement rates:

    a. Quarterly

    b. Semiannually

    c. Annually

    d. Biannually

27. Most U.S. hospitals contract with Blue Cross and Blue Shield and are referred to as:

    a. Member hospitals

    b. Cost outliers

    c. Swing-bed hospitals

    d. Acute care hospitals

28. The designated spaces on the UB-04 are called:

    a. Blocks

    b. Data elements

    c. Form locators

    d. Code indicators

29. The revised universal claim form for current use in inpatient hospital claims is the:

    a. CMS-1500

    b. UB-82

    c. UB-92

    d. UB-04

30. The process by which a patient can participate in choices about his or her healthcare is commonly referred to as:
   a. Informed consent
   b. Preauthorization
   c. Release of information
   d. Registration

31. An individual who has the legal authority to speak on a patient's behalf is called a:
   a. Volunteer
   b. Fiscal intermediary
   c. Covered entity
   d. Surrogate

32. The manual(s) used for inpatient diagnostic coding is(are) the:
   a. CPT-4
   b. HCPCS
   c. ICD-9-CM, Volume 3
   d. ICD-9-CM, Volumes 1 and 2

33. The manual(s) used for inpatient procedural coding is(are) the:
   a. CPT-4
   b. HCPCS
   c. ICD-9-CM, Volume 3
   d. ICD-9-CM, Volumes 1 and 2

34. Coders must distinguish key elements or words in the patient's hospital health record that identify the:
   a. Prime diagnosis
   b. Primary diagnosis
   c. Principal diagnosis
   d. Chief diagnosis

35. The "sections" in ICD-9-CM Volume 3 are organized by:
   a. Anatomy sites
   b. Surgical specialty
   c. Disease or condition
   d. Principal diagnoses

36. A table or search engine that maps the relationships and equivalencies between two or more data formats is called a:
   a. Rubric
   b. Code set
   c. Crosswalk
   d. Equivalency array

37. What type of codes is found in the Index to External Causes?
   a. V codes
   b. E codes
   c. Discontinued codes
   d. HCPCS codes

38. The hospital claim form may report how many significant procedures other than the principal procedure?
   a. 2
   b. 5
   c. 8
   d. 10

380

39. The payment system implemented in 2000 and used by the Centers for Medicare and Medicaid Services (CMS) to reimburse for hospital outpatient services is called the:

a. Ambulatory payment classification system

b. Hospital outpatient prospective payment system (HOPPS)

c. Registered health payment system

d. Vertically integrated payment system

40. HOPPS (or OPPS) allows for temporary payment of new technologies, drugs, devices, and biologicals for which no ambulatory payment classification (APC) payment rate is available, called:

a. Rubrics

b. Outliers

c. Pass-throughs

d. Crosswalks

True/False

Place a "T" in the blank preceding the sentence if it is true; place an "F" if it is false.

_____ 1. Clinics generally provide outpatient services only.

_____ 2. Ambulatory surgery centers (ASCs) are facilities where surgeries are performed that do not require hospital admission.

_____ 3. ASCs treat patients who already have seen a healthcare provider and patients who have not.

_____ 4. Because ASC patients are not formally admitted to the hospital, ASCs are among the more loosely regulated healthcare facilities.

_____ 5. A subacute care facility provides a level of maintenance care where there is no urgent or life-threatening condition that requires medical treatment.

_____ 6. A nursing home can qualify as an SNF.

_____ 7. Licensed hospitals must provide care within the minimum health and safety standards established by state rules and regulations.

_____ 8. All hospitals *must* seek accreditation by nationally recognized accrediting agencies.

_____ 9. Hospitals accredited by The Joint Commission are considered to be in compliance with most of Medicare's "Conditions of Participation for Hospitals."

_____ 10. Privacy and confidentiality issues are not as important in hospitals compared with physicians' offices.

_____ 11. HIPAA Privacy Rule is not intended to prohibit providers from talking to other providers and to their patients.

_____ 12. Each state's Medicaid program determines the method it uses to pay for hospital inpatient services.

_____ 13. An NAS is no longer necessary for most outpatient procedures.

_____ 14. Inpatient TRICARE payments are calculated using the same PPS as Medicare.

_____ 15. Preauthorization is necessary for inpatient hospitalization and some outpatient procedures and diagnostic testing.

_____ 16. Most private insurers negotiate contracts with facilities regarding hospital inpatient payment methods on a month-to-month basis.

_____ 17. The hospital billing process begins when the patient is discharged from the facility.

_____ 18. The principal diagnosis is defined as the condition determined after study to be chiefly responsible for the patient's admission to the hospital.

_____ 19. In determining the principal diagnosis, Uniform Hospital Discharge Data Set definitions take precedence over the coding conventions in the ICD-9-CM Volumes 1 and 2.

Chapter **18** **Hospital Billing and the UB-04**

_____ 20. ICD-9-CM Volume 3 codes are presented in alphabetic order.

_____ 21. V codes are used only in physicians' offices and outpatient clinics.

_____ 22. V codes indicate the reason for the encounter.

_____ 23. An E code can *never* be a principal (first-listed) code.

_____ 24. ICD-9-CM procedure codes (Volume 3) are required for inpatient hospital Part A and Part B claims.

_____ 25. Hospitals submitting claims electronically must do so in a format that is HIPAA-compliant.

Short Answer

1. Discuss the function of today's modern hospital.

_____

2. List and discuss emerging issues in healthcare.

_____

_____

_____

3. The Accreditation Association for Ambulatory Health Care expects substantial compliance with all applicable standards assessed through at least one of three ways. What are they?

_____

_____

_____

4. Discuss, in your own words, what The Joint Commission's Medical Staff Standard MS.6.9 requires.

_____

_____

5. Define a "covered entity," and list the three types of organizations fall under this classification.

_____

_____

_____

6. Some types of practices (i.e., discussions) are considered to be permissible under the HIPAA Privacy Rule, if reasonable precautions are taken to minimize the chance of inadvertent disclosures to others who may be nearby. List these allowed practices.

_____

_____

_____

7. List four methods in which health insurance professionals and other healthcare workers can demonstrate the basic principles of medical ethics.

_____

_____

_____

_____

8. List the major hospital payers, and tell how a health insurance professional can acquire the most recent guidelines for submitting claims.

_____

_____

_____

9. For states to receive matching federal funds, Medicaid programs must offer certain basic services to the categorically needy populations. List these services.

_____

_____

_____

10. List the four methods by which Blue Cross and Blue Shield's fees for facility services are established.

_____

_____

_____

_____

11. Discuss the basic function of the National Uniform Billing Committee.

_____

_____

_____

12. List the information patients typically must provide at the time of hospital registration.

_____

_____

_____

13. Informed consent typically includes a discussion of several elements. List at least four of these elements.

_____

_____

_____

_____

14. If more than one diagnosis meets the criteria for principal diagnosis, what should the coder do?

_____

_____

15. When symptoms are listed with a comparable diagnosis or contrast with the diagnosed condition, what should the coder use?

_____

_____

16. What is the purpose of the new HIPAA edit?

_____

_____

17. In 1996, CMS implemented the Correct Coding Initiative. What function does this initiative serve?

_____

_____

18. List at least six common hospital billing errors.

_____

_____

_____

_____

_____

_____

19. List at least four advantages of submitting hospital claims electronically.

_____

_____

_____

_____

20. Name six exceptions to the HIPAA electronic claims submission requirement.

_____

_____

_____

_____

_____

_____

CRITICAL THINKING ACTIVITIES

A. Brittany Weston was asked by a former coworker how hospital billing differs from that performed in the small, two-physician office they previously worked in together. Assume you are Brittany. Create a dialogue or a critical thinking paragraph of how you might explain these differences.

B. The text discusses two basic payment systems—Medicare's PPS, using diagnosis-related groups for inpatient hospitalization, and the outpatient prospective payment system (HOPPS or OPPS), using APCs. Compare and contrast these two payment systems, citing how are they similar and how they are different.

C. Experts say that two of the most common hospital billing problems are (1) receiving incorrect insurance information and (2) failure to acquire the necessary preauthorization/precertification. How might these problems be avoided or minimized?

D. How might the "emerging issues" discussed in Chapter 18 affect today's hospitals?

PROJECTS/DISCUSSION TOPICS

A. Create a chart or a bulletin board display showing the various types of healthcare facilities and the nature of care provided in each.

B. Your group will be assigned a specific healthcare profession common to today's modern hospitals, such as a medical records technician, a registered health information technician, a hospital coding specialist, or hospital claims specialist. Research the Web (or other available reference sources), and find out what the scope of practice is, what courses and training you would need, the necessary certification or credentialing, and any other information that would be helpful to get started and succeed on this career path.

C. Discuss the process of accreditation, and why it is important for hospitals to be accredited.

D. Generate a 1-page patient handout for inpatients outlining Broadmoor Medical Center's billing policies. You may use the Internet to locate sample policies by existing facilities, if desired, or visit a local hospital.

E. Discuss the major differences between "primary" and "principal" diagnoses.

F. Locate a comprehensive health insurance policy (from the Internet, from a local insurance company such as Blue Cross and Blue Shield, or from your own policy), and outline its hospital inpatient coverage.

385

A. Maria Franklin saw Dr. Lucero at Broadmoor Medical Clinic on 10/03/20XX for complaints of nausea, vomiting, and diarrhea. Dr. Lucero documented the condition in Ms. Franklin's health record as *probable gastroenteritis*. We learned in Chapter 12, however, that in this scenario the health insurance professional would code the nausea, vomiting, and diarrhea, but *not* the gastroenteritis because it is described as *probable* and is not yet confirmed. The diagnosis on the CMS-1500 form would be the symptoms, rather than probable gastroenteritis. Dr. Lucero subsequently admits Maria to the hospital. For inpatient facility billing, coding of signs or symptoms (especially as the principal diagnosis) is not a routine practice because many payers would not pay for or would question inpatient admissions coded with signs and symptoms only. What would the health insurance professional use as the principal diagnosis on the UB-04? Discuss.

B. Hillas Archer, who is having an outpatient hernia repair at Broadmoor Medical Center, also has diabetes and coronary artery disease. What is the principal diagnosis? Should Mr. Archer's diabetes and coronary artery disease also be coded on the UB-04? Discuss.

C. Fig. 18-1 is a sample statement from The Children's Hospital of the King's Daughters. There are 12 numbered areas on the form. John Doe's father is in your office asking for an explanation of the bill. Explain the information in each of these 12 areas to him.

1. _____

2. _____

3. _____

4. _____

5. _____

6. _____

7. _____

8. _____

9. _____

10. _____

11. _____

12. _____

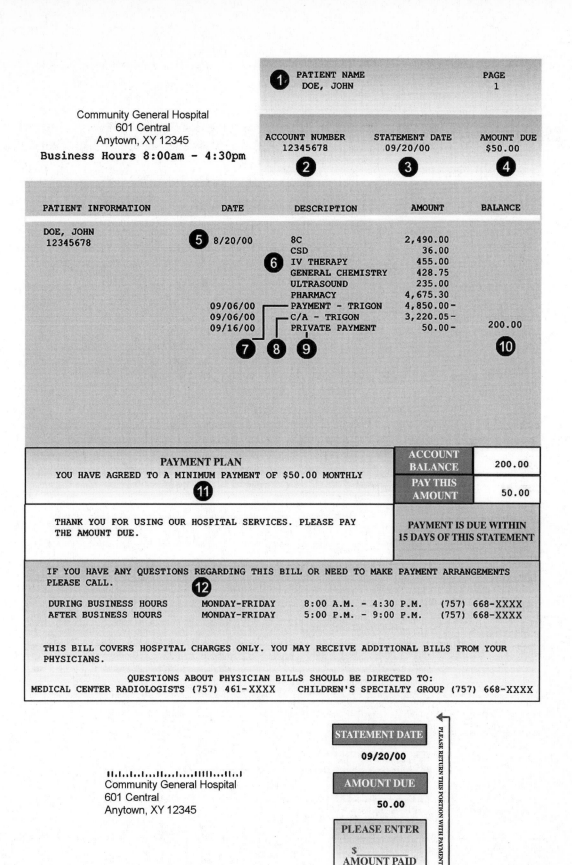

Fig. 18-1 Community General Hospital bill.

D. In the sample statement shown in Fig. 18-2, explain each of the 16 entries to an inquiring patient. (Suggestion: Use a classmate to play the role of an "inquiring patient.")

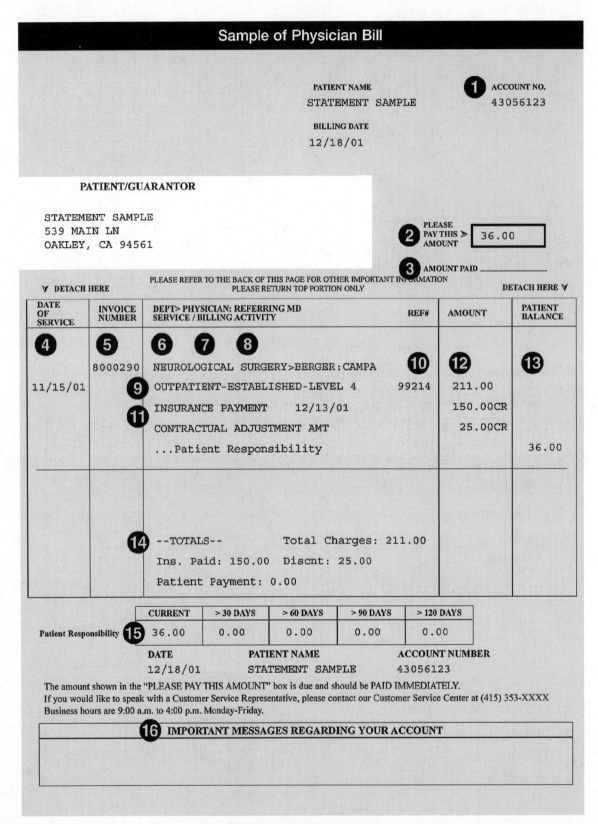

Fig. 18-2 Sample physician bill.

E. **Coding from Inpatient Hospital Records:** Choose the correct series codes from the following case studies.

1. A 10-year-old boy with hemophilia is admitted with severe blood loss anemia resulting from uncontrolled bleeding. He is given clotting factor and 6 U of whole blood. What codes would be assigned?
   a. 286.0, 99.06, 99.03
   b. 285.1, 286.0, 99.06, 99.03
   c. 286.0, 285.1, 99.06, 99.03

2. A 65-year-old black woman with type 2 diabetes is admitted in a diabetic coma. She has nephritic syndrome resulting from the diabetes and gangrene of several toes. What codes would be assigned?
   a. 250.30, 581.81, 785.4
   b. 250.30, 250.41, 581.81, 785.4
   c. 250.30, 250.40, 581.81, 250.70, 785.4

3. A 78-year-old white man was admitted with an infected partial hip prosthesis. The prosthesis was removed, and the patient underwent a total hip arthroplasty. What codes would be assigned?
   a. 996.66, 81.53
   b. 996.67, 81.51
   c. 996.67, 81.53, 81.51

INTERNET EXPLORATION

A. The National Committee on Vital and Health Statistics (NCVHS) has developed a set of data elements with standardized definitions that can be used to collect and produce standardized data for inpatient and outpatient hospitalization. Log on to the following website for more information on the NCVHS Core Health Data Elements Report: **http://www.ncvhs.hhs.gov/ncvhsr1.htm**

B. For informative articles on hospital billing, go to the CMS website at **http://www.cms.hhs.gov,** and key "hospital billing" in the search box. Peruse this list of articles, and choose one that interests you. Prepare a brief oral presentation/written report on your article of choice.

C. Log on to the American Health Information Management Association website at **http://www.ahima.org,** and click on "Schools/Jobs" or "Professional Development" to learn more about career opportunities in health information technology/management.

There are three Performance Objectives for Chapter 18. You will follow a patient's complete hospital experience from admission to discharge and billing. To complete these objectives satisfactorily, use the health records of patient Julius R. Flowers and the blank forms presented in Figs. 18-3 through 18-8. After you have completed each Performance Objective, remove the scoring sheet from the workbook, and attach your completed exercise to it for submission.

Special Notes

Broadmoor Medical Center is a participating provider for Medicare and Blue Cross and Blue Shield.

All patients have a current release of information on file.

All claims are assigned.

Dr. R.L. Jones is the operating surgeon.

Provider Block	
Broadmoor Medical Clinic 4353 Pine Ridge Drive Milton, XY 12345-0001 Clinic NPI X100XX1000 Telephone: 555-656-7890 Fax: 555-656-7899	Clinic EIN # 42-1898989 Dr. R.L. Jones NPI 1234567890 Dr. Marilou Lucero NPI #2907511822 Group # GRW0000 Date claims 1 day after hospital discharge

Performance Objective 18-1—Completing a Preadmission Form

Conditions: Student will complete a preadmission form (Fig. 18-3) using the information listed on the patient information sheet (Fig. 18-4).

Supplies/Equipment: Pen/typewriter, patient record; preadmission information form

Time Allowed: 30 minutes

Accuracy Needed to Pass: 90%

Procedural Steps	Points Earned	Comments
Evaluator: Note time began: _____		
1. Carefully read and study the Patient Information Form for Mr. Flowers. (0)		
2. Complete all required information on the Preadmission Form. (40)		
3. Proofread the form for accuracy, legibility, and completeness. (10)		
Optional: May deduct points for taking more time than allowed.		

Total Points = 50

Student's Score: _____

Evaluator: _____

Comments: _____

_____

_____

_____

_____

Broadmoor Medical Center

4353 Pine Ridge Drive
Milton, XY 12345-0000

Everything for life℠

PRE-ADMISSION INFORMATION FORM

Phone: 555-656-XXXX   Fax: 555-656-XXXX

SURGERY ☐ Yes ☐ No   ACCIDENT ☐ Yes ☐ No   PREGNANCY ☐ Yes ☐ No   OTHER _____

DATE OF ADMISSION OR DUE DATE _____ PRIMARY CARE PHYSICIAN / PHYSICIAN NAME _____

LAST NAME _____ FIRST NAME _____ MIDDLE INITIAL _____

DATE OF BIRTH _____ MAIDEN NAME _____ PRIMARY LANGUAGE _____ SEX M / F

ADDRESS _____ CITY _____ STATE _____ ZIP _____

PHONE _____ RELIGION _____ HOUSE OF WORSHIP _____

MARITAL STATUS _____ SOCIAL SECURITY # _____ OCCUPATION _____

☐ I am currently unemployed

EMPLOYER'S NAME _____ EMPLOYER'S ADDRESS _____

CITY _____ STATE _____ ZIP _____ PHONE _____

PATIENT'S RACE   ☐ Hispanic   ☐ Non Hispanic   ☐ Unknown

PATIENT'S ETHNICITY   ☐ White   ☐ Black   ☐ Native American   ☐ Asia / India / Pacific Isles   ☐ Other

NEWBORN'S RACE (if applicable)   ☐ Hispanic   ☐ Non Hispanic   ☐ Unknown

NEWBORN'S ETHNICITY (if applicable)   ☐ White   ☐ Black   ☐ Native American   ☐ Asia / India / Pacific Isles   ☐ Other

EMERGENCY CONTACT / NEXT OF KIN

LAST NAME _____ FIRST NAME _____ MIDDLE INITIAL _____

ADDRESS _____ CITY _____ STATE _____ ZIP _____

HOME PHONE _____ WORK PHONE _____ RELATIONSHIP _____

PATIENT'S INSURANCE INFORMATION

☐ PPO   ☐ HMO   ☐ EPO   ☐ POS   ☐ Medicare   ☐ MediCal   ☐ Other   ☐ I am currently uninsured

INSURANCE COMPANY NAME _____

ADDRESS _____ CITY _____ STATE _____ ZIP _____

PHONE _____ GROUP # _____ POLICY # _____

HMO MEMBER # _____ MEDICAL GROUP NAME _____

PRIMARY CARE PHYSICIAN OR PHYSICIAN NAME _____

MEDICARE # _____ MEDICAL CIN # _____

EFFECTIVE DATES _____ SUBSCRIBER'S DATE OF BIRTH _____

SPOUSE'S INFORMATION (if applicable)

LAST NAME _____ FIRST NAME _____ MIDDLE INITIAL _____ PHONE _____

DATE OF BIRTH _____ SOCIAL SECURITY # _____

EMPLOYER _____ OCCUPATION _____

EMPLOYER ADDRESS _____ CITY _____ STATE _____ ZIP _____

SPOUSE'S INSURANCE INFORMATION (if applicable)

☐ PPO   ☐ HMO   ☐ EPO   ☐ POS   ☐ Medicare   ☐ MediCal   ☐ Other   ☐ My spouse is currently uninsured

INSURANCE COMPANY NAME _____

ADDRESS _____ CITY _____ STATE _____ ZIP _____

PHONE _____ GROUP # _____ POLICY # _____

HMO MEMBER # _____ MEDICAL GROUP NAME _____

PRIMARY CARE PHYSICIAN OR PHYSICIAN NAME _____

MEDICARE # _____ MEDICAL CIN # _____

EFFECTIVE DATES _____ SUBSCRIBER'S DATE OF BIRTH _____

UPON ARRIVAL IN ADMITTING, PLEASE HAVE YOUR VALID PHOTO ID AND INSURANCE CARD READY. PATIENT'S DEDUCTIBLE AND EST. CO-PAY ARE REQUESTED AT TIME OF ADMISSION. ALL MAJOR CREDIT CARDS ACCEPTED.

Fig. 18-3 Preadmission information form.

Chapter **18** **Hospital Billing and the UB-04**

PATIENT INFORMATION SHEET

Today's date: __10/12/20XX__

HEAD OF HOUSEHOLD

Head of household: __JULIUS R. FLOWERS__ Occupation: __RETIRED FARMER__

Social Security # __098-87-6655__ Employer's name __N/A__

Sex: __M__ Date of birth __03/29/1933__ Employer's address __N/A__

Address: __25387 GLENBROOK ROAD__ Employer's City, St: __N/A__ Zip ____

City, St: __MILTON, XY__ Zip __12345__ Employer's phone # __N/A__

Home phone # __555-656-0110__

PATIENT INFORMATION

Patient's legal name __JULIUS R. FLOWERS__ Nickname __JUBE__ Relationship to head of household __SAME__

Date of birth __03/28/1933__ Age ____ Sex __M__ Marital Status __MARRIED__

Employer name __N/A__ Social Security # __098-87-6655__

Employer address __N/A__ Employer phone # __N/A__

City, St: __N/A__ Zip ____ Worker's Compensation Carrier (If applicable) __N/A__

Referring Physician __TEREZ__ Allergies __SULFA DRUGS__

EMERGENCY INFORMATION

Other contact not living with you: __BETHANY PORTER__ Home phone# __555-656-4433__ Work phone# __555-659-8818__

Address __8614 PARKWAY__ City __MILTON__ St __XY__ Zip __12345__

Patient relationship to other contact __DAUGHTER__ If patient is a child, parent name ____

INSURANCE INFORMATION

Primary insurance __MEDICARE__ Subscriber ____

ID # __098876655A__ Relationship to subscriber __SELF__

Secondary insurance: __BCBS SENIOR BLUE (MEDICARE SUPPL)__ Subscriber __JULIUS R. FLOWERS__

ID # __006SPF4491__ Relationship to subscriber __SELF__

OTHER FAMILY MEMBERS: SAME ADDRESS

Name __BEVERLY T. FLOWERS (WIFE; RETIRED TEACHER)__ & PHONE NO. Date of birth: __05/20/1939__

Name ____ Date of birth: ____

Name ____ Date of birth: ____

Name ____ Date of birth: ____

I understand that it is my responsibility that any incurred charges are paid.

To the extent necessary to determine liability for payment to obtain reimbursement, process claim forms, I authorize the release of any medical information necessary to process claims.

I hereby assign all medical and/or surgical benefits, to include major medical benefits to which I am entitled, including Medicare, private insurance, and other health plans to Broadmoor Medical Center.

This assignment will remain in effect until revoked by me in writing, a photocopy of this assignment is to be considered as valid as an original. I hereby authorize said assignee to release all information necessary to secure the payment.

Signed __Julius R. Flowers__ Date __10/12/20XX__

If patient is a minor, parent or guardian signature.

Fig. 18-4 Patient information sheet.

Performance Objective 18-2—Completing a UB-04 Claim Form

Conditions: Student will complete the required sections of a UB-04 claim form (Fig. 18-5) using the information listed in the patient record for Julius Flowers (Fig. 18-6), patient information sheet (see Fig. 18-4), and hospital billing summary (see Fig. 18-8).

Supplies/Equipment: Pen/typewriter, patient record, UB-04 claim form

Time Allowed: 45 minutes

Accuracy Needed to Pass: 90%

Procedural Steps	Points Earned	Comments
Evaluator: Note time began: _____		
1. Carefully read and study the documents from Mr. Flowers' record. (0)		
2. Using the information in the patient record, complete the required sections on the UB-04 form. (60)		
3. Proofread the form for accuracy, legibility, and completeness. (10)		
Optional: May deduct points for taking more time than allowed.		

Note: Student must complete the following form locaters: **1, 3b, 5, 6, 8b, 9a-d, 10, 11, 12, 38, 42, 43, 44, 46, 47, 50, 58, 60, 63, 69**.

Total Points = 70

Student's Score: _____

Evaluator: _____

Comments: _____

_____

_____

_____

_____

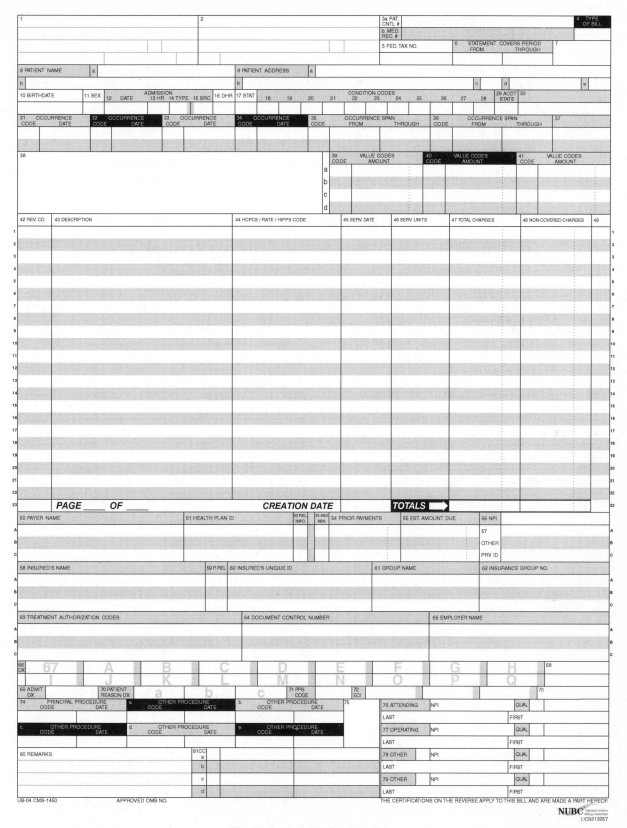

Fig. 18-5 Blank UB-04 claim form.

Chapter **18 Hospital Billing and the UB-04**

PATIENT ER RECORD

PATIENT NAME: Julius R. Flowers   DOB: 03/28/1933
DATE: 10/12/20XX   RECORD NO: 2910388
PRIMARY CARE PHYSICIAN: R.L. Jones, MD

S: Mr. Flowers is a 74-year-old Native American, English-speaking male who was admitted to Broadmoor Medical Center through the Emergency Department at 7:45 a.m. today after sustaining a head injury from a fall down the porch steps at his home, hitting the right side of his head. Patient's wife reported that the patient suffered a brief loss of consciousness—but "only a minute or so." After the fall, he seemed confused but was able to walk with some help. The ambulance was called, and he was transported to Broadmoor Medical Center.

O: Upon admission to the Emergency Department, Mr. Flowers exhibited weakness and tingling to the left upper extremity, mild headache, and confusion. There was some bruising and minor bleeding above his right ear. Denied double vision and nausea. Reflexes were diminished on the left; balance and gait were unsteady. Patient's ability to answer questions was somewhat compromised, as he was somewhat incoherent. His wife answered most of the questions regarding the details of the accident. B/P: 112/68; Pulse: 66. PERRLA. Patient is currently on Captopril, 25 mg., bid. **He is allergic to all SULFA DRUGS.** A CT scan was ordered.

A: Subdural hematoma

P: Surgical evacuation of subdural hematoma

(s)   Emelio R. Terez, MD
      Emergency Room Physician

Fig. 18-6 Patient record (Flowers).

Conditions: Student will complete a hospital billing form (statement) (Fig. 18-7) using the information listed on the hospital billing summary (Fig. 18-8). Assume that Medicare paid all but the first $952, which his Medigap policy paid. List only the total charges using the date of discharge, the payments, and the balance due, if any. Statement date should be the day after the last payment was received.

Supplies/Equipment: Pen/typewriter, patient record, preadmission information form

Time Allowed: 30 minutes

Accuracy Needed to Pass: 90%

Procedural Steps	Points Earned	Comments
Evaluator: Note time began: _____		
1. Carefully read and study information and forms associated with this Performance Objective.		
2. Enter all pertinent information on the form provided in Fig. 18-7. (10)		
3. Calculate the total charges for patient's hospitalization. (5)		
4. Medicare payment date: 11/12/XX (5)		
5. Medigap payment date: 12/02/XX (5)		
6. Current balance, if any (5)		
7. Proofread the form for accuracy, legibility, and completeness.		
Optional: May deduct points for taking more time than allowed.		

Total Points = 30

Student's Score: _____

Evaluator: _____

Comments: _____

_____

_____

_____

_____

HOSPITAL BILLING FORM (STATEMENT)

Broadmoor Medical Center

4353 Pine Ridge Drive
Milton, XY 12345-0000

Phone: 555-656-7890 Fax: 555-656-6890

THIS IS YOUR HOSPITAL BILL			
Patient Name & Address	**Account #**	**Primary/Secondary Insurance(s)**	

Dates of Service	**Activity**	**Amount**	**Balance**

Statement Date: **Due Date:**   **Balance Due:**

If you have billing questions, telephone 555-656-7890 Ext: 3210

Fig. 18-7 Hospital billing form.

```
HOSPITAL BILLING SUMMARY

Patient Name: Flowers, Julius R.        Acct. # 200200546

Discharge Date: 10/16/20XX at 11:45 a.m.

Hospital Charges:

Rev CD    Description            HCPCS/Rates    Serv Units    Total Charges

121       2-Bed Room (Med/Surg)    $2010.00          4          $8040.00
250       Pharmacy                                                 187.45
260       IV Therapy                                               144.90
272       Sterile Supplies                                          65.00
301       Lab/Chemistry                                           2314.12
305       Lab/Hematology                                           201.30
351       CT Scan                                      1           612.50
424       Phys. Therapy/Eval.                                      176.00
450       Emergency Room                               2           562.25
730       EKG                                                      105.00


Primary Payer:                   Medicare
Provider No.                     0976540
Treatment Authorization Code     36378833
Principal Diagnosis Code         431.1
```

Fig. 18-8 Hospital billing summary.

APPLICATION EXERCISES

Health Insurance Professional's Notebook

- Blank UB-04 form
- Current guidelines for completion of the UB-04
- Typical sample forms associated with patient hospitalization

Online Course Assignment/Activities (Evolve)

Chapter Check List

Student name: _____

Chapter completion date: _____

1.	Record	Your start time and date: _____
2.	Read	The assigned chapter in the text
3.	View	PowerPoint slides (if available)
4.	Complete	Exercises in the Workbook as assigned
5.	Compare	Your answers to the answers posted on the bulletin board/website/handout
6.	Correct	Your answers
7.	Complete	All tests and required activities
8.	Read	Assigned readings (if any)
9.	Complete	Chapter performance objectives (competencies), if any
10.	Evaluate	Chapter performance, and submit to your instructor
11.	Record	Your ending time and date: _____
12.	Move on	Begin next chapter as assigned

PERFORMANCE EVALUATION

Evaluate your classroom performance. Complete the self-evaluation and submit it to your instructor. When your instructor returns this form to you, compare your self-evaluation with the evaluation completed by your instructor.

Skill	Student Self-Evaluation			Instructor Evaluation		
	Good	Average	Poor	Good	Average	Poor
Attendance/punctuality						
Personal appearance						
Applies effort						
Is self-motivated						
Is courteous						
Has positive attitude						
Completes assignments in timely manner						
Works well with others						

Student's Initials: _____

Date: _____

Instructor's Initials: _____

Date: _____

Points Possible: _____

Points Awarded: _____

Chapter Grade: _____

Appendix
Blank Forms to Be Reproduced

The Appendix contains sample blank forms to be reproduced for applicable Student Workbook exercises:

- A blank CMS-1500 (08/05) form
- A blank ledger card

Blank electronic forms also can be found in the Electronic Forms file on the Student CD bound into this Workbook.

1500

HEALTH INSURANCE CLAIM FORM

APPROVED BY NATIONAL UNIFORM CLAIM COMMITTEE 08/05

| | PICA | | | | | | | | | | PICA | |

1. MEDICARE (Medicare #) **MEDICAID** (Medicaid #) **TRICARE CHAMPUS** (Sponsor's SSN) **CHAMPVA** (Member ID#) **GROUP HEALTH PLAN** (SSN or ID) **FECA BLK LUNG** (SSN) **OTHER** (ID)

1a. INSURED'S I.D. NUMBER (For Program in Item 1)

2. PATIENT'S NAME (Last Name, First Name, Middle Initial)

3. PATIENT'S BIRTH DATE MM DD YY **SEX** M F

4. INSURED'S NAME (Last Name, First Name, Middle Initial)

5. PATIENT'S ADDRESS (No., Street)

6. PATIENT RELATIONSHIP TO INSURED Self Spouse Child Other

7. INSURED'S ADDRESS (No., Street)

CITY STATE

8. PATIENT STATUS Single Married Other

CITY STATE

ZIP CODE TELEPHONE (Include Area Code) ( )

Employed Full-Time Student Part-Time Student

ZIP CODE TELEPHONE (Include Area Code) ( )

9. OTHER INSURED'S NAME (Last Name, First Name, Middle Initial)

10. IS PATIENT'S CONDITION RELATED TO:

11. INSURED'S POLICY GROUP OR FECA NUMBER

a. OTHER INSURED'S POLICY OR GROUP NUMBER

a. EMPLOYMENT? (Current or Previous) YES NO

a. INSURED'S DATE OF BIRTH MM DD YY **SEX** M F

b. OTHER INSURED'S DATE OF BIRTH MM DD YY **SEX** M F

b. AUTO ACCIDENT? YES NO PLACE (State)

b. EMPLOYER'S NAME OR SCHOOL NAME

c. EMPLOYER'S NAME OR SCHOOL NAME

c. OTHER ACCIDENT? YES NO

c. INSURANCE PLAN NAME OR PROGRAM NAME

d. INSURANCE PLAN NAME OR PROGRAM NAME

10d. RESERVED FOR LOCAL USE

d. IS THERE ANOTHER HEALTH BENEFIT PLAN? YES NO *If yes*, return to and complete item 9 a-d.

READ BACK OF FORM BEFORE COMPLETING & SIGNING THIS FORM.

12. PATIENT'S OR AUTHORIZED PERSON'S SIGNATURE I authorize the release of any medical or other information necessary to process this claim. I also request payment of government benefits either to myself or to the party who accepts assignment below.

SIGNED _____ DATE _____

13. INSURED'S OR AUTHORIZED PERSON'S SIGNATURE I authorize payment of medical benefits to the undersigned physician or supplier for services described below.

SIGNED _____

14. DATE OF CURRENT: MM DD YY ILLNESS (First symptom) OR INJURY (Accident) OR PREGNANCY(LMP)

15. IF PATIENT HAS HAD SAME OR SIMILAR ILLNESS. GIVE FIRST DATE MM DD YY

16. DATES PATIENT UNABLE TO WORK IN CURRENT OCCUPATION MM DD YY FROM TO MM DD YY

17. NAME OF REFERRING PROVIDER OR OTHER SOURCE 17a. 17b. NPI

18. HOSPITALIZATION DATES RELATED TO CURRENT SERVICES MM DD YY FROM TO MM DD YY

19. RESERVED FOR LOCAL USE

20. OUTSIDE LAB? YES NO $ CHARGES

21. DIAGNOSIS OR NATURE OF ILLNESS OR INJURY (Relate Items 1, 2, 3 or 4 to Item 24E by Line)

1. |___ . ___ 3. |___ . ___

2. |___ . ___ 4. |___ . ___

22. MEDICAID RESUBMISSION CODE ORIGINAL REF. NO.

23. PRIOR AUTHORIZATION NUMBER

24. A. DATE(S) OF SERVICE						B. PLACE OF SERVICE	C. EMG	D. PROCEDURES, SERVICES, OR SUPPLIES (Explain Unusual Circumstances)		E. DIAGNOSIS POINTER	F. $ CHARGES	G. DAYS OR UNITS	H. EPSDT Family Plan	I. ID. QUAL.	J. RENDERING PROVIDER ID. #
From MM	DD	YY	To MM	DD	YY			CPT/HCPCS	MODIFIER						
1														NPI	
2														NPI	
3														NPI	
4														NPI	
5														NPI	
6														NPI	

25. FEDERAL TAX I.D. NUMBER SSN EIN

26. PATIENT'S ACCOUNT NO.

27. ACCEPT ASSIGNMENT? (For govt. claims, see back) YES NO

28. TOTAL CHARGE $

29. AMOUNT PAID $

30. BALANCE DUE $

31. SIGNATURE OF PHYSICIAN OR SUPPLIER INCLUDING DEGREES OR CREDENTIALS (I certify that the statements on the reverse apply to this bill and are made a part thereof.)

SIGNED _____ DATE _____

32. SERVICE FACILITY LOCATION INFORMATION

a. NPI b.

33. BILLING PROVIDER INFO & PH # ( )

a. NPI b.

NUCC Instruction Manual available at: www.nucc.org

APPROVED OMB-0938-0999 FORM CMS-1500 (08/05)

405

STATEMENT

BROADMOOR MEDICAL CLINIC
4353 Pine Ridge Drive
Milton, XY 12345-0001
Telephone: 555-656-7890

DATE	PROFESSIONAL SERVICE DESCRIPTION	CHARGE		CREDITS			CURRENT BALANCE	
				PAYMENTS	ADJUSTMENTS			

Due and payable within 10 days.   **Pay last amount in balance column**

407

Appendix   **Blank Forms to Be Reproduced**